W9-BSH-267

Chronic Fatigue Syndrome, Fibromyalgia and Other Invisible Illnesses

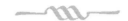

PRAISE FOR DR. KATRINA BERNE'S CLASSIC EARLIER WORK ON CHRONIC FATIGUE SYNDROME, "RUNNING ON EMPTY"

Without flinching, Katrina Berne describes the emotional, physical, and cognitive onslaught of this disease. She explains both the science and the impact of CFIDS, making a mysterious, invisible disease visible and understandable. Dr. Berne employs an array of devices to depict life with CFIDS: descriptive metaphors, excerpts from her own personal journal, and compassionate vignettes that tell the tales of other PWCs and their feelings. Her insights into the experience and trauma of CFIDS will touch many chords inside people with the disease and those who care for them. And her exploration of what PWCs have lost is riveting and frightening. Fortunately, Dr. Berne pursues the difficult issue of "How do I live with CFIDS?" with the same vigor, wisdom, sympathy, and humor that she uses to explain the nature of the disease. The tools are here for PWCs, their families, their friends, and even their physicians to develop new scripts. After reading *Running On Empty* you walk away feeling full. It is authoritative but friendly, personal, and easily accessible. It is the single most useful book on CFIDS to date.

> — *Marc Iverson, president, The CFIDS Association of America (now former president)*

From the standpoint of a physician who has been ill with CFIDS for four years, I highly recommend *Running on Empty* to health care providers and patients.

> — *Sara S. Reynolds, M.D., AAFP*

We as patients should introduce this book to our health care providers to help educate them about CFIDS. Your book is a valuable reference material at meetings. It truly empowers us to be our own health care advocates.

> — *S. O. H., former support group leader*

Running on Empty is my second "Bible." You have literally saved my life, marriage, and family.

> — *L. B., PWC*

In her award-winning book, Berne gives a thorough and often poignant overview of this devastating yet poorly understood illness. Combining current medical knowledge of CFIDS with the results of patient interviews and entries from her personal journal, she discusses its physiological, psychological, and social aspects. . . .

This book, however, is more than a self-help book for CFIDS patients and a reference book for health-care professionals. It is insightful commentary on the devastating effects of chronic, debilitating illness.

— *American Medical Writer's Association Journal*

This work is truly a landmark compendium of present knowledge in the field. For the physician, the book presents an historical summary, review theories of pathogenesis and outlines current therapeutic strategies. Patients are presented with a complete, readable, and comprehensible self-study course in CFS. The author has intertwined experimental data with hard science to produce the most complete overview of CFIDS to date. It will undoubtedly serve as a catalyst for future research and as a ready reference for patients and families of those suffering from CFIDS.

— *Daniel Peterson, M.D.*

The appendices are full of helpful information on CFIDS national organizations, consumer resources, books and other publications, sources of financial aid, and tips for organizing a support group. Highly recommended for public and health care libraries.

— *Library Journal*

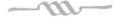

Ordering

Trade bookstores in the U.S. and Canada please contact:

Publishers Group West
1700 Fourth Street, Berkeley CA 94710
Phone: (800) 788-3123   Fax: (510) 528-3444

Hunter House books are available at bulk discounts for textbook course adoptions; to qualifying community, health care, and government organizations; and for special promotions and fund-raising. For details please contact:

Special Sales Department
Hunter House Inc., PO Box 2914, Alameda CA 94501-0914
Phone: (510) 865-5282   Fax: (510) 865-4295
E-mail: ordering@hunterhouse.com

Individuals can order our books from most bookstores,
by calling **(800) 266-5592**, or from our website at
www.hunterhouse.com

Chronic Fatigue Syndrome, Fibromyalgia

and Other Invisible Illnesses

THE COMPREHENSIVE GUIDE

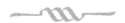

Katrina Berne, Ph.D.

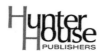

Copyright © 2002 by Katrina H. Berne, Ph.D.
All rights reserved. No part of this publication may be reproduced or transmitted
in any form or by any means, electronic or mechanical, including photocopying
and recording, or introduced into any information storage and retrieval system
without the written permission of the copyright owner and the publisher of this
book. Brief quotations may be used in reviews prepared for inclusion in a magazine or newspaper or for broadcast. For further information please contact:

Hunter House Inc., Publishers
PO Box 2914
Alameda CA 94501-0914

Library of Congress Cataloging-in-Publication Data
Berna, Katrina H.
Chronic fatigue syndrome, fibromyalgia, and other invisible illnesses : the
comprehensive guide / Katrina Berne.— 3rd ed., rev.
p. cm.
Second ed. Under title: Running on empty.
Includes bibliographical references and index.
ISBN 0-89793-280-3 (paper)
1. Chronic fatigue syndrome. 2. Fibromyalgia. I. Berne, Katrina H. Running on
empty. II. Title.
RB150.F37 B47 2001
616'.0478—dc21   2001039721

Project Credits

Cover Design: Jil Weil
Book Production: Hunter House
Copy Editor: Mali Apple
Proofreader: John David Marion
Indexer: Kathy Talley-Jones
Acquisitions Editor: Jeanne Brondino
Associate Editor: Alexandra Mummery
Editorial and Production Assistant: Emily Tryer
Sales and Marketing Assistant: Earlita K. Chenault
Publicity Manager: Sara Long
Customer Service Manager: Christina Sverdrup
Warehousing and Shipping: Lakdhon Lama
Administrator: Theresa Nelson
Computer Support: Peter Eichelberger
Publisher: Kiran S. Rana

Printed and Bound by Transcontinental Printing

Manufactured in Canada

9 8 7 6 5 4 3   Third Edition   03 04 05 06

Contents

*Readers wishing to contact the author may reach her through
her website,* **www.LivingWithIllness.com**

Important Note

The material in this book is intended to provide a review of information regarding chronic fatigue syndrome, fibromyalgia syndrome, and other chronic disorders. Every effort has been made to provide accurate and dependable information. The reader should be aware that health-care professionals have differing opinions and approaches to treatment, and advances in medicine and scientific research may render some of the information outdated.

Therefore, the publisher, author, editors, and reviewers cannot be held responsible for any error, omission, or dated material. Any treatments described should be undertaken only under the guidance of a licensed health-care practitioner. The author and publisher assume no responsibility for any outcome of the use of any of these treatments in a program of self-care or under the care of a licensed practitioner.

If you have a question concerning your care or treatment or about the appropriateness or application of the treatments described in this book, consult your health-care professional.

Some of the therapies, treatments, or products mentioned in this book have been trademarked. Where the author and publisher were aware of a trademark claim, the designations have been printed with initial capital letters.

Dedication

FOR ELDON HUSTED, MPH

Foreword

As we proceed into the twenty-first century, there is a growing realization among clinical scientists that the group of problems commonly referred to as "medically unexplained symptoms" are not so inexplicable after all. Two so-called medically unexplained symptoms are debilitating persistent fatigue and unremitting widespread pain. When these symptoms fail to be explained in terms of conventional investigations, the labels of chronic fatigue syndrome (CFIDS) or fibromyalgia (FM) are commonly used to describe such conditions. This new book by Katrina Berne, the author of *Running On Empty*, is a comprehensive overview of contemporary information regarding these two syndromes. It provides a compassionate insight into the wide clinical spectrum of both disorders and describes complicated scientific concepts at a level intelligible to the average reader. The overall theme of successfully coping with both CFIDS and FM is to maintain the delicate balance of body and mind that is referred to as "homeostasis." Dr. Berne's training as a clinical psychologist is evident in the way that she successfully deals with these issues.

Many patients with fibromyalgia and chronic fatigue syndrome are disillusioned with the quality of medical care they receive, especially the lack of compassion of many health-care providers. As a physician who frequently lectures on these topics, I am pleased to report there is an increasing interest in both of these disorders, but this interest is often tempered by therapeutic apathy. Most primary care physicians want to know "What do I do now that I have made the diagnosis?" To quote from Dr. Berne's book,

> *When physicians lack a biomedical model that explains patient complaints, they revert to psychiatric diagnoses: depression, somatization disorder, or malingering. They are trained to cure people and that's what they like to do. When they can't fix what's wrong, they become frustrated, their professional identities threatened. We don't*

get better, we don't go away; we just keep coming back with same old complaints and additional new ones.

This frustration on the part of physicians is compounded by the dictates of a managed care system that financially penalizes physicians who take too much time with an individual patient or order too many "unnecessary" tests. It is my philosophy that all patients with chronic fatigue and fibromyalgia should have potentially treatable causes of their symptoms investigated if the history and/or physical examination suggests any of the following disorders: anemia, hyper/hypothyroidism, hemochromatosis, hepatitis C, Lyme disease, HIV and other chronic infections, major depression, any of the autoimmune disorders (e.g., lupus or multiple sclerosis), Addison's disease, autonomic dysfunction with low blood pressure, and primary sleep disorders (e.g., sleep apnea, narcolepsy, periodic limb movement disorder).

Unfortunately, the frustrations of the medical profession with these disorders often results in patients developing an "existential crisis" that further aggravates the mind-body imbalance. To quote from Norman Cousins (taken from Dr. Berne's book):

Illness is always an interaction among both mind and body. It can begin in the mind and affect the body, or it can begin in the body and affect the mind, both of which are served by the same bloodstream. Attempts to treat most mental diseases and as though they were completely free of physical causes and attempts to treat most bodily diseases as though the mind were in no way involved must be considered archaic in the light of new evidence about the way the human body functions.

Some twenty-one years later, research scientists are validating Mr. Cousins's claims with innovative new technologies of functional brain scanning, measurement of neurotransmitters (brain signaling molecules) in the cerebrospinal fluid, and the psychoneuro-immunological effects of acute and chronic stress. In 1991, chronic fatigue syndrome researcher Jay Goldstein stated: "CFS represents the final common pathway for multifactorial disorder with a limbic system encephalopathy causing autonomic dysfunction and subtle neuroendocrine derangements."

An exciting finding of the past two years may help confirm and explain the loose ends of Dr. Goldstein's hypothesis: the role of cytokines as the possible mediator of the numerous bodily insults that seem to set off FM and CFIDS. Cytokines are small bioactive molecules released from one cell that influence (stimulate or depress) the activity of itself or other cells. Cytokines can be found in the blood, inflammatory fluids, and the cerebrospinal fluid. They are the molecules responsible for the "sickness response"—the fever, fatigue, and achiness that accompany many infections. Until just recently, they were considered to be produced mainly by immune cells such as lymphocytes and macrophages. However, research by Linda Watkins (University of Colorado at Boulder) and others has demonstrated that some cytokines are produced by a specialized type of brain cell called a "glial cell." The production of cytokines deep within the brain and spinal cord can activate neuro-transmitters involved in the production of pain impulses and also lead to a "sickness response" with resulting fatigue and malaise. Cytokines such as IL-6 are potent stimulators of the hypothalamic pituitary stress response that also modulate the activity of the auto-nomic nervous system.

As you read Dr. Berne's book, you will learn that there appear to be many triggers that can initiate the onset of both CFIDS and FM. An important new finding is that cytokine release from glial cells can be initiated by such diverse events as infections, physical trauma, emotional trauma, exposure to toxins, depression, and autoimmune diseases. Viruses and other infectious agents that gain access to the central nervous system would be expected to be espe-cially adept at stimulating glial cells to release cytokines. One such agent is the virus responsible for AIDS; thus it is not surprising that HIV-infected patients complain of profound fatigue and about one-third develop fibromyalgia. Presumably, then, there are as yet undiscovered infectious agents that can initiate the cascade of events that culminate in the development of symptoms characteris-tic of chronic fatigue syndrome or fibromyalgia. A large body of research to date has concentrated on finding such infections, but no one agent has ever been implicated in the causation of CFIDS or FM. They may wreak their damage and then disappear, so by the time researchers seek them out the hunt is predestined to fail. The central message of the emerging cytokine story is that not only is a single causative agent unnecessary to explain the causation of CFIDS and FM, but noninfectious triggers, such as physical trauma, repetitive physical stresses, emotional distress, and concomitant inflammatory disorders (e.g., multiple sclerosis and lupus) could also result in similar syndromes. Cytokines, then, are emerging as strong candidates for mediators of the "final common pathway" postulated by Dr. Goldstein in 1991. Once the body's homeostasis (i.e., internal balance) is out of kilter, achievement of equilibrium will be hindered by any of the numerous insults that can result in cytokine secretion.

Once the cytokine switch has been "turned on," the body appears to develop a new set-point for any stressor in terms of increased reactivity. In most people the set-point does not change, and they do not develop persistent fatigue or widespread pain. Why an unfortunate group of individuals develops a new set-point is going to be a major challenge to researchers in the coming years. Almost certainly they will find not one but an array of genes that predispose to the development of FM and CFIDS, maybe even elucidating why one individual has symptoms of mainly fatigue, while another has distressing and persistent pain. I predict that they will also determine that a succession of life-stressors (e.g., infections, injuries, surgeries, autoimmune disorders, and unhappy relationships) sets up the genetically predisposed individual to eventually develop CFIDS or FM. It may be that the *initial* insult, which leads to the development of chronic fatigue or fibromyalgia in the first place, has long since passed, but the symptoms continue to be driven by *secondary* insults to which the patient is now sensitized. Thus eliminating or minimizing these secondary insults is critically important in reestablishing the necessary homeostasis of mind and body. The successful self-management of chronic fatigue and fibromyalgia demands an informed patient utilizing a holistic approach to coping with chronic illness. To this end, it is pertinent to quote Dr. Andrew Weil: "We know health well in its absence." Dr. Berne adds:

> *Apart from being merely the absence of illness, however, the term 'wellness' connotes harmony of body, mind, and spirit, and an appropriate style of living and self-care—proper nutrition, rest, and exercise. We seek magic remedies in our instant-fix society. But the wellness we seek eludes us; it cannot be purchased or easily achieved. We are impatient for relief but forced to accept that there is no quick fix, and no one fix. The only reliable 'treatment' is self-care—seeking*

balance, slowing down. Medical professionals can help us augment the healing process, and we must dismiss notions of magical panaceas.

There is not currently, and there may never be, a "magic fix" for fibromyalgia or chronic fatigue. The author of this book has experienced chronic fatigue syndrome, understands the frustrations of both patients and physicians, and has researched the scientific literature to produce a comprehensive, accurate, and above all readable guide to understanding CFIDS and FM. This is a book for patients and their friends and loved ones; it offers practical advice on how to achieve the harmony of mind, body, and spirit that is necessary to survive and even overcome the debilitating effects of chronic fatigue and widespread pain. In a nutshell, this book provides the essentials to becoming an informed patient.

— Professor Robert M. Bennett, M.D., FRCP, FACP
Oregon Health and Science University
Portland, Oregon
August 2001

Foreword

Through her own professional and personal experience with chronic fatigue syndrome (CFS or CFIDS) and fibromyalgia syndrome (FMS), Dr. Berne has developed an intimate and thorough knowledge of these diseases. The horror, frustration, and anger produced by the disabling condition are graphically portrayed, yet balanced by the reality of palliative treatment and hope for future research.

Most Americans have heard of CFS and FMS or know someone suffering from these diseases. However, the fledgling scientific literature of CFS and FMS has reached few patients and even fewer physicians. While patients are acutely aware of the potentially disabling power of these diseases, most researchers and physicians continue to view them as trivial anthills on the mountain of medicine.

While scientific research will ultimately yield answers to the many unknowns of CFS and FMS, this work is truly a landmark compendium of present knowledge in the field. For the physician, the book presents an historical summary, reviews theories of pathogenesis, and outlines current therapeutic strategies. Additionally, and perhaps more importantly, the author reifies the debilitating, disabling effects of the disease and contradicts the common perception that they are trivial or even nonexistent. Postulated etiologies challenge medical researchers to intensify their efforts.

Patients are presented with a complete, readable, and comprehensible self-study course in CFS and FMS. Chapters dedicated to self-help and adjustment to chronic disease are particularly critical for patients suffering from an incurable, long-lasting disease. Common pitfalls of self-diagnosis and self-treatment are clearly illustrated. Families and friends can find insight into the symptoms and reactions to symptoms that alter the physical functioning and personalities of their loved one. The author also suggests realistic and functional solutions to improve interpersonal relationships and to preserve the family structure. An extensive bibliography directs those interested in historic and current publications to scientific and lay literature. Physicians, patients, and their families are provided with a current list of support groups, research organizations, and governmental agencies.

Finally, society at large is confronted with the desperate need for recognition of these worldwide health problems. Lack of research funding, lack of national interest on the part of federal and private research agencies, and physician misinformation and apathy combine to retard discovery into the pathogenesis and treatment of these disorders. Hopefully, this book will serve to unite and stimulate a broad base of support and research.

CFS and FMS are fraught with systematic difficulties including diagnostic and therapeutic confusion due in large part to unknown or unproved etiologies and pathogenesis. This creates frustration for the physician as well as the patient and often leads to a dysfunctional and unsatisfactory patient/physician relationship. Dr. Berne strives to look beyond knowledge gaps and expose the poorly defined disease processes in terms of their functional impact on the physical and mental health of the patient. Numerous real-life examples compel the physician to accept the seriousness of these diseases, while patients are reassured that they are not alone in the morass of signs and symptoms. The author has intertwined experiential data with hard science to produce the most complete overview of CFS and FMS to date. It will undoubtedly serve as a catalyst for future research and as a ready reference for patients and families of sufferers.

— *Daniel L. Peterson, M.D.*
Incline Village, Nevada
1992, updated 2001

Preface

In the not-so-distant past, most people were unfamiliar with chronic fatigue syndrome and fibromyalgia. Despite growing familiarity with the names of these illnesses, most people do not really know what the illnesses are about. When a person with chronic fatigue syndrome (CFS) or fibromyalgia syndrome (FMS) mentions a symptom, particularly fatigue or pain, others are likely to exclaim, "I think I have your illness, too!"—betraying their unwitting insensitivity and ignorance. The media, the medical profession, and the public may now lend a somewhat sympathetic ear to our ailments, but they still don't "get it." The extent of their understanding depends upon their sources of information and proximity to those with the disorders; however, they can never truly understand what it's like in the trenches. We simply don't have words in our vocabulary to describe this experience.

The uninitiated have difficulty comprehending the invisibility of the disorders, the large number of symptoms spanning virtually every body system, and the unpredictability and suddenness of symptom exacerbations. One moment we feel reasonably okay, and the next we are flat on our backs, or dizzy, or unable to respond appropriately to simple questions. Difficulty processing input of all kinds leads to "irritable everything," as input becomes distorted, exhausting, and overwhelming: light, noise, touch, chemical odors, conversation...the list goes on. Fearful of being judged, we make understandable but self-defeating attempts to hide or downplay our symptoms for fear of being labeled crazy people, malingerers, or hypochondriacs and thus often succeed in convincing others we are "fine," one of the many catch-22s associated with chronic illness.

Unfortunately, the names chronic fatigue syndrome and fibromyalgia are not particularly helpful. The term fibromyalgia, although inaccurate, at least sounds credible. The name chronic fatigue syndrome lends itself to a misinterpretation of the illness, since fatigue is only one among many symptoms and not usually the most debilitating or disabling one. Lack of consistent research findings clouds the issue of renaming the disorders. We know that both CFS and FMS are characterized by dysregulation of numerous body systems, but test results are inconsistent and abnormalities do not occur with equal frequency in all patients.

We search for *the* cause, *the* pathogen, *the* successful treatment, and *the* cure, but illness is not simply the product of simple cause and effect. CFS and FMS are most likely multifactorial illnesses. Years of research have yielded few conclusions but increasingly sophisticated questions. The answer to *any* question about CFS or FMS begins with, "I don't know; the research is inconclusive, but one particular theory is...." Every theory regarding these common, devastating, and poorly understood illnesses is met by numerous opinions and no clear consensus. The experts have no answers.

We know that the symptoms and abnormalities of CFS and FMS overlap substantially, but we do not understand the relationship between the two disorders. They may be distinct illnesses, overlapping entities, or two among many that comprise a spectrum of illnesses.

When I wrote the first edition of *Running on Empty* in 1991, I drew upon all available resources, which amounted to a handful of articles. In 1994, a sizeable amount of research literature and patient-generated information made the first revision a substantial task. Now, in 2001, papers, books, sticky notes, journals, and files obscure every surface in my office. The amount of literature generated within the past five years is enormous. I am astonished, confused, grateful, angry, and overwhelmed with the wide disparity among findings and the lack of a common meeting ground. I try to simplify my life, my work, and my thinking—with disappointing results; my brain is as cluttered as my office. This book represents an attempt to organize a huge amount of information into its simplest common denominators—and they're not simple, either.

I have broadened the scope of this book to include other poorly understood, possibly overlapping chronic disorders with common features. What are the relationships among these disorders? What factors cause and perpetuate them: genetics, environment, toxins, pathogens, emotional traumata, or—most likely—a combination of factors?

The field of medicine has made tremendous strides in treating and often curing acute illnesses but has been far less successful in dealing with chronic disorders, which may begin to develop years before any symptoms appear, rendering causal and perpetuating factors extremely difficult to identify. In most cases, cause, pathophysiology, treatments, and cure elude us. In cases where diagnostic markers exist, they are often inconsistent. Chronic illness remains a mystery and a challenge to modern medicine.

— *Katrina Berne*
September, 2001

Acknowledgments

I am fortunate to have an abundance of bright, sensitive, and caring people in my life. My "in-house" editor and husband, Eldon Husted, has been an unfailingly steadfast partner, proofreader, cook, and errand runner, offering suggestions, encouragement, and emotional support. He believes in me even when I don't believe in myself and makes quite a convincing case. My mother, Claire Berne, and my grown children, Karen Bertiger and Jeffrey Bertiger, have been mainstays during times of difficulty as well as triumph, offering love, understanding, and friendship despite the fact that we're related.

My friends, too numerous to mention (and perhaps preferring to enjoy their anonymity), have been loyal and caring above and beyond the call of duty, listening (or giving the appearance of listening) to my complaints and celebrating my successes. Undoubtedly the brightest, funniest, and most perceptive people on the planet, they provide generous humor and sanity fixes.

Dr. David Payne helped with medical terminology, concepts, and suggestions as well as unconditional friendship and support, even on the (infrequent) occasions when I didn't do my best work. Drs. Daniel Peterson and Robert Bennett willingly added one more task to their overflowing calendars to review this book and write introductory pieces. Kristin Thorson, Stephanie Hopkins, and Robin Long once again proved their resourcefulness with an abundance of ideas and materials.

The staff at Hunter House has been helpful, encouraging, and committed to this project. In 1991, publisher Kiran Rana recognized CFS (then dubbed "yuppie flu") as a serious disorder long before it was acknowledged as a "real" illness and took a leap of faith by publishing *Running on Empty: Chronic Fatigue Immune Dysfunction Syndrome*. Jeanne Brondino, acquisitions editor, was exceptionally patient and understanding as a six-month project turned into a thirty-month process. Alexandra Mummery, associate editor, supplied timely answers to my many questions and cheered me on. Mali Apple, who did an excellent job of editing this text, cleaned up evidence of my cognitive dysfunction. Having been warned about the callousness and insensitivity of publishing houses, I am pleased to report at least one glowing exception.

Many readers took the time to send letters, providing valuable feedback and encouragement; I regret that due to illness and time constraints, I was frequently unable to respond to their wonderful letters. Likewise, I would like to thank my patients, who have been my teachers and sources of inspiration.

PART ONE

What These Illnesses Are

1

Changed Lives

Jane awoke one morning feeling fluish, with a sore throat, tender lymph nodes, malaise, and achiness. She stayed in bed, assuming she had a minor illness that would resolve in a few days or weeks. An active, energetic, Type A accountant, she assumed she would soon resume her previous responsibilities and activity level. "It's just a bug," she told herself. "I'll be fine in a few days." A week later she had to force herself to resume her busy schedule. She felt exhausted and a bit off balance and spacey, as if her head were filled with cotton. She returned to the office and was embarrassed to admit that tasks that had once been second nature had somehow grown into major challenges. She developed the habit of periodically sneaking off to a storage room to lie down. Sick, frightened, and uncertain, Jane attempted to pass herself off as well. Ultimately, she realized her coping efforts were insufficient and that she was unable to continue her job.

Two years later Jane still spends most of her time in bed. Debilitated by her lingering illness, she is unable to fulfill her former responsibilities at work or home. Her former leisure-time activities—jogging, hiking, racquetball, and dinner parties—have dwindled to almost nothing. Her once-spotless house is in chaos, and she has gained a significant amount of weight although her eating habits have not changed. She often feels helpless and depressed, wondering why she is unable to recover. Several doctors have attributed her symptoms to depression and stress, and Jane is beginning to feel crazy and lazy, almost believing that it's "all in her head," since her medical test results have all been normal.

"Logically, I know this isn't my fault," she says. "I'd never have given up my job, which I loved, my income, my friends, and activities just to stay in bed feeling awful." Minor household chores and basic personal grooming require almost superhuman effort. Jane feels guilty about neglecting her responsibilities, but her symptoms increase when she pushes herself. "I don't understand what happened to me. I'm not myself anymore. I always took care of everything and everyone, and now I can't even function. Numbers don't make a whole lot of sense to me anymore."

Jane wonders whether her life will ever return to normal. "I can handle anything as long as I understand it, but I can't make sense out of feeling like this. My mind can't focus; I ache all over. I'm letting everyone down, and I'm frightened. What's wrong with me? What if I never recover?" Having researched her symptoms, Jane believes she has chronic fatigue syndrome but has not yet received a medical diagnosis.

Rob worked in a chemical plant for fifteen years before he began to notice odd sensations. "I started getting wobbly and lightheaded. Noise bothered me. Light bothered me. I have allergies now, never had them before. And I get sick a lot. I worked around a lot of chemicals, no big deal, but suddenly it *was* a big deal. I had to quit my job because I couldn't stand to be around the stuff. The company doc didn't have much to say; he just listened and wrote down a few notes. He said I'd get over it, whatever it was. He was dead wrong.

"I don't see the guys from work any more. They don't say it, but I know they think I'm wacko." So did the second doctor he saw, who ran a few tests and told Rob there was nothing wrong with him; Rob just needed to change his attitude. By then Rob was having blinding headaches that lasted for days. "I got sick and dizzy from the smell of gasoline, bleach, insecticides—so many chemicals I can't count them all. I couldn't go to the mall or the movies or any crowded, noisy places. I couldn't drink alcohol anymore, and certain foods make me sick. I'm a real wimp now."

A third doctor told Rob he was depressed and prescribed medication. Another was understanding but baffled. "By then I was having headaches almost every day and my muscles hurt. I thought, this can't be. I've seen four doctors, and they can't find anything wrong. I must be a nut case, just like everyone thinks. I get hot, then cold. I get weak, and I drop things." Rob didn't see any doctors for a long time, but then he read a newspaper article about chemical sensitivities. "A support group hooked me up with a good doctor who diagnosed me with environmental illness and fibromyalgia. I thought those illnesses were a lot of bull—until I got them. Now I feel sorry for anyone who has to go through this."

Driving to work one day, Lydia braked for a red light and was hit from behind by another car. She sustained whiplash and soft-tissue injuries. Over a period of months, the pain spread to her shoulders and back, and she developed frequent headaches, although she did not initially relate these symptoms to the relatively minor collision. "The pain got worse, and I ached from head to toe. I couldn't sleep and began to have daily headaches and a lot of other symptoms. My HMO doc said I might have fibromyalgia, but he just told me to take ibuprofen when it got bad. He didn't understand why I had so many other symptoms, like irritable bowel, 'brain fog,' and insomnia. I had to pay out-of-pocket to see a rheumatologist, who put the picture together. It's posttraumatic fibromyalgia, and he thinks I might have lupus, too."

Lydia describes constant pain and exhaustion. She reports, "My brain isn't working right. I can't balance my checkbook or remember my friends' names. Even little things take a huge mental effort." She is often unable to follow movie plots or concentrate on what she reads. "I read a few pages and don't remember what I've read. I read it again, and it doesn't even look familiar."

Lydia was able to keep her job for two years after the accident, but as the pain, fatigue, and cognitive problems grew more severe, her productive hours dwindled. She is able to work part-time at home at her own pace but does little else. "I spend most of my time in bed or in my recliner, and I have difficulty getting comfortable. I have to move around a lot or the pain becomes unbearable. I only leave the house for medical appointments, physical therapy, and occasional errands—and they wipe me out." Her symptoms flare in cold weather, when the weather changes, following exertion, and sometimes for no apparent reason.

Lydia says, "At the time, I thought the accident was no big deal. I never imagined it could change my life so drastically and permanently. I've read about fibromyalgia, everything I could get my hands on, but I don't think I've ever really accepted it."

"My doctors think I'm a big fake," says fourteen-year-old Sandra. "They said I'm missing too much school and my parents shouldn't let me stay home, like they're babying me. I don't have energy like the other kids, and the school has threatened my parents: 'If you don't send her to school, you're breaking the law.' I can't even sit up most of the time and I can't think right; I don't understand my textbooks or remember anything I read. I used to get straight As. I hate being like this, and I'm being blamed for it. It is totally unfair."

Sandra's parents initially believed the doctor's diagnosis of school phobia and forced Sandra to attend school, watching her become sicker each day. They now realize she is too ill to attend but have been threatened by the school administration.

Sandra has seen nine physicians. "Most of them were clueless," she reports. "Finally, one doctor told me I have chronic fatigue syndrome and that I should rest a lot, but there's no treatment for it and I might not ever get better. That really bummed me out." She has recently seen a more supportive physician who has provided appropriate treatment and educational materials. "I hate being sick, but at least now there's a name for what I have and medicine that helps. Most of my friends have stuck by me, but some are history. It really hurt when they'd roll their eyes like I'm faking or whatever. But I can't really blame them for not understanding; I look okay, but I'm too sick to do the stuff I used to do. We'd be listening to music, and suddenly I'd yell, 'Turn it off!' The noise really got to me, but they didn't understand. It's really hard to live like this."

After battling the school system, Sandra's parents report that she is able to attend two classes per day, is excused from physical education, and is home-tutored for her other classes. Sandra's health remains unpredictable; she looks forward to school but is often is too ill to attend even for a few hours. She enjoys getting together with one or two friends but sometimes doesn't want to see anyone. "Too exhausting," she says. "Nobody gets it. *I* don't get it. I'm scared because I don't know what will happen to me in the future. I don't even know if I *have* a future."

Luke complains of weakness and bodywide pain. He has frequent migraine-like headaches and can't seem to get a good night's sleep. Looking back on his life, he cannot remember ever feeling well. "I never had as much energy as the other kids. My parents thought I was lazy, and I believed them. My legs used to hurt, and the doctor said I had growing pains. I thought everyone felt like I did, achy and tired, only they handled it better." Luke now recalls his mother's constant fatigue: "She'd fall asleep in the middle of the day, wherever she was. She never complained, but I knew she took pain pills when it got really bad. She was up all night doing who knows what, and now I understand what she went through."

Over the past few years, Luke has developed increasing pain in his muscles and joints. "I hate to admit this, but doing the least little thing makes me feel like I've climbed a mountain. I ache and sometimes can barely get out of bed, and I haven't done anything out of the ordinary. I have no stamina. I was diagnosed with fibromyalgia when I was twenty-six, and by then I'd had it for twenty-six years—my whole life!" His pain vacillates, but he is never pain free. Like his mother, he doesn't complain much, but those close to him know when he's having a rough day. "He can't get comfortable," says his wife Linda. "He loves to play with the kids but often he can't. He comes home from work and crashes. Some of our friends think he's weird or faking, but I know better." Luke regularly attends a support group, "mostly for moral support, to remind me I'm not the only one who lives this way and that I'm not crazy. I'm fortunate to have a wife and family who understand." Facing a future that is unlikely to be different from the past, Luke adopts a stoic façade that belies his chronic pain.

Jane, Rob, Lydia, Sandra, and Luke share common symptoms and life issues. They and millions like them have encountered disbelief and ridicule. Each has tried to conquer the symptoms; each has failed. Medical treatment offers some symptom relief, but there is no known cure for fibromyalgia syndrome (FMS) or chronic fatigue syndrome (CFS). Both disorders are poorly understood, invisible, chronic illnesses that affect multiple body systems. Overlapping symptoms and abnormalities call into question whether these are two overlapping illnesses, unrelated illnesses, or variants of the same illness.

In addition, these disorders resemble and overlap with many other chronic illnesses. Some are regarded as immune disorders or autoimmune disorders; some are related to known pathogens. Symptoms may be constant or cyclical. Some people with CFS/FMS improve over time, others stay about the same, and some become progressively worse. Research into these poorly understood illnesses has been inconclusive due in part to inadequate funding and contradictory study results. Years of research have left us with more questions than answers.

This book is about CFS and FMS: similarities and differences, symptoms, diagnosis, exacerbations and remissions, possible causal factors, treatment, and coping. The term CFS/FMS is used in discussions of their commonalities; the terms CFS and FMS are used separately when information applies to one but not necessarily the other.

No term is adequate for those with these illnesses. Because the terms "sufferers" and "victims" are objectionable, I have chosen the term "patient" by default.

2

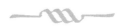

Chronic Fatigue Syndrome

CFS is probably the most severe end of a spectrum of fatiguing
illnesses with a similar pathogenesis.
— *Paul Levine, M.D.*

Chronic fatigue syndrome (CFS) is a complex illness characterized by incapacitating fatigue (experienced as exhaustion and
extremely poor stamina), neurological problems, and a constellation
of symptoms that often resemble such other disorders as fibromyalgia, mononucleosis, multiple sclerosis, Lyme disease, and postpolio
syndrome. Onset may be abrupt or gradual, often following a flulike
illness or stressful events. It was originally believed that abrupt
onset characterized two-thirds of cases; in retrospect, many patients
are able to identify preexisting symptoms of lesser severity, with a
trauma triggering full-blown illness. Patients experience multisystem symptoms—notably fatigue, pain, and cognitive dysfunction—
with symptoms and their severity varying among patients.

CFS is characterized by a broad range of physiological, cogni-
tive/neurological, and emotional symptoms that persist over time.
The most profound symptoms include severe exhaustion, worsened
by exertion; neurological/neurocognitive problems; muscle and
joint pain; flulike symptoms; new-onset headaches; and sleep disorders. CFS patients frequently manifest environmental sensitivities,
sleep disorders, irritable bladder and irritable bowel syndromes, and
intolerance to temperature changes. These symptoms tend to wax
and wane but are often severely debilitating, usually persisting for
years.

Symptoms vary from person to person and fluctuate in severity
over time. Cases span those who are able to work a full workweek
but do little else to those who are bedfast and completely reliant

upon others. Some patients become well, others improve, and a minority worsens over time.

Fatigue is a symptom of a wide range of disorders, including acute and chronic infections, end-stage neoplasia (abnormal cell growth), renal insufficiency, congestive heart failure, depression, and multiple sclerosis. Although fatigue is prominent in CFS, only about 1 percent of people in the general population with persistent fatigue meet the diagnostic criteria for chronic fatigue *syndrome*. Those with unexplained fatigue of at least six months' duration who do not experience the CFS constellation of symptoms are considered to have "idiopathic fatigue," that is, fatigue of unknown cause. (Streeten 1998).

Described by one patient as a "mystery waiting for a miracle," CFS has no known cause, with a combination of predisposition and infectious, environmental, immunological, neurohormonal, and psychiatric factors playing a role. Although viewed by skeptics as the manifestation of an underlying psychological disorder such as depression, anxiety, or somatization disorder, CFS is a debilitating illness involving symptoms and abnormalities of the immune system, circulatory system, central nervous system, and hypothalamic-pituitary-adrenal (HPA) axis, and is associated with a number of infectious agents. No specific diagnostic test for CFS exists.

CFS crosses all age, gender, and socioeconomic lines, appearing in children, male and female adults, the elderly, and all socioeconomic groups and races. The one time stereotypical CFS patient—the Caucasian, active, middle-aged woman—has not stood up under scrutiny. Until publication of a study by Jason, Richman, and colleagues (1997), incidence in minority groups was underrepresented in prevalence studies. All segments of the population, including children, are at risk, but women in their middle years seem to be most susceptible.

Although sporadic, or endemic, cases occur more frequently than those associated with epidemics, they are poorly documented. Outbreaks of illnesses with CFS-like characteristics have been described since at least the 1700s with some accounts dating back as far as 1400 B.C. Outbreaks have been documented in cooler countries rather than those with tropical climates: England, Scotland, Canada, Switzerland, Japan, Iceland, Australia, New Zealand, Germany, and South Africa. Names for past outbreaks around the

world often reflected suspected causes, symptoms, or outbreak locations: the English sweats (with which Anne Boleyn, wife of King
Henry VIII, was believed to suffer), neurasthenia, myasthenia,
Akureyri or Iceland disease, Royal Free disease, (epidemic) neuromyasthenia, vegetative neuritis, low natural killer cell disease,
postviral fatigue syndrome, chronic Epstein-Barr virus, yuppie flu,
and chronic fatigue immune dysfunction syndrome. The names
CFS and myalgic encephalomyelitis (ME), used in other English-
speaking countries, are often used synonymously. Most outbreaks
were briefly noted in the medical literature and forgotten; only
recently have the links among them been explored.

In the early 1980s, a large portion of the population of Incline
Village, Nevada, was stricken with an unusual illness. Drs. Daniel
Peterson and Paul Cheney treated many of these patients and in
1985 called upon the Centers for Disease Control and Prevention
(CDC) to investigate the outbreak. The CDC (Gary P. Holmes,
M.D., and colleagues) initially denied the existence of an epidemic,
but later claimed they had taken the illness seriously and believed it
to be related to Epstein-Barr virus (EBV). In 1988, the CDC, taking
the position that the illness was not caused by EBV, renamed it
"chronic fatigue syndrome," issuing a case definition. The apparently disinterested CDC essentially turned its back on the devastation in Incline Village and elsewhere.

On a name-change petition, Hillary J. Johnson, author of
Osler's Web, commented that the name "chronic fatigue syndrome"
was selected

> *by a small group of politically motivated and/or poorly informed*
> *scientists and doctors who were vastly more concerned about costs to*
> *insurance companies and the Social Security Administration than*
> *about public health. Their deliberate intention—based on the corre-*
> *spondence they exchanged over a period of months—was to obfus-*
> *cate the nature of the disease by placing it in the realm of the psychi-*
> *atric rather than the organic. The harm they have caused is surely one*
> *of the greatest tragedies in the history of medicine.*

In 1994, a new research definition was published by the CDC
recommending a stepwise approach to diagnosis, starting with a
clinical evaluation of "self-reported persistent or relapsing fatigue
lasting six or more consecutive months." Other conditions that

explain chronic fatigue, excluding a diagnosis of CFS, include previous, unresolved conditions, major depressive disorder with psychotic or melancholic features, bipolar affective disorders, schizophrenia, delusional disorders, dementias, anorexia nervosa, bulimia, substance abuse within two years prior to onset, and severe obesity. Conditions that may coexist with CFS include other illnesses that cannot be confirmed by lab tests, including fibromyalgia, anxiety or somatoform disorders, nonpsychotic or nonmelancholic depression, neurasthenia, multiple chemical sensitivity disorder, fatigue-producing conditions that are or have been adequately treated, and any single finding that is not sufficiently strong to suggest one of the exclusionary conditions. Presence of any of these conditions would not rule out a diagnosis of CFS.

According to the CDC's 1994 research definition, a case of CFS is defined by the presence of

1. clinically evaluated, unexplained persistent or relapsing chronic fatigue of new or definite onset (not lifelong) that is not the result of ongoing exertion; is not substantially alleviated by rest; and results in substantial reduction in previous levels of functioning, and

2. concurrent occurrence of at least four symptoms, which must have persisted or recurred during at least 6 consecutive months following the onset of fatigue: short-term memory impairment, sore throat, tender cervical or axillary lymph nodes, muscle pain, multi-joint pain without joint swelling or redness, headaches of a new type, unrefreshing sleep, and post-exertional malaise lasting over 24 hours. (Fukuda, Straus, et al. 1994)

Jason, Richman, and colleagues (1997) note flaws in the 1994 definition, which excludes some cases of CFS but may characterize other disorders as well. Criteria are assessed at only one point in time, based only on presence but not severity of symptoms. Individuals who do not have "new or definite onset" (vague terms) are excluded. Symptoms must begin after the onset of fatigue, yet this is not always the case in CFS. Contrary to the criteria, fatigue may be alleviated to some degree by rest, and fatigue may be precipitated by only minimal exertion. Although neurological and neurocognitive symptoms are hallmarks of the disorder, they are downplayed, with an overemphasis on infectious-type symptoms. One perplexing flaw is the lack of a definition for fatigue and an inability to assess it. Criteria are not standardized among countries, making study results difficult to compare. Since the case definition is undergoing revision, development of an internationally accepted definition would be advantageous.

Intended by the CDC to be a restrictive research tool to identify a homogeneous group, the CDC definition is frequently misused as the standard for clinical diagnosis and disability determination. No clinical criteria or definition exists.

CFS: A DIFFERENT LEAGUE OF FATIGUE

The name of an illness has a profound impact upon those who suffer from it, upon how the uninformed perceive it, and upon medical research and treatment.

— *John Herd, CFS patient and advocate*

Chronic fatigue syndrome (CFS) is a silly name for a serious illness, clearly inappropriate since fatigue is associated with many chronic disorders and is common in the healthy population. The name, insulting to patients and to physicians and researchers involved in the study and treatment of CFS, does not reflect the severity or associated abnormalities of the syndrome, making patients easy candidates for dismissal by the medical profession, media, and the uninformed. Resulting misconceptions leave family members baffled and make sufferers the brunt of jokes and snide remarks.

CFS has been called a committee definition rather than a disease or a syndrome, and the consensus of medical professionals, researchers, and patient groups is that CFS should be renamed. Some maintain that no accurate alternative exists at this time since cause and pathophysiology of the illness remain unknown.

In a giant step backward, a 1996 report of the Joint Working Group of the Royal Colleges of Physicians, Psychiatrists and General Practitioners on Chronic Fatigue Syndrome in the United Kingdom recommended that the term "myalgic encephalomyelitis" be dropped and replaced with "chronic fatigue syndrome" in the UK. Dr. Stephen Straus of the National Institutes of Health called the report "the finest contemporary position statement in the field."

Suggested alternate names include chronic fatigue and immune dysfunction syndrome (CFIDS); chronic immune dysfunction syndrome (CIDS); myalgic encephalomyelitis (ME) or its variant, myalgic encephalopathy; myoencephalopathy; Ramsay's disease; chronic immunologic-neurologic disorder; multisensory sensitivity syndrome (MUSES); dysregulation spectrum syndrome (DSS); multiple immune dysfunction syndrome (MIDS); and neuroendocrine immume disorder (NEID). Everyone agrees that the term "fatigue" (the "f" word) needs to be dropped because it falsely characterizes and oversimplifies the disorder, recognizing only one symptom among many. David Bell, M.D., considers the word "fatigue" inappropriate since it is defined as a response to exertion that is relieved by rest, whereas CFS "fatigue" may result from little or no exertion and is not substantially relieved by rest.

Byron Hyde, M.D., differentiates CFS and myalgic encephalomyelitis (ME) on the basis of the CFS definition's emphasis on flulike or infectious symptoms, but this distinction relates to differing criteria rather than distinctions between disorders.

Patients have written letters, staged forums, and signed petitions to change the name. The CDC agreed to study the matter but later announced that the adoption of a new name is premature. In a catch-22, the present name trivializes the illness, thereby discouraging research funding needed to uncover the pathophysiology of the disorder, which would help determine a more accurate name. A new name for the disorder should reflect the nature and severity of the illness, eliminate the "f" word or any other individual symptom, sound scientifically credible, and not imply cause or pathophysiology, which remain speculative. A new name must serve us well in the long term, making further revision unnecessary, and ideally should meet international approval.

CAUSE

The cause of CFS may vary among patients and is probably multifactorial, involving pathogen(s), genetic predisposition, age, gender, stressful events (e.g., infections, surgery, childbirth, emotional trauma, periods of intense stress), and exposure to environmental toxins. Suspects for the causative agent(s)—there may be none or more than one—include viruses and other infectious agents. Most

Persons With CFS (PWCs) do not meet criteria for preexisting psychiatric diagnoses, indicating that psychopathology is not causal, as contended by skeptics.

Calling it "the most complex disease I have ever studied," Jay Goldstein, M.D., regards CFS as "the final common pathway of a multifactorial psychoneuroimmunologic disorder with a limbic encephalopathy causing autonomic dysfunction and subtle neuroendocrine derangements" (1991). That is, disruption in normal brain functioning is the cause of most or all CFS symptoms, although the causes of the brain abnormalities are not currently known. Defining CFS as a psychoneuroimmunologic disorder addresses the interactions among behavior, the immune system, and the central nervous system.

ONSET

Sudden onset of chronic illness is unusual, making CFS an exception. Susan commented, "For no apparent reason, my life fell flat on its face." Patients with an abrupt onset of symptoms generally assume they have a "normal" or self-limiting illness that will last a week or two without realizing that it is the beginning of a long-term illness. Abrupt onset is said to characterize about three-fourths of cases, and some patients are able to specify the date and place the illness began. "My medical history reeks of good health, but one day I got sick and never recovered," says Mike. However, onset in others may follow a long period of mild symptoms with full-blown illness triggered by trauma: infection, surgery, or difficult life events. Often the illness begins with flulike symptoms and frequent infections, interspersed with intervals of feeling relatively well. As the illness progresses, other symptoms emerge, particularly in the neurocognitive realm, often reported as the most difficult aspect of the illness that causes the greatest degree of disability. Kyle expresses confusion about her illness. "I may have been sick for five years and not really known it. I [had] pneumonia, depression, inability to concentrate. Later I had every kind of medical test in the world. I still didn't know what was wrong with me, but my brain is shot. Once sharp, it can no longer focus or reason."

CFS may not be diagnosed unless the symptoms have been present for six months or longer. Patients may be given appropriate medical treatment, including recommendations for rest, symptomatic treatment, and encouragement to schedule a follow-up visit if symptoms do not resolve. As patients wonder, "What could be wrong with me? Why don't I get better?" their physicians may be saying, "You've just worn yourself out. Relax. Get a little rest and go back to work," or "You're too stressed. Get some exercise."

"When I developed CFS," says Paula, "I was working and taking a few classes. Suddenly I couldn't function or think clearly, couldn't keep up at school, and forgot how to do things I knew how to do. At first I thought it was the flu and it would go away, but it didn't go away. I was fine one day and not fine the next—just that quick."

Yolanda, a recently remarried mother of three children, was attending law school when unusual symptoms began to appear—fatigue, "brain fog," equilibrium and anxiety symptoms, numbness, shakiness, exhaustion, insomnia, allergic and viral-type problems—worsening over a period of years until "I totally fell apart. I couldn't stay alert. I would fall asleep and be in another zone; I was in a fog. It was really scary." Yolanda felt fine for short periods of time but inevitably crashed. Special arrangements were made to help her complete school, but she has never become well enough to work.

In her book *Living with Chronic Illness,* Cheri Register describes the initial phase of chronic illness: the waxing and waning of symptoms, difficulty obtaining a diagnosis, attempts to attribute these symptoms to a psychological cause, and determination to chase the illness away by changing habits and behavior. She describes numerous, frustrating contacts with medical professionals in her attempt to obtain a specific diagnosis.

Fear inevitably accompanies the onset of unusual, unexplained symptoms. People wonder if they're going crazy or whether they will die. One patient recalls, "Because I felt so horrible, I figured it was going to kill me, whatever it was." And another: "I just couldn't go any more. That wasn't like me. I could always do whatever was necessary. My body didn't work right; I was scared." The common thread is a feeling of being out of control, captive of an unknown, frightening, invisible force that came out of nowhere.

DEMOGRAPHICS

Dennis Jackson, Ph.D., called CFS an "equal opportunity attacker" because it crosses all barriers—age, nationality, gender, lifestyle, socioeconomic group, and occupation. Females are believed to out-number males by 2:1 or 3:1. Female preponderance is common in autoimmune diseases, a category that may include CFS. CFS has a greater-than-average incidence in health care workers. Several studies indicate average age at onset is 37, with most patients in their middle or "prime" years, ages 25–50 (potentially devastating to the workforce). About 75 percent of patients are aged 20–49; 50 to 60 percent are 30–49. This age range may be inaccurate because the illness is probably underdiagnosed in children and the elderly.

The true prevalence of CFS remains unknown, with each suc-cessive study finding increased numbers. According to a Chicago-based study by Jason, Richman, and colleagues (1999), the total number of patients remains unknown but is conservatively one mil-lion, with fewer than 10 percent of cases diagnosed. CFS emerges as a serious health concern, much more common than AIDS or breast or lung cancer in women.

Problems estimating the true prevalence of CFS include differ-ing criteria; shifting case definitions; exclusion of children, the eld-erly, and those in remission; varying methods of collecting data; misdiagnosis with other disorders; and different prevalence rates in specific groups of individuals or geographic locations. True preva-lence has been estimated at two to ten million cases in the United States alone. It seems that the number of new cases is on the rise, but this has not been scientifically studied.

SYMPTOMS

Symptoms tend to wax and wane but are often severely debilitating, lasting for years. Symptom type and severity vary from patient to patient and in each individual over time.

General or physical symptoms include profound fatigue worsened by exertion; frequent infections; new-onset headaches; allergies of new onset or increased severity; sensitivities to foods, odors, or chemicals; sore throat; swollen or tender lymph nodes; fevers; night sweats; weight change, usually gain without a change in eating habits; muscle and joint aches; irritable bladder; irritable bowel (gas, alternating constipation and diarrhea, nausea, and abdominal pain); rashes; shortness of breath on minimal or no exertion; heart palpitations; chest pain; cough; urinary tract problems; and decreased sex drive.

Neurological symptoms, a hallmark of CFS, include sleep disorders; sensory disturbances (including vision changes and sensitivity to bright light, odors, chemicals, foods, medicines, and temperature changes); pain; multiple tender points; dysequilibrium (balance problems, "spaciness," and disorientation); altered perception; cognitive problems ("brain fog," difficulty with concentration and memory, impaired calculation ability and word usage); seizure-like episodes or "blackouts"; unusual and disturbing nightmares; altered spatial perception; numbness and tingling in the extremities; and alcohol intolerance.

Emotional problems associated with CFS include depression, which may be accompanied by suicidal ideation or attempts; anxiety with or without panic attacks; mood swings; irritability; "rage attacks"; and personality changes. Depression may be both endogenous (chemically caused) and exogenous (caused by external events). Although patients often *feel* crazy, many of the emotional changes they experience are secondary to the illness. Most did not experience such problems prior to the onset of CFS.

EFFECTS

CFS affects one's lifestyle and self-image considerably. Although some persons with CFS are able to work full- or part-time, others are too ill to work at all. In addition to occupational issues, CFS results in numerous, significant changes and losses in relationships, identity, self-esteem, and the ability to engage in previously enjoyed activities, to handle finances, to plan ahead, to think clearly, and to exercise good judgment.

Patients generally feel poorly understood by others, experiencing self-doubt as well as relationship conflicts. It is impossible for those without CFS to understand the true impact of the illness and the havoc it can wreak. Because patients invariably appear healthier than they feel, those with whom they come into contact are not immediately aware of CFS-related limitations and often expect them to behave "normally"—that is, to be active and to handle the same responsibilities as in the past. It is difficult for patients to communicate the degree of their physical impairment and emotional pain to others, and as a result many relationships are disrupted. In addition, the patient copes daily with lowered self-esteem, a very restricted activity level, an inability to predict health fluctuations, and feelings of powerlessness and worthlessness due to the inability to function as in the past. Many have based their self-esteem on *what they were able to do* rather than on *who they were and are,* leading to changing roles and identity problems that must be addressed. The emotional fallout of CFS can be as devastating as the symptoms themselves.

DIAGNOSIS

It's always been said that this is an illness of exclusion, that everything else must be ruled out before the diagnosis of chronic fatigue syndrome can be made. That is not true. The pattern of symptoms is unique; there is no other illness in general medical practice that looks like this one.

— *David Bell, M.D.*

The *Merck Manual of Diagnosis and Therapy,* known as "the most widely used general medical textbook in the world," lists CFS among hundreds of recognized diseases and conditions. The CDC announced that in 2002, the US ICD diagnostic code for CFS will be changed from 780.71 ("General symptoms—Malaise and fatigue") to G93.3 ("Other disorders of the brain"). The World Health Organization established the latter code in 1992 to encompass myalgic encephalomyelitis and postviral fatigue syndrome.

No diagnostic laboratory test exists for CFS. Diagnosis is based on symptoms, findings on clinical exams, length of time ill, degree of impairment, and by ruling out other illnesses with similar symptoms. At one time, an Epstein-Barr antibody test was regarded as a diagnostic test but is no longer used since the elevated Epstein-Barr antibodies found in most patients also occur in the general population.

When standard test results and a cursory physical examination are normal, physicians may attribute symptoms to psychological causes or "a bug." Resulting treatment is inadequate.

Many patients see numerous doctors before being diagnosed. CFS is both underdiagnosed (when patients' symptoms are not understood or taken seriously by their doctors) and overdiagnosed (when fatigue is caused by other factors).

Although most routine laboratory tests yield normal results, abnormalities emerge on more specialized testing of immune functioning, brain imaging, neurocognitive testing, sleep studies, tilt table testing, endocrine and metabolic function, treadmill or bicycle ergometry, presence of abnormal urinary metabolites, cardiac and respiratory abnormalities, and cell wall abnormalities. The most significant finding to date, and a potential marker for the illness, is abnormality in the 2-5A synthetase/RNaseL antiviral pathway, the body's primary defense against viruses. Unfortunately, the presence of abnormalities varies among individuals and probably in each individual over time. This variation may be the result of the CFS population being nonhomogeneous, testing at only one point in time, fluctuations of the illness in each individual, and/or variability among study protocols and laboratory procedures.

David Bell, M.D., takes issue with reports of "normal" physical examinations: "Virtually all [CFS] patients will have abnormalities on physical exam, but on average the patient will look pretty healthy. What the doctor is thinking is that the physical exam is not abnormal enough to explain why someone says they can be up only two hours a day. The degree of reported activity restriction is so dramatic physicians frequently just don't believe it's possible."

COURSE OF THE ILLNESS

The severity of the illness varies considerably among patients and in individual patients across time. Some are mildly affected and can carry on a modified activity schedule; others are extremely debilitated but able to function at least minimally; and many are completely disabled, bedbound, or housebound. Most cases fall between the extremes, with the illness following a waxing and waning cycle.

Patricia Fennell, Ph.D., and colleagues (1999) have identified four stages of CFS:

Crisis: Onset may unfold over a period of years. Denial, a coping mechanism, gives way to crisis as symptoms linger without explanation. Isolation and bewilderment, vocational difficulties, and lack of family support develop.

Stabilization: Initial relief following diagnosis is replaced by disappointment and desperation as additional difficulties develop. Fears about the future and decreased self-esteem accompany difficulty keeping a regular work schedule and losses within one's social network. A sense of control begins to emerge as one learns to cope with symptoms and life changes.

Resolution: Illness plateau characterized by relapses interspersed with attempts to normalize. Further vocational and social problems are accompanied by feelings of abandonment by friends and significant others.

Integration: Continuation of plateau or symptom improvement may occur. Many lose faith in the medical profession, realizing that they may remain ill indefinitely. Use of new coping mechanisms and a search for meaning lead to adaptation, new pursuits (vocational, educational, volunteer, or personal), reassessment of priorities and values, and spiritual development.

Early stages of CFS may be characterized by flulike symptoms (e.g., non-exudative pharyngitis, fevers, body pain, malaise, "brain fog," and lymphadenopathy) and frequent infections, interspersed with intervals of feeling relatively well. As the illness progresses, the flulike symptoms may abate as other symptoms emerge. The fluctuations in illness and levels of functioning often become less pronounced over time. Cognitive and other neurological difficulties usually emerge as the illness progresses, and often these are reported by patients as the most difficult aspect of the illness, causing the highest degree of disability.

EXACERBATIONS

Exacerbations may occur in the presence or absence of identifiable triggers. Symptoms are often worsened by changes in weather or temperature; exertion; physical, emotional, or cognitive stress; and toxic exposure. For those who are disabled by CFS, ongoing, protracted adversarial situations with disability insurance carriers causes a marked exacerbation of symptoms, which may continue and even intensify after the matter is resolved.

CONTAGION

The mode of transmission is unknown. Multiple cases of CFS in families are common, and those afflicted are usually genetically related (blood relatives) rather than nonblood relatives such as spouses. Some researchers suspect that the risk for partners increases over time due to repeated exposure, while others believe that the risk of contagion is high only in the early stages of the disease. However, there is no direct evidence that CFS is contagious or transmissible. Genetic predisposition and/or exposure to environmental agents may explain the route by which the disease is contracted. Anecdotal evidence indicates an increased incidence of autoimmune disorders in close relatives of patients.

Because of the uncertainties regarding contagion, patients are advised not to be blood or organ donors. Some experts believe that immunizations may challenge an already disrupted immune system; others assert that flu shots pose no danger and are advisable. Because the transmissibility of the illness has not been determined, some physicians advise against sharing eating utensils and drinking glasses or kissing on the mouth and recommend the use of condoms for those who are sexually active with more than one partner. Most physicians feel that such precautions are unnecessary, so it is up to the individual to decide whether precautions are appropriate.

Several practitioners have noted an increased prevalence of CFS in spouses/partners of patients in perhaps 10 percent of cases. The risk of contagion to a spouse seems highest in the first year of the illness, and affected spouses often have less severe symptoms.

CFS AND PREGNANCY

Pregnant CFS patients often experience a temporary remission of symptoms beginning several weeks after conception and lasting until several weeks after delivery. This may be attributable to increased blood volume, changes in hormone levels, or altered immune function. Those considering pregnancy should bear in mind that they will have to curtail the use of medications during pregnancy and breast-feeding. They must address the unknown possibility of an infectious agent being transmitted in utero or via breast-feeding, the possibility of genetic predisposition in the child, and the difficulties of energy-intensive infant and toddler care. Although the rate of first-trimester miscarriage is higher than normal, babies of CFS patients usually thrive and do well. This topic is not well studied, and all information is anecdotal.

PETS

Although it is rare for one species to share illness with another, an informal study of patients with pets in Charlotte, North Carolina, indicated that half of the pets were ill (Cheney 1991). Anecdotal reports link domestic animals, particularly dogs and cats, with CFS. Tom Glass, D.D.S., Ph.D., investigated reports of CFS-like illness in household pets, finding that a large proportion of the group had pets, often several. In cases where significant contact occurred between patients and their pets, many respondents indicated that the pets had CFS-like neurologic, neuromuscular, and rheumato-logic symptoms, often prior to their owners' illness. No evidence of any specific disease entity was found. Symptoms in pets included weakness, lethargy, sleep disorders, tremors, myalgia (muscle pain), arthralgia (joint pain), palsy, anxiety, depression, balance problems, gastrointestinal symptoms, photophobia, visual problems, tooth/gum disease, and blood disorders, with a high incidence of tumors, leukemia, and lymphoma. Rigorous systematic studies have not yet been conducted.

TREATMENT

CFS is presently treatable but not curable. Rest and lifestyle modifi-cation are consistently rated as the most helpful treatments. For-merly active patients find that moderating their activity levels falls somewhere between inconvenient and impossible. However, it is absolutely necessary to adapt by making appropriate lifestyle changes. The worst thing patients can do is push too hard, inviting relapses and possibly prolonging the course of the illness.

Treatment must be tailored to the individual, since no univer-sally helpful therapies exist. Treatment is generally symptom-focused and is changed over time as necessary. Current therapies include prescription drugs, vitamins and supplements, lifestyle modification, dietary changes, rest therapy, exercise as tolerated, and adjunctive therapies. As in the case of all poorly understood debilitating illnesses, patients may fall prey to spurious claims of cures by unscrupulous individuals touting treatments that may be ineffective and even dangerous. Patients are advised to become well-educated consumers of health services.

Psychotherapy is often helpful for addressing adjustment issues and developing coping skills. Practical approaches (e.g., education, emotional support, problem-solving and cognitive behavioral therapy as opposed to insight-oriented therapy) seem to be most helpful. Individual or group psychotherapy is helpful for dealing with the emotional devastation that invariably accompanies CFS: illness-imposed limitations, anger, losses, depression, relationship and family issues, and lifestyle alterations. Instruction in relaxation and stress-reduction techniques can also be helpful. It is essential to work with a CFS-knowledgeable physician with an educated and open-minded approach to treatment. Most support groups provide referral lists of recommended professionals.

PROGNOSIS: IS THERE LIFE AFTER CFS? DO PEOPLE RECOVER?

The prognosis is variable, with most patients remaining symptomatic over time. The recovery rate has been estimated at 4 to 12 percent, including those in remission who continue to run the risk of relapse. However, these figures may be inaccurate and misleading, as follow-up study results depend upon anecdotal reports from physicians and patients. Physicians may interpret discontinuation of treatment as recovery, when, in fact, the opposite may be true. Patients may become less symptomatic due to lifestyle modification and coping strategies and hence may overestimate their degree of wellness. Patients contacted only once may be having a particularly good or bad day, and some may feel the need to present favorably to please the interviewer or physician. Some patients improve in some ways but worsen in others. Surprisingly, many who report complete recovery continue to experience symptoms. Perhaps the greatest difficulty in estimating recovery is that patients who have become asymptomatic may still be vulnerable to future relapses.

The prognosis cannot be assessed in individual cases. Degree of recovery seems to be associated with the length of time ill but not with type of onset, severity, abnormalities, presence of psychiatric diagnoses, demographics, treatments, lab test results, or number of symptoms. Recovery episodes can occur at any time during the course of CFS but are most likely during the early years, with chances of complete recovery diminishing markedly after the first few years of illness. Those who have become fully disabled often remain disabled for many years.

Many patients improve gradually over time. The majority continue to have chronic moderate-to-severe symptoms over time, with a small subgroup recovering fully and another small subgroup becoming sicker. Emotional adjustment often improves independently of the course of the illness.

The prognosis is considered more favorable in children and adolescents as compared with adults. Some fully recover, and the majority regain the ability to study or work full-time despite remaining symptomatic. A third, smaller group remains significantly ill.

STILL A MYSTERY

At a 12 May 1995 congressional briefing, Mark Loveless, M.D., an infectious disease specialist and head of the AIDS and CFS Clinic at Oregon Health Sciences University, testified that a CFS patient feels every day effectively the same as an AIDS patient feels two months before death.

CFS has significantly affected us individually and collectively. By afflicting those in their most productive years, CFS presents a serious threat to the nation's workforce. The loss of workers, the mounting medical and research expenses, the increasing number of disability cases, and cumulative disability payments from Social Security and private insurers are potentially devastating to our national economy.

Also devastating are the divorce and suicide rates among patients. The divorce rate for chronically ill persons is an astounding 75 percent. Although the suicide rate has not been determined, it is significantly higher than in the general population. Because many patients (including children and adolescents) feel overwhelmed, misunderstood, depressed, and hopeless, suicide is often contemplated and sometimes attempted as an alternative to a life of desperation and pain.

Inadequate research funding has been a problem from the start. Additionally, funds allocated to CFS by congress were misspent by the Centers for Disease Control and Prevention (CDC) on other projects. An agency audit revealed that from 1995 through 1998, only about $10 million of an allocated $23 million was spent on CFS research.

The CDC added CFS to the list of "Priority 1 New and Reemerging Infectious Diseases" in 1995. The National Institutes of Health (NIH), the CDC, and the National Institute for Allergy and Infectious Diseases (NIAID) have published pamphlets for physician and patient education. The responses of these agencies sound good, but they have often printed inaccurate information and given numerous indications that they do not consider this illness a priority.

Subtypes of CFS, which have not been well identified or studied, may account for variability of study results. Subtypes may be based on patient history, type of onset, triggering/causal factors, symptoms at onset, symptom patterns, severity, response to medications, accompanying diagnoses, or laboratory test abnormalities.

Patients are encouraged to play an active role in treatment and to obtain current, accurate information. There is cause for hope. The medical community is becoming increasingly sensitive to CFS and those afflicted; researchers are searching for causes, treatments, and cures; and a significant number of patients do recover—at least to some degree. Meanwhile, self-care, education, medical treatment, and emotional support remain the most precious resources of persons with CFS.

3

Fibromyalgia Syndrome

Fibromyalgia syndrome (FMS) is a common, debilitating disorder of widespread musculoskeletal pain, sleep disturbance, fatigue, and additional somatic symptoms. FMS affects muscles, joints, tendons, ligaments, and other soft tissues, most frequently causing pain in the neck, shoulders, back, and hips. Most patients with FMS state that they hurt all over, with the pain varying in severity and migrating to various body sites over time. The pain is described as aching, burning, and radiating and is accompanied by stiffness, burning, twitching, numbness or tingling of the extremities, and the type of ache that typically follows muscle exertion. Multiple tender points in specific areas, usually where muscle attaches to bone, are considered the hallmark of the disorder and form the basis of diagnosis. Although FMS is treatable, its cause and cure remain unknown. FMS is not progressive or life-threatening but usually persists indefinitely. Robert Bennett, M.D., has called it "the commonest cause of widespread pain," and its cost to society is steep in terms of lost productivity, disability, and medical expenses.

The pain is believed to be of central origin, stemming from an amplification of pain processing and defects in pain inhibition in the central nervous system (CNS)—a phenomenon called "central sensitization." Although the CNS shows no structural injury or lesion, its function is impaired, causing hyperalgesia (heightened pain response to a stimulus that normally causes only minor pain and allodynia (pain sensation in the absence of a painful stimulus).

The term "fibromyalgia syndrome" is preferred to "fibromyalgia" as better describing the disorder, which is characterized by a constellation of symptoms and dysfunction in multiple body systems, including neuroendocrine and immunologic abnormalities. "Fibro" refers to connective tissue, "myo" signifies muscle, and "algia" means "pain." The term "fibromyalgia" has been criticized because it refers to muscle disorders that do not adequately characterize the syndrome and because FMS pain is largely attributable to central nervous system abnormalities rather than structural changes in muscles.

HISTORY

Fibromyalgia is not a new disorder, but awareness of the illness has increased and its incidence is probably higher than in the past. It has been known by other names, including fibrositis, fibromyositis, neurasthenia, and myofascial pain syndrome. Since it is a noninflammatory illness, terms ending with *-itis* (signifying inflammation) are no longer used. The term "fibromyalgia" was introduced in 1976, and the disorder has been described but known by other names since the seventeenth century or earlier, possibly back to the time of Hippocrates, who suffered diffuse musculoskeletal pain.

Despite the World Health Organization's acceptance of fibromyalgia syndrome as a legitimate illness in 1992, many physicians continue to maintain that it does not exist. Like CFS, FMS is chronic and has no visible symptoms. Media and government attention have been underwhelming, with the illness largely ignored or disparaged.

PREVALENCE

Fibromyalgia is one of the most common diagnoses made by rheumatologists. FMS shows no apparent ethnic bias and exists in most countries of the world. Worldwide incidence is estimated at 1 to 12 percent of total population, although diagnostic criteria vary. United States prevalence estimates are 4 to 7 million, or as many as 10 million. By contrast, 15 million people in the United States are believed to have osteoarthritis and 2 million to have rheumatoid arthritis.

Although women in their middle years (20 to 50) seem to be most commonly afflicted, FMS is seen in men, children, and the elderly. FMS is more common in women by an estimated ratio of 5:1 to 20:1. The diagnosis may not be made until the condition has been present for many years, and average age at the time of diagnosis is 34 to 53. About 60 percent of cases are diagnosed by rheumatologists and 31 percent by internists or family practitioners.

A family history of FMS is found in about 30 percent of patients, suggesting a genetic component to the illness, although the precise genetic mechanism is not yet known. Family members without chronic pain have been found to have taut, ropy muscles similar to those of FMS patients.

Reports comparing symptom severity in men and women conflict, with some indicating equal severity and others greater or lesser severity. This discrepancy may result in part from men's reluctance to seek medical attention. In males, FMS is often accompanied by sleep apnea.

ONSET

"My car was rear-ended while I was stopped at a red light," recalls Lonnie. "I went to the doctor even though I was basically okay, just to cover all the bases." Although the pain in her neck and back was mild, she took muscle relaxants and pain medication as prescribed. The pain became worse rather than better over the following weeks, and she continued treatment, expecting a successful outcome. She developed new symptoms over a period of months, experiencing bodywide achiness, fatigue, and cognitive problems. Lonnie says, "I began to make stupid mistakes at work, forgetting how to do things I had done practically forever. I couldn't concentrate or make decisions." Unable to keep up with job responsibilities, she was soon forced to take a leave of absence. Additional unusual symptoms began to develop: stiffness, migrating pain, sensitivity to perfumes and chemical odors, inability to think clearly, and gastrointestinal upset. Thinking she had lost her mind, Lonnie described these symptoms to her rheumatologist, who diagnosed posttraumatic fibromyalgia. To this day, she remains incredulous that a minor accident could result in chronic, debilitating illness, especially because "I know so many people who have been involved in major collisions with severe injuries who have *not* gone on to develop FMS." She is grateful to her knowledgeable and supportive physician.

Mark says, "My mother fell asleep regularly at the breakfast table, to the point that it became a family joke. She was knocked out by almost any major exertion and seemed to be in pain most of the time," although she stoically attempted to conceal her pain. "That's just the way she was," he says. "We never really talked about it. I had a lot of achiness as a kid but was told I had growing pains. Looking back, I think we both had fibromyalgia, and so did some of my cousins. It seemed normal in my family to ache, and nobody made a big deal about it." It became a big deal in adulthood, when Mark's active, stressful lifestyle exacerbated his pain level and sleep disorder. Mark says, "I spent a long time just lying around in isolation, waiting to feel better, but that never happened. The best thing I ever did was become active in our local support group." Mark began a multidisciplinary treatment program and has cut back on his work schedule. "I'm luckier than most because my work schedule is very flexible. I'm still sick, but at least I feel productive."

The onset of FMS may be abrupt or gradual, beginning in childhood in up to 28 percent of patients. Onset may follow a trauma or an injury (e.g., motor vehicle accident or sports injury); repetitive motion; or emotional or physical stress including major life changes, toxic exposure, infectious or flulike illness, surgery, or development of another disorder such as lupus or rheumatoid arthritis. It typically begins with a focal point of pain that becomes generalized, with a triggering event leading to the development of full-blown FMS. The triggering event may be considered a causal factor, or a catalyst that triggers FMS along with other factors. The prevalence of FMS in family members may indicate a predisposition, although alternative explanations have been considered.

The average age at onset is twenty-five to forty-five years, although FMS may begin at any age. Those with childhood onset may not realize they have a disorder, especially when their complaints are dismissed or if they cannot remember a time when they were not symptomatic.

SYMPTOMS

The hallmark symptom of FMS is pain that varies in intensity and may migrate to different body sites. It is described as deep muscle aching, burning, shooting, throbbing, and stabbing. Pain and stiffness are often worse in the morning and with repetitive motion. Most fibromyalgics complain of fatigue, nonrestorative sleep, and decreased energy. Pain may be accompanied by headaches (tension and/or migraine), irritable bowel and bladder, sleep disorders, tinnitus (ringing in the ears), numbness, light-headedness, and cognitive dysfunction. Sensation may be decreased in some parts of the body, most often the extremities. Range of motion is often limited. Reaching, twisting, bending, and other types of motion may not be possible due to muscle tightness and spasms. FMS is not associated with loss of muscle tone, muscle wasting or deterioration, or local inflammation (redness and swelling). When these symptoms exist, they are attributed to concomitant illnesses.

Additional symptoms include the following:

Abnormal sensory processing: sensitivities to sensory stimuli (light, noise, mildly painful stimuli, scents and odors, foods).

Cognitive dysfunction: Concentration and short-term memory are most often impaired. Problems may also occur with word finding, calculations, comprehension, motor speed, sustaining a train of thought, and ability to express ideas in words.

Equilibrium problems: dizziness, unsteady gait, clumsiness, and balance problems.

Fatigue: Ranging from mild to severe, FMS fatigue is described as a feeling of being drained or weighted down, with mental fatigue or "fibro-fog"—difficulty thinking clearly, focusing, and concentrating.

Headaches: migraine, muscle tension, or a combination of types, on an intermittent, frequent, or constant basis, and ranging in severity from mild to incapacitating.

Irritable bladder: discomfort with frequent need to urinate, sometimes associated with pain on voiding and often misdiagnosed as infection.

Irritable bowel syndrome (IBS): alternating diarrhea and constipation, abdominal cramping and gas, and nausea.

Multiple sensitivities: to medicines; odors; environmental chemicals including cleaning agents, petroleum products, pesticides, and herbicides; light; noise; and certain foods. Abnormal sensory processing may lead to sensory overload in the presence of multiple stimuli, intensifying symptoms.

Neurally mediated hypotension (NMH): dysregulation of the complex series of events that regulates blood flow, involving communication between the brain and the heart, with blood pooling in the lower part of the body and insufficient oxygen traveling to the brain, causing presyncope (a feeling of faintness), light-headedness, and fatigue.

Pain: primarily related to abnormalities in pain processing by the central nervous system rather than in the muscles themselves.

Sleep disorders: a significant factor in pain exacerbation, fatigue, cognitive dysfunction, and other symptoms. Several aspects of sleep may be abnormal:

- alpha-delta intrusion, in which deep (slow-wave) sleep is disrupted by bursts of near-awakening;
- nonrestorative, unrefreshing sleep, described by patients as "just skimming the surface of sleep" and "waking up feeling as if I've been run over by a Mack truck";
- difficulty falling asleep despite feeling exhausted;
- difficulty maintaining sleep due to several interrupting factors, including pain and frequent urination;
- unusual, disturbing dreams, sometimes related to certain medications;
- sleep apnea: breathing disturbance during sleep;
- bruxism: clenching or grinding of the teeth;
- periodic limb movement during sleep (PLMS, formerly called myoclonus): involuntary jerking of the limbs;
- restless leg syndrome (RLS): an uncomfortable condition characterized by paresthesias (abnormal sensations such as crawling, tingling, itching, and other odd sensations in the extremities, usually the legs) and a need to move the legs, somewhat relieved by walking or stretching. RLS is most common at night;
- altered circadian rhythms (being "out of synch" with the rest of the world, with alertness and energy best at night);
- unusual sensations, such as dysesthesias (unpleasant sensations) and feelings of numbness, pain, or tingling in the extremities;
- stiffness of the muscles, especially upon awakening;

‣ temporomandibular joint dysfunction (TMD): pain in the joint of the jaw near the ears that may lead to generalized facial and head pain;

‣ weakness.

Symptoms are exacerbated (worsened) by lack of sleep, poor quality sleep, cold and damp environments, exertion, repetitive motion, or with no apparent trigger. Hormonal states may affect FMS symptoms, with intensification of premenstrual and menopausal symptoms. As with CFS symptoms, FMS symptoms may subside after six to eight weeks of pregnancy, often returning six to eight weeks following delivery.

FMS may be accompanied by other conditions, including mitral valve prolapse, Raynaud's phenomenon, and pain disorders (e.g., rheumatoid arthritis, systemic lupus erythematosus (SLE), low back pain, Sjögren's syndrome, and osteoarthritis); however, most people with these disorders do not have FMS. Robert Bennett, M.D., estimates that about 75 percent of patients diagnosed with chronic fatigue syndrome also meet the criteria for diagnosis of FMS.

DIAGNOSIS

Primary care physicians estimate that complaints of musculoskeletal pain or inflammation account for about one of every seven patient visits, in most cases resolving with short-term treatment. FMS pain, in contrast, does not resolve but worsens over time and is accompanied by additional symptoms. A diagnosis of FMS is often not made until the condition has been present for many years.

Important diagnostic tools include a thorough history, including medical records and history of injuries; a thorough physical examination; and the patient's report of current complaints (pain characteristics, onset, location, frequency, duration, severity, and accompanying symptoms).

Although FMS is not a diagnosis of exclusion, testing for other illnesses characterized by pain and fatigue is appropriate. A review of organ systems and conditions associated with rheumatologic disorders can help narrow the diagnostic possibilities. Rule-outs are suggested by symptoms in individual cases and may include osteoarthritis, rheumatoid arthritis, lupus, ankylosing spondylitis, endocrine/metabolic disorders, neoplastic disorders, infections, primary sleep disorder or psychiatric conditions, and other neuromuscular diseases, such as autoimmune disorders, polyneuropathy, Chiari I malformation or cervical spinal stenosis, polymyositis, nodular fasciitis, metabolic myopathies, and myasthenia gravis.

The workup is much like that for CFS, with emphasis on the ANA, a blood test for inflammatory conditions. As with other pain disorders, laboratory tests and X-rays are usually normal. An accurate tender point examination (see the map of tender points on the next page) is essential to diagnosis; unfortunately, this technique is not taught in most medical schools. These points are tender on palpation and may feel like "knots." By contrast, trigger points are those that cause pain in other body locations.

Sedimentation rate may be elevated. Hormone levels should be checked, either to rule out problems or to indicate co-occurrence. FMS often co-occurs with CFS, hypothyroidism, and inflammatory disorders.

Diagnostic criteria published by the American College of Rheumatology in 1990 specify widespread pain affecting the left and right sides of the body, above and below the waist, that has persisted for at least three months, with pain on digital palpation in at least eleven of eighteen specified tender points when 4 kilograms of force is applied (about 9 pounds of pressure, enough to whiten the fingernail or to cause pain when the finger is pressed against the forehead). These bilateral points cluster around the neck, shoulder, chest, hip, knee, and elbow regions, in most cases where muscle narrows and attaches to bone (the occiput, low cervical, trapezius, supraspinatus, second rib, lateral epicondyle, gluteal, greater trochanter, and the fat pad inside the knee). A positive tender point examination is an objective finding; it is reproducible and can be measured if necessary with a dolorimeter, a device that ensures application of exactly 4 kilograms of pressure. The experienced physician will also detect abnormalities in muscle tissue, felt as nodules or tight bands. Fibromyalgia pain is not limited to these specified sites.

These criteria are not intended to be applied rigidly. Fewer tender points may be found on an initial exam, and the basis for diagnosis may include associated symptoms such as morning stiffness, fatigue, sleep disturbance, numbness or tingling in the hands and feet, or chronic headaches.

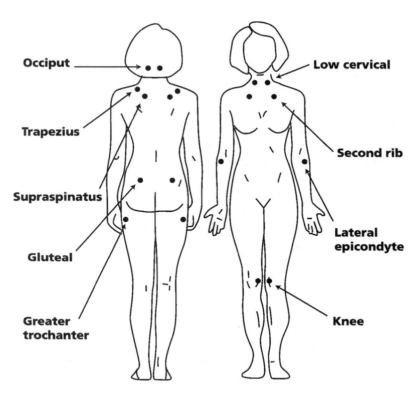

No laboratory test can confirm a diagnosis of FMS. Routine blood work and X-rays are usually normal, often leading to an incorrect diagnosis of masked depression, somatization disorder, or malingering. Psychological testing has proven these diagnoses largely unfounded. Sophisticated immune and endocrine tests and brain scans may yield abnormal results but are not routinely performed because they are costly, results vary over time and among laboratories, and they reflect abnormalities that are not treatable.

Children typically have similar symptoms with fewer tender points. They often experience sleep disorders and diffuse pain, although headache, general fatigue, and morning stiffness may not be present.

TYPES OF FIBROMYALGIA

FMS is a heterogeneous illness, meaning that not all patients experience the disorder in the same way. The subtypes of FMS are referred to as primary, secondary, and posttraumatic. Primary FMS exists in the absence of other connective tissue or immune disorders. Secondary or concomitant FMS occurs along with a primary underlying illness, often a connective tissue disease. Although FMS symptoms may be more prevalent or severe, the underlying illness is considered primary if it was present before the onset of FMS. (Differentiation between primary and secondary FMS is not used in the 1990 American College of Rheumatology diagnostic criteria.) Many FMS patients have no underlying disorders while others have associated conditions.

Posttraumatic fibromyalgia results from trauma or soft tissue injury, most commonly sustained in automobile accidents, sports, recreation, or work accidents due to either sudden injury or repetitive motions over time. Additional triggers include surgery, head injury, and pregnancy. A typical sequence begins with pain subsequent to an injury, usually in the neck, shoulders, or back. Over time, pain may develop in other regions of the body, accompanied by sleep disorder. Although one expects to recover from the injury, local pain may become widespread over a period of months to years. In examining 2,000 patient records, Mark Pellegrino, M.D., found that posttraumatic onset characterized 65 percent of his FMS patients. In this group, 52 percent resulted from vehicle accidents, particularly whiplash; 31 percent from work injuries; and 17 percent from another type of trauma. It is more likely that those with traumatic neck injuries, as opposed to other types of injuries, will develop FMS. Pellegrino identifies the key features of generalized posttraumatic fibromyalgia as absence of previous pain complaints prior to trauma, a trauma that caused pain to develop, persistence of pain for at least six months, and characteristic tender points that continue in follow-up medical exams.

The pathologic mechanism that ultimately leads to FMS is unknown. One hypothesis maintains that localized changes cause alterations in muscles and pain pathways, resulting in amplification of pain signals traveling through the central nervous system to the brain, causing disordered sensory processing that affects the entire nervous system and results in a diffuse pain disorder.

Regional FMS is localized to a specific area of body, often the site of an injury, and is characterized by fewer than eleven tender point responses. Over time, regional FMS may develop into gener-alized FMS as pain spreads and additional symptoms develop.

Subtyping of patients has been attempted on the basis of symp-toms, genetic predisposition, cause, rheumatic disease overlap, CNS and neuroendocrine disorders, behavioral disorders, and psy-chiatric history. Identification of such subgroups might result in identification of specific treatments for each group. Inconsistencies among symptoms and lab test results may occur when subgroups are lumped together in studies.

OTHER PAIN SYNDROMES

FMS may lie on a spectrum of complex pain disorders. Other disor-ders may need to be ruled out, since they can co-occur with FMS. Musculoskeletal pain syndromes are classified as inflammatory and noninflammatory. Inflammatory conditions include rheumatoid arthritis, ankylosing spondylitis, Reiter's syndrome, psoriatic arthri-tis, systemic lupus erythematosus, scleroderma, polymyositis, vas-culitis, infectious arthritis, and sarcoidosis. Noninflammatory pain disorders include osteoarthritis, cervical spine syndrome, traumatic arthritis, tumors, and neuropathic joints.

Arthritis is characterized by joint inflammation, possibly related to imbalance in body chemistry or immune system problems. Of an estimated one hundred types, the most common are osteoarthritis and rheumatoid arthritis.

Osteoarthritis (OA), the most common form of arthritis, is the break-down of joint cartilage with symptoms of pain and stiffness. OA is common in fingers, hips, knees, and spine and most prevalent in women and men ages fifty to ninety. Increasingly common with age, osteoarthritis afflicts nearly twenty-one million Americans, more prevalent in men up to age forty-five and more common in women thereafter. Although its cause is unknown, OA is associated with heredity, injury, repeated overuse (often in the work setting), and obesity. Diagnosis is based on physical exam, symptom patterns, rul-ing out other disorders, X-rays, and joint aspiration. Treatment is individualized, and a comprehensive program includes medication, physical and occupational therapy, aerobic exercise, weight control, and surgery in severe cases.

Rheumatoid arthritis (RA) is characterized by inflammation of the synovium, the membrane lining a joint. Symptoms of RA are stiffness and swelling in multiple joints, which may be "hot" and red, typically the hands, wrists, and feet. Onset generally occurs between the ages of thirty and fifty, and the disorder is more common in women.

Septic arthritis refers to joint infections involving pain and swelling.

Gout, caused by a buildup of uric acid crystals in the joint fluid, begins with the sudden onset of burning pain, stiffness, and swelling, usually in the big toe, ankle, wrist, knee, and elbow. It is most common in men over thirty and rare in women before menopause.

Bursitis and tendonitis result from irritation caused by injuring or overusing a joint. Bursitis affects the small sac that helps muscles move easily; tendonitis affects the tendons that attach muscle to bone.

Carpal tunnel syndrome (CTS) affects the carpal tunnel, which is a narrow passageway of bone and ligament in the wrist through which pass some of the finger tendons and the median nerve; it controls sensation in the fingers, thumb, and some hand muscles. Repetitive motions associated with repeated use of the hand or wrist may cause swelling of the wrist tendons, pressing nerve against bone. Symptoms include numbness, tingling, pain in the hand and fingers (with the little finger unaffected), pain radiating up the arm, and loss of function. CTS is diagnosed by nerve conductance tests and is treated with injections, splint or wrist support, and surgery.

Disc herniation can cause shooting pains in an arm or a leg. It is diagnosed by magnetic resonance imaging (MRI) or nerve conductance tests and treated with rest, medications, and surgery.

Low back pain can result from back strain or injury and from certain types of arthritis. Therapies include pain relievers, anti-inflammatory drugs, exercise, heat or cold, joint protection, and self-pacing of activities.

Complex regional pain syndrome (CRPS), sometimes referred to as "reflex sympathetic dystrophy," is characterized by intense pain in an arm or a leg, usually triggered by injury at that site. A specialized bone scan is used for diagnosis, and treatment often involves sympathetic blocks.

Polymyalgia rheumatica (PMR) is a condition of chronic hip and shoulder pain that is treated with steroids.

Multiple sclerosis (MS), or progressive demyelinization, does not typically cause pain but, like FMS, involves muscle twitching and numbness and tingling sensations. MS is diagnosed by MRI and sometimes a spinal tap.

Myositis is an autoimmune disorder characterized by chronic muscle inflammation that may appear in association with other rheumatic diseases. Subtypes are polymyositis, dermatomyositis, and juvenile myositis. An illness found in all age groups, myositis is most common in children between ages 5 and 15 and adults between 30 and 60. More women than men are afflicted. Symptoms of weakness and sometimes pain, warmth, and swelling develop, most commonly in the hips and shoulders, but skin and internal organs may also be affected. Although its cause is unknown, genetic predisposition, certain drugs, immune abnormalities, trauma (including chemical exposure), and infection may play a role. Onset may be gradual or abrupt. The course of the disorder often includes unpredictable flares and remissions. Diagnosis involves ruling out similar disorders, blood tests for autoantibodies and muscle enzymes, electromyogram (EMG), MRI, and muscle biopsy. Treatment is individualized according to symptoms, commonly including medication, rest, and exercise.

Myofascial pain syndrome is pathophysiologically distinct from FMS. Lacking a case definition, its hallmark is the presence of trigger points, "hyper-irritable [foci] within skeletal muscle and the surrounding fascia," according to Stephen Glacy, M.D. "Trigger points can develop in response to various types of trauma, such as repetitive injuries or a motor vehicle accident." (Those who define the syndrome more loosely do not include the requirement of trigger points.) Trigger points are localized and discrete; some are superimposed on tender points and located over a palpable band of taut muscle, often associated with sudden overload or longtime use.

A trigger point has been defined as "an irritative focus within a muscle that is painful to palpation, results in referred pain, induces shortening of the muscle, and causes pain on muscle contraction." (Bennett 1993) Trigger points are common, but most heal spontaneously. However, they may become self-perpetuating, with spasms leading to physiological changes (Glacy 1997). Inflammatory substances build up and muscle cell degeneration may occur, creating an increasing pain spiral in the absence of effective intervention. Unlike a tender point, in which pain is felt at the site of palpation, trigger point palpation produces pain in other body sites, often with accompanying sensations of numbness, tingling, or a feeling of "electricity," and the muscle may jump or twitch. Arm and hand pain, for example, may be related to neck and shoulder trigger points. Pain associated with trigger points may be exacerbated by emotional stress, repetitive use, or poor body mechanics.

Myofascial pain is treated with medication, stretching exercises, rest, trigger point injections, a technique known as "spray and stretch" (see page 264 in Chapter 14), massage or physical therapy, including myofascial release, muscle relaxation techniques, heat and cold, and hydrotherapy. Finding the exact trigger point for an area of pain requires expertise. Trigger point injections are often "peppered" throughout the area, followed by muscle stretching to the fullest range of motion.

ABNORMALITIES

No consistent laboratory findings are specific to fibromyalgia, but prevalent hypothalamic, immune, and neurological abnormalities debunk the once-prevalent notion that emotional factors play a primary role in causing FMS symptoms. It remains unknown whether these findings represent cause, effect, or an endless feedback loop that perpetuates the disorder. Abnormalities vary from one patient to another and may fluctuate over time.

FMS may begin with a chronically overactivated stress-cortisol state. Over time, as the system gradually "tires," a low cortisol response to stress may be produced. In turn, continuing stressors may increase the release of certain cytokines (chemical messengers between cells) that cause pain, fatigue, cognitive impairment, and other problems, while inhibiting the cytokines that promote positive functions such as sleep and tissue repair.

Studies of hormonal, metabolic, and brain chemical activity in fibromyalgia patients reveal numerous abnormalities that are all consistent with disturbances in central nervous system processing, including abnormal functioning of the hypothalamic-pituitary-adrenal (HPA) axis and abnormalities found in brain scans; neuropsychological testing; immune tests; neurotransmitter and hormone levels; and muscle, sleep, and oxygen/energy mechanisms. Abnormal processing of input causes amplification of pain signals; as a result, normally neutral stimuli are perceived as being extremely painful.

◆◆ Endocrine and Neuroendocrine Abnormalities ◆◆

Pituitary-adrenal abnormalities include altered levels of cortisol, catecholamines, growth hormone, and thyroid hormone, causing autonomic nervous system (ANS) dysfunction. The ANS regulates involuntary functions such as breathing, blood pressure, and bladder and bowel function, and imbalances can cause or exacerbate many FMS symptoms, such as headache, sleep disorder, irritable bowel, and circulatory disorders.

An abnormal stress response may cause the abnormal levels of growth hormone (GH) and cortisol. Somatomedin C (also called insulin-like growth factor, or IGF-1), a hormone produced by the pituitary gland in the brain during deep sleep, communicates information about pain-producing stimuli to the brain. Elevated somatomedin C levels in the cerebrospinal fluid (CSF) may disrupt sleep and cause a heightened sensitivity to pain following even mild muscular activity.

Usually absent in the CSF of adults, nerve growth factor (NGF) is elevated in the CSF of FMS patients. NGF signals the synthesis of substance P, among other proteins, leading to hyperalgesia, or lowered pain threshold (the smallest sensation of pain one can recognize) and increased pain sensitivity.

Growth hormone, typically secreted during stage 4 sleep, is decreased in FMS.

Hypothyroidism (underactive thyroid), abnormal levels of estrogen and progesterone, and low levels of cortisol and adenosine triphosphate (ATP) have been found in FMS patients.

Dehydroepiandrosterone (DHEA), a steroid secreted by the adrenal glands, is often low, possibly due to decreased immunoglobin A (IgA), a chemical that stimulates DHEA production. DHEA also decreases over time as part of the normal aging process.

Oxytocin, the hormone that induces labor, regulates blood flow, and may enhance energy, cognition, and gastrointestinal function, may be low.

N-methyl-D-aspartate (NMDA) receptors, believed to be pain amplifiers, are elevated in persons with FMS. Ketamine, a medication used to improve pain threshold and muscle endurance, is an NMDA receptor agonist whose effectiveness supports the theory of disordered sensory processing in FMS.

◆◆ Neurotransmitter Abnormalities ◆◆

Neurotransmitters are brain chemicals that act as messengers between neurons. In FMS, neurotransmitter dysfunction can contribute to increased pain sensitivity.

Substance P (SP) is a neurotransmitter related to injury and pain modulation in a sequence of chemical reactions called nociception. Although found in normal levels in the blood, SP is elevated three- to fourfold in the spinal fluid of those with FMS. Found at nerve endings in areas of inflammation, SP is known to be elevated in other pain disorders and appears to stimulate central sensitization. Although research has not established a correlation between SP levels and pain severity, Jon Russell, M.D., refers to elevated SP as the "most dramatic and consistent biochemical finding" in FMS.

Serotonin (5HT) is related to mood, deep sleep, well-being, and pain perception. Low serum (blood) levels of serotonin in FMS may be due to insufficient tryptophan, its precursor.

Norepinephrine, a hormone associated with mood and pain, is elevated.

Levels of endorphins (morphine-like chemicals produced by the body) are low in FMS and other pain disorders.

Opioid receptors (cell-membrane proteins that regulate the function of endorphins) may be decreased in body tissues.

◆◆ Brain Scan Abnormalities ◆◆

SPECT (single photon emission computed tomography) scans show hypoperfusion (reduced blood flow) to certain parts of the brain (thalamus, caudate nuclei, and anterior cingulate cortex), particularly following application of an acute pain stimulus, indicating altered sensory processing. Elevated substance P often correlates with regional hypoperfusion. Abnormal functional MRI, or fMRI (a measure of neural activity that reflects cerebral blood flow and metabolism and allows the study of the brain's reaction to stimuli), is often found in FMS. Limbic system dysregulation may relate to abnormal pain processing.

♦♦ Immune Abnormalities ♦♦

Like CFS, FMS is characterized by general upregulation (overreaction) of the immune system. Abnormalities include elevation of certain cytokines, decreased natural killer (NK) cell numbers and activity, T-cell activation, elevated viral antibody titers, new onset of or increase in existing allergies, and increased levels of such immune chemicals as interleukin-2 (IL-2) and interleukin-6 (IL-6). According to Russell Wilson, Ph.D., antipolymer antibodies (APAs), usually low in patients with connective tissue diseases, may be increased in FMS, correlating with reduced pain tolerance.

♦♦ Pathogens ♦♦

Pathogens such as viruses, bacteria, and parasites may be present in patients with FMS.

♦♦ Sleep ♦♦

Both quality and duration of sleep may be disturbed. Decreased deep sleep is associated with disruption of the HPA axis, likely affecting secretion of growth hormone and prolactin. Additionally, abnormal melatonin levels at night may disrupt circadian rhythms, the body's internal clock.

♦♦ Muscle Abnormalities ♦♦

Numerous studies have described muscle abnormalities, but findings are inconsistent. Some studies indicate microspasm of muscle bundles, abnormalities in muscle blood flow, muscle tissue abnormalities, compromised capillary microcirculation, ischemia (decreased blood supply) with hypoxemia (oxygen deficiency), decreased intramuscular levels of ATP and phosphocreatine, increased anaerobic metabolism with accumulation of metabolic products, decreased muscle strength, decreased physical fitness, edema, increased mast cells and fluid content, increased interstitial fluid, increased fat content, degeneration of muscle fibers, degenerative changes, abnormal mitochondria (the "energy factories" within cells), variation in fiber size, ragged fibers, "moth eaten" Type I fibers, atrophied Type II fibers, glycogen deposits, and bandlike compression of muscle fibers. Muscle metabolism is usually normal, and electromyogram (EMG) studies are not significantly abnormal.

CAUSE

The cause of FMS remains unknown but contributory factors may include trauma, repetitive strain injury, infection, environmental factors, psychosocial stress, disordered muscle pathology, and abnormalities in immune, endocrine, and neurologic functioning.

FMS is a stress-associated but not a stress-caused disorder. Although depression is associated with FMS, it does not cause the disorder. Depression is a natural response to constant pain and inability to obtain restful sleep, among other symptoms. Since serotonin modulates mood, among other functions, low levels of this neurohormone might well cause depression in FMS as well as CFS. Posttraumatic stress syndrome has been hypothesized to play a role in the development of CFS and FMS, perhaps by changing aspects of brain organization or creating disruption of prolonged stress responses, but this theory remains controversial.

◆◆ Central Pain Mechanisms ◆◆

In patients with FMS, pain signals to the brain are amplified by defects in pain processing, and inhibitory pain mechanisms do not function normally. FMS pain is due to abnormal sensory processing by the central nervous system as evidenced by

‣ Abnormal diffuse noxious inhibitory control (DNIC): FMS patients have an abnormal response to repeated stimulation as compared to people without the disorder.

‣ Secondary hyperalgesia, or pain in healthy, uninjured tissues. In response to electrical nerve stimulation, pain responses last longer (even when the source of pain is discontinued) and may be referred to other body sites in FMS patients.

‣ Hyper-responsive somatosensory induced potentials: FMS is associated with altered neurological processing of nociceptive (painful) stimuli.

Chemical intolerance is a state in which various substances cross-sensitize with one another in the body, leading to an amplified response to small amounts of stimuli—such as various chemicals, fumes, odors, and pain—that others tolerate without any reaction. Chemical intolerance may be a biochemical link between CFS and FMS, in which the brain's abnormal amplification of signals or stimuli induces unusual neurological sensations including pain.

◆◆ Perpetuating Factors ◆◆

Reactivation of latent viruses, sleep abnormalities, dysregulation of the HPA axis, and other stressors may perpetuate the illness. In turn, the chronic pain and sleep disturbance experienced by FMS patients are stressors that feed a vicious cycle.

TREATMENT

Although incurable, FMS is treatable. The absence of a universally successful therapeutic regimen presents a challenge to both patient and physician. An individualized, comprehensive, multidisciplinary treatment approach combines traditional and nontraditional therapies to achieve maximal relief.

An integrated treatment program combines the use of pharmaceutical drugs (such as sleep modifiers, analgesics, anti-inflammatories, antidepressants, and muscle relaxants) and physical modalities (such as physical therapy, craniosacral therapy, acupuncture, trigger point therapy, occupational therapy, osteopathic or chiropractic manipulation, heat, and massage). Treatment of sleep disorders takes top priority, since sleep problems contribute to other FMS symptoms. Medication for pain relief should begin with milder agents, progressing to stronger medications as necessary. Nonsteroidal anti-inflammatory drugs (NSAIDs) may help somewhat, but stronger agents such as opioids are often used.

Self-help strategies include adaptive lifestyle changes, conservation of energy, frequent rest periods, stretching, exercise as tolerated, proper nutrition, judicious use of dietary supplements, attention to ergonomics, use of self-therapies such as application of heat and ice, avoidance of aggravating factors, stress reduction, and emotional support. Support, education, and treatment are of primary importance. Copious information is available from support groups, books, articles, and online resources. It is helpful for patients to develop realistic expectations regarding the course of the illness, prognosis, and treatment.

Patients are advised to identify and minimize factors that increase pain, such as drafts, muscle tension, repetitive motion, and remaining in one position for long periods. A gentle exercise routine should be carefully established, beginning with stretching and adding other activity as tolerated. Stretching helps to increase range of motion and decrease pain when done to the point of resistance but short of producing pain. Stretches should initially be held for short periods of time, working up to about one minute. A cautious approach to exercise begins with a few minutes of walking or water exercise, adding minutes gradually while remaining vigilant for signs of relapse during or following exertion. Several short periods of exercise over the course of the day are preferable to a single lengthier one. Prolonged vigorous exercise is usually poorly tolerated.

Psychotherapy may be helpful for illness acceptance and adjustment, lifestyle management and coping skills, support, secondary anxiety and depression, and dealing with illness-related issues, such as lowered self-esteem, difficulty with making decisions, and altered family dynamics. Cognitive therapy involves challenging irrational beliefs that give rise to the feelings of inadequacy, hopelessness, and helplessness that often accompany the illness. Coexisting anxiety and depression are treated with medication and psychotherapy.

COURSE OF THE ILLNESS

The location and severity of pain may vary over time, and pain may migrate from one area to another. Some patients experience constant bodywide pain that varies in severity. One patient commented, "I wake up each morning wondering what's going to hurt today." FMS symptoms may be intermittent, disappearing and reappearing; fluctuating, with constant pain that sometimes abates; or persistent and progressive over time.

Exacerbating triggers include changes in weather, barometric pressure, and humidity; cold or drafty environments; heat; inactivity or overactivity; repetitive motions, eccentric motions, and sustained motor tasks; sensory overload (excessive light, noise, odors, and other stimuli); hormonal fluctuations (premenstrual and meno-pausal states); stress or trauma (physical, emotional, or cognitive); disrupted sleep; the experience of emotions such as depression, anxiety, and anger; environmental sensitivities; poorly tolerated medications; poor nutrition; and food sensitivities, particularly to sugar, caffeine, nicotine, alcohol, and aspartame. Symptoms may wax and wane unpredictably in the absence of an identified trigger.

EFFECTS

When asked whether she was depressed, Monique said, "Of course I'm depressed. I hurt all the time, my friends and family don't understand my symptoms, I can't work, and I have no social life. Who wouldn't be depressed?" The toll of living with chronic pain and other debilitating symptoms disrupts virtually all aspects of an individual's life. In addition to presenting difficult symptoms, FMS reduces one's quality of life, affecting finances, social activities, hobbies, relationships, and the ability to work or attend school, and causing alienation by those who do not understand.

According to studies, the majority of FMS patients view their health as fair to poor. Many have difficulty with or are unable to perform routine daily activities, and tasks usually take a longer time than expected.

Others often do not and cannot comprehend the difficulties of living with chronic, unrelenting, and debilitating pain. Although everyone has experienced pain at one time or another, most pain is acute and transitory rather than prolonged and complicated, as it is in FMS. Others may have difficulty believing that a large number of varied symptoms are part of the disorder. Because the symptoms are invisible, others may not even believe that an individual with FMS is really ill. Many symptoms are difficult to explain. "My husband doesn't understand that sometimes I can't be touched," says Marguerite. "He thinks I'm rejecting him. He just doesn't get it."

Occupational impairment is often present in FMS. Some patients are able to maintain employment status despite decreased function, some change or modify their jobs, and others are unable to work at all. The rate of disability is about 15 to 30 percent, with some estimates as high as 40 percent. Those diagnosed with both CFS and FMS report more numerous and severe symptoms, with a greater likelihood of becoming disabled.

The extent of the damage may be mitigated by compassionate and skilled medical care, social support, coping mechanisms, spirituality, a sense of humor, a life philosophy, and following an appropriate course of treatment.

PROGNOSIS

Fibromyalgia is considered a persistent condition that is not degenerative or fatal. Some patients are disabled by their symptoms while others are able to continue to work and function reasonably well. Although most patients do not fully recover, the illness may follow a waxing and waning cycle, with half to two-thirds of patients reporting some improvement over time, somewhat attributable to management and coping skills. Gradual improvement may take place, with periods of significant remission lasting months or even years, although many patients experience little or no symptomatic improvement over time. Postmenopausal patients tend to be more debilitated, often faring less well than others. More than half of all patients report their health as only fair or poor on follow-up studies. Although symptoms are persistent, appropriate treatment and management provide relief. Lifestyle management techniques result in symptom improvement, but it remains unproven whether any specific intervention alters the course of the illness.

4

FMS and CFS: Identical, Overlapping, or Distinct Disorders?

I've had CFS for eight years but have recently begun to have body-wide aching as well as localized pain," says Katie. "Ever since I stopped running fevers and having a sore throat, the doctors have been calling it fibromyalgia."

"I have been achy and fatigued for years, but now I'm much worse," Jerry reports. "I've been more fatigued than most people all my life." Symptoms of achiness, allergies, and fatigue present since childhood have worsened. "I've never been this sick before. After surgery and my divorce, my old symptoms got worse, and new ones have developed."

Pat described the onset of bone-crushing fatigue, bodywide pain, gastrointestinal distress, and "brain fog," sometimes called "fibrofog." Always present, the symptoms vary in severity, especially with weather changes and exertion.

John has developed memory lapses, impaired concentration, and difficulty thinking clearly, reporting, "I feel so stupid when I can't find the right word, do simple math, or recall the names of my medications." Fear has set in—of the unrelenting symptoms and an uncertain future.

What is Jerry's diagnosis, or Pat's, or John's: CFS, FMS, both, or neither? That would depend upon the specialty of the diagnosing physician, the patient's history, abnormal lab test results, and findings in an office exam. In such cases, there is no definitive answer. Rarely have the three groups—those diagnosed with FMS, those with CFS, and those with both—been compared. Researchers and practitioners differ in their views of the overlap among these groups.

▶ Many experts now feel that there is such a large overlap between the vast majority of patients with Chronic Fatigue Syndrome (CFS) and Fibromyalgia (FM) that they are probably different expressions of the same disorder. [The] majority of CFS patients have significant fibromyalgia-like symptoms, and most FM patients also have chronic fatigue.
    — Scott Rigden, M.D.

▶ It remains this author's opinion that fibromyalgia and CFIDS are disorders reflecting varying clinical expressions of similar or even the same epiphenomenon.
    — Michael Goldberg, M.D.

▶ [CFS and FMS] are very similar overlapping disorders.
    — Don Goldenberg, M.D.

▶ There is considerable overlap between CFS and FM and many people have both. There is evidence for similar abnormalities but there are some significant differences as well.
    — Paul Levine, M.D.

▶ Chronic fatigue syndrome and fibromyalgia, as with the other fatigue-related disorders, are highly overlapping syndromes that may share common aspects of pathophysiology.
    — Andrew Lloyd, M.D.

According to researchers Dedra Buchwald, M.D., and Anthony Komaroff, M.D., CFS and FMS overlap by as much as 75 percent. The disorders share common symptoms, demographics, sleep physiology, and abnormalities in neurological, immune system, and endocrine function. They may begin differently but ultimately share a final common pathway, and may be attributable to different causal factors. When symptoms fit the patterns for both disorders, CFS and FMS may be diagnosed concurrently. The boundaries, if any, are unclear.

In considering research regarding similarities and differences between CFS and FMS, one must take into account methodology, survey instruments, settings from which cases are identified, and the case definitions applied.

CFS and FMS may be

▶ distinct: unrelated

▶ identical: two names for the same disorder

▶ overlapping: sharing certain characteristics, or two different expressions of the same disorder, or the result of different causes or triggers leading to a final common pathway

▶ two subtypes of one umbrella illness

▶ part of a spectrum of illnesses that includes both

The similarities and differences require further study before a definitive answer can be found. In the meantime, "lumpers" study the disorders together, and "splitters" regard them as separate entities. To complicate matters further, both disorders are homogeneous, with a number of subtypes. Those diagnosed with both have highest symptom prevalence and severity as well as the highest rate of disability either because they have severe cases of an illness or two illnesses simultaneously.

SIMILARITIES BETWEEN CFS AND FMS

The following similarities have been noted in CFS and FMS, although many studies yield contradictory findings:

▶ Approximately 75 percent of those diagnosed with CFS meet FMS criteria; 58 percent of females with FMS and 80 percent of males with FMS meet CFS criteria.

▶ Both overlap with other disorders, such as allergies, tension headaches, periodic limb movement disorder, migraines, autoimmune disorders, dysmenorrhea, irritable bladder, and irritable bowel.

▶ Treatment is similar or the same.

▶ Increased incidence is found in blood relatives.

▶ Most patients were healthy before onset of the illness.

▶ Most routine lab tests yield normal results.

▶ The populations are similar; CFS and FMS are most common among women in their middle years.

▶ Strenuous activity and physical, emotional, or cognitive stress trigger relapses.

‣ The course of illness is chronic and persistent, with symptoms occurring steadily or in waxing and waning cycles.

‣ Prognosis is poor, with full recovery unlikely but improvement possible.

‣ Secondary psychological problems occur, including depression, anxiety, mood swings, and irritability.

‣ Symptoms are exacerbated after exertion, possibly more so in CFS.

The disorders share numerous abnormalities (explained in Chapters 8 and 9), including the following:

‣ Multiple body systems are affected.

‣ Muscle pathology is present.

‣ Pain threshold is decreased.

‣ Central nervous system (CNS) abnormalities are often present, including decreased levels of neurotransmitters such as serotonin and norepinephrine and decreased neuropeptide Y.

‣ Disordered sensory processing produces increased sensitivity to pain stimuli and sensory input (light, sound, odors, chemicals, medications, and foods).

‣ Blood flow to certain areas of the brain is diminished.

‣ Abnormalities occur in both branches of the nervous system: sympathetic and parasympathetic.

‣ Neuroendocrine disturbances are common, for example, disordered hypothalamus and ACTH stimulation and abnormal levels of prolactin and growth hormone.

‣ HPA axis dysfunction, such as low cortisol levels, characterizes both disorders.

‣ Abnormal brain scans—such as MRI, functional MRI, and SPECT—are found in both.

‣ Immune abnormalities include increased cytokines, decreased natural killer (NK) cell function, elevated viral titers, enhanced T-cell activation, and altered interleukin/cytokine levels.

‣ Cardiac abnormalities are present.

‣ Abnormal tilt table test results frequently indicate orthostatic intolerance.

▶ Sleep abnormalities are significant and nearly universal.

▶ Tender points are present in all FMS and many CFS patients.

◆◆ Common Symptoms in CFS and FMS ◆◆

The following symptoms are commonly found in both disorders:

General symptoms: fatigue, usually worsened by exertion or stress; decreased activity level; allergies; symptoms worsened by temperature extremes or changes in weather; and sensitivity to medications

Pain: headache, muscle pain, twitching, weakness, joint pain, and eye pain

Gastrointestinal symptoms: abdominal cramps, nausea, esophageal reflux (heartburn), frequent diarrhea and/or constipation, bloating, and intestinal gas

Neurological symptoms: disordered sensory processing, light-headedness, feeling "spaced out," faintness, vertigo or dizziness, numbness or tingling sensations, tinnitus (ringing in one or both ears), noise sensitivity, dysequilibrium (difficulty with balance), and staggering gait (clumsy walking, bumping into things)

Neurocognitive symptoms: calculation difficulties (e.g., basic math, balancing checkbook), word-finding difficulty, frequently saying the wrong word, concentration problems, memory disturbance, losing train of thought midsentence, comprehension deficit, difficulty following written or oral instructions, and difficulty judging distances

Sleep disturbance: unrefreshing or nonrestorative sleep, difficulty falling asleep, difficulty staying asleep, altered sleep/wake schedule (alertness and energy best late at night), and sleep phase disturbance

Emotional symptoms: depression, anxiety, panic disorder, irritability, and mood swings

Other symptoms: night sweats, feeling cold often, cold extremities, dryness of eyes or mouth, frequent thirst, symptoms worsened by air travel, temporomandibular joint dysfunction (TMD), chest pain, painful and frequent urination, bladder pain, worsening of premenstrual syndrome (PMS), decreased libido (sex drive), rashes, and vivid or disturbing dreams or nightmares

The table below combines information from several studies and surveys on the prevalence of symptoms in the two disorders. The percentages of patients within each disorder and between the two vary widely, possibly because symptoms are underreported or overreported or vary among patient populations or types of surveys. Patients do not necessarily experience these symptoms all the time.

Symptom Prevalence in FMS and CFS

Symptom	% FMS	% CFS
Cognition		
Cognitive problems (general)	40–90	80–100
Confusion, inability to think clearly	75–100	—
Concentration deficit	70–85	70–100
Short-term memory deficit	70–85	80–90
Losing train of thought (e.g., midsentence)	75–85	80–90
Aphasia (e.g., word-finding difficulty)	70–75	75–95
Comprehension deficit	45–65	80–90
Dyscalculia (calculation difficulty)	45–55	75–80
Attention deficit	40–90	75–85
Frequently saying the wrong word	30–60	50–70
Long-term memory deficit	25–45	50–60
Difficulty following written instructions	25–40	70–75
Difficulty speaking	15	60–75
Difficulty following oral instructions	35–60	80–90
Easy distractibility	—	
Dental and Periodontal (Gum)		
Periodontal disease	5–20	10–25
Aphthous ulcers (canker sores)	5–30	10–25
Pain in teeth, loose teeth, and endodontal problems	—	—
Dermatologic (Skin)		
Skin changes	70–80	—
Systemic yeast/fungal infection	30–80	—
Fungal infection of skin and nails	70	—
Rash or flushing of face	30	35–45
Skin changes, including recurrent sores	20–80	30–40
Skin rash	15–50	35–55
Butterfly rash (lupus-like)	25	—
Tendency to bruise easily	25	—
Eczema or psoriasis	10–20	20–30
Hair loss	0–10	20–50

Symptom Prevalence in FMS and CFS

Symptom	% FMS	% CFS
Fatigue		
Fatigue	65–100	95–100
Postexertional fatigue	80–90	up to 100
Activity level less than 50 percent of pre-illness level	70	100
Gastrointestinal		
Irritable bowel	30–75	50–90
Abdominal cramps	50–55	40–60
Nausea	30–45	60–90
Bloating, intestinal gas	60–80	60–75
Frequent diarrhea or constipation	60–70	50–70
Esophageal reflux (heartburn)	40–55	30–45
Vomiting	0–5	15–30
Infectious or Flulike Illness		
Flulike onset	50	—
Recurrent flulike illness	45	70–85
Fevers, chills, sweats, or feeling hot often	20–70	60–95
Recurrent illness and infection	15–50	70–85
Malaise	80	—
Painful or swollen lymph nodes	20–50	50–80
Hoarseness	20	50
Cough	10–20	40–50
Sore throat	40–50	60–80
Swelling of nasal passages	—	—
Metabolic		
Weight gain	50–70	50–80
Weight loss	20–30	—
Increased appetite or food cravings	50–55	50–70
Decreased appetite	20–25	25–40
Hypoglycemia or hypoglycemia-like symptoms	—	—
Neurological		
Dysequilibrium, spatial disorientation, dizziness, vertigo	25–90	40–90
Light-headedness, "spaciness"	70–85	75–90
Photosensitivity	65–90	—
Muscle twitching, involuntary movements	15–70	55–80
Shortness of breath	60–70	30–80
Paresthesias (e.g., numbness and tingling)	65–90	25–75
Tinnitus	40–45	60–80
Difficulty judging distances (e.g., when driving)	30–35	40–65

Symptom Prevalence in FMS and CFS

Symptom	% FMS	% CFS
Spatial disorientation	10–20	60–70
Fainting (syncope) or presyncope	20–50	50–70
Low blood pressure	20–30	60–85
Difficulty swallowing	55–60	—
Frequent sighing	35–55	40–60
Heart palpitations	30–70	40–60
Episodic hyperventilation	40–45	—
Tremor or trembling	15–30	25–40
Staggering gait	40–50	60–85
Coordination problems, clumsiness	60	—
Strange taste in mouth (bitter, metallic)	25	—
Seizure-like episodes	10–70	—
Seizures	—	—
Ocular (Eyes and Vision)		
Changes in visual acuity (ability to see well)	45–70	70–80
Accommodation difficulty (switching focus)	30–45	65–80
Eye pain	55–75	30–60
Visual disturbances	45–55	—
Blind spots in vision	5–15	20–25
Pain and Associated Sensations		
Muscle pain	100	65–95
Meet tender point criteria	100	55–70
Headache	60–90	75–95
Chronic headache	50	50
Morning stiffness	60–100	—
Joint pain	80	70–80
Muscle weakness	20–80	45–95
Chest pain	45–70	40–55
Migraines	15–50	—
Sinus pain	56	—
Temporomandibular joint dysfunction (jaw pain or locking)	15–75	20–25
Pressure at the base of the skull	30	—
Eye pain	30–60	—
Earache	20	—
Allodynia (feeling pain in response to neutral stimulus)	—	—
Carpal tunnel syndrome	—	—
Pyriform muscle syndrome, causing sciatica	—	—
Pressure sensation behind eyes	—	—

Symptom Prevalence in FMS and CFS

Symptom	% FMS	% CFS
Psychological and Psychiatric		
Irritability	60–90	70–90
Emotional lability (mood swings)	30–70	70–90
Depression	15–85	65–90
Anxiety	5–75	55–90
Personality change	20–30	45–75
Panic attacks	20–30	20–40
Rage attacks	30	25–35
Phobias (irrational fears)	15–20	15–30
Isolative tendencies	—	—
Sensitivities and Allergies		
Sensitivities to medicines, inhalants, odors, and foods	10–70	25–90
Noise sensitivity	45–60	75–85
Photosensitivity (sensitivity to light)	30–40	65–90
Medication sensitivity	30–60	50–90
Alcohol intolerance	30–50	45–75
Severe or increased allergies	40–75	45–70
Food sensitivity or intolerance	45	60–70
Alteration of taste, smell, or hearing	10–50	60–65
Multiple chemical sensitivities	15–70	—
Sleep Disorders		
Sleep disorder (general)	70–95	65–100
Sleep problems	80–95	up to 100
Unrefreshing, nonrestorative sleep	85–100	85–100
Difficulty falling asleep	80–90	60–90
Difficulty staying asleep, frequent awakenings	80	75–80
Vivid or disturbing dreams, nightmares	30–45	50–60
Altered sleep/wake schedule	35–45	65
Restless leg syndrome	15–70	60–70
Temporary paralysis after sleeping	20	—
Sleep apnea	—	—
Thermoregulation		
Fevers, chills, or sweats	69–95	—
Heat or cold intolerance	95	75–80
Exacerbation with temperature extremes or weather changes	80–90	70–80
Subnormal body temperature	30–35	55–65
Cold extremities	40–70	40–60

Symptom Prevalence in FMS and CFS

Symptom	% FMS	% CFS
Feeling cold often	45–50	40–60
Raynaud's phenomenon	20–30	—
Urogenital		
Bladder pain or painful urination	20–95	50–90
Increased or severe PMS, dysmenorrhea	20–90	10–70
Swelling, fluid retention	70–80	55–70
Frequent urination	45–60	65–70
Decreased libido	45–50	60–75
Endometriosis	25	15
Impotence	—	—
Vulvodynia	—	—
Other		
Dry eyes or mouth	70–90	50–90
Frequent thirst	60	70–75
Symptoms worsened by air travel	20	30–40
Mitral valve prolapse	20–75	10–30
Antithyroid antibodies	20–30	—
Thyroid inflammation	—	—
Serious cardiac rhythm disturbances	—	—

This list is based upon information reported by Drs. David Bell, Paul Cheney, Hugh Fudenberg, Don Goldenberg, Jay Goldstein, Carol Jessop, Anthony Komaroff, Bruce Massau, Robert Olin (as quoted in the Fibromyalgia Newsletter), and Daniel Peterson, and three surveys: one in Kansas City, Missouri, and two in the Phoenix, Arizona, area. Symptoms are grouped into categories for convenience. Spaces indicate that data were unavailable.

POSTULATED DIFFERENCES BETWEEN CFS AND FMS

FMS is more commonly diagnosed than CFS. (This distinction may be based on higher prevalence of FMS, greater credibility afforded FMS in the medical community, or because fibromyalgia is a more acceptable term.)

Abrupt onset of CFS is often characterized as "viral" or "infectious," whereas abrupt onset of FMS often follows injury or other physical trauma, although infection or injury may precede either disorder.

❖❖ Symptoms More Prevalent in CFS ❖❖

Chronic fatigue syndrome is more strongly associated with these symptoms:

▶ greater fatigue

▶ exercise intolerance (although this has been challenged)

▶ flulike symptoms, including recurrent flulike illness, sore throat, tender or swollen lymph nodes, and low-grade fever (although some CFS patients have no flulike symptoms and some FMS patients do)

▶ changes in vision (which may be underreported in FMS), such as changes in visual acuity (frequent changes in ability to see well) and difficulty with accommodation (switching focus from one thing to another)

▶ sensitivities: sensitivities to odors (cleaning products, exhaust fumes, colognes, hair sprays); alcohol intolerance; alteration of taste, smell, or hearing; and photophobia (light intolerance)

▶ neurological/neurocognitive symptoms: difficulty speaking (slowness, stuttering, moving mouth to speak), attention deficit, and spatial disorientation (may be underreported in FMS)

▶ emotional symptoms: phobias and personality changes

▶ other symptoms: decreased appetite, recurrent sores, hair loss, shortness of breath, feeling hot often, low body temperature, low blood pressure, heart palpitations

❖❖ Symptoms More Prevalent in FMS ❖❖

These symptoms are more commonly associated with fibromyalgia syndrome:

▶ presence of tender points and trigger points

▶ allodynia (strong pain responses to stimuli that would not normally be painful)

❖❖ Other Differences Between CFS and FMS ❖❖

Several other significant distinctions can be made between the two disorders:

▶ CFS has been reported in epidemic form; FMS has not.

‣ CFS symptoms wax and wane on a more frequent basis.

‣ The rate of disability is higher in CFS.

Although they share numerous abnormalities (more fully explained in Chapters 8 and 9), there are significant differences:

‣ Substance P, a neurotransmitter associated with pain signal transmission, is elevated in FMS but less likely to be elevated in CFS.

‣ Abnormal RNaseL is common in CFS, with a much smaller percentage of the defective form of this enzyme among those with FMS.

‣ Vasopressin is low in CFS but high in FMS.

‣ Hypoperfusion, as measured by SPECT scan, differs between the disorders, although findings vary within each disorder.

‣ Higher plasma 5-HIAA levels are found in CFS.

In a study of individuals attending two CFS/FMS seminars in Scottsdale, Arizona, in 1997–98, subjects were asked to fill out questionnaires. A total of 91 responses was obtained from 29 people diagnosed with CFS, 27 diagnosed with FMS, and 35 patients diagnosed with both disorders. The results are shown in the table on pages 60–61. Results in the three groups are remarkably similar on all parameters except type of onset, most prevalent symptoms at onset, specialty of diagnosing physician, present work status, and course of the illness.

WHY DON'T WE KNOW THE ANSWER?

The scientific community cannot yet give us a definitive answer to the question of the relationship between CFS and FMS for many reasons:

‣ **Diagnostic criteria vary,** making comparison difficult. Studies have been done using different illness criteria (who has CFS and/or FMS, and who does not). Criteria have been developed in various countries, all definitions have their limitations, and the criteria do not match each other. Some are intentionally restrictive, having been developed for research purposes rather than clinical diagnosis. Many people who have the disorders may not fit the criteria exactly and so are not counted. Others

CFS/FMS Questionnaire Responses

Symptom	CFS	FMS	CFS and FMS
Average age of respondent	46	49	47
Average age at onset of illness	39	39	39
Average number of doctors seen before a diagnosis was made	4.5	5.3	5.8
Specialty of the diagnosing physician	Family practitioner (40%) Internist (35%)	Rheumatologist (56%) Family practitioner (38%)	Rheumatologist (37%) Family practitioner (30%)
Number of major life events (stressors) in the year prior to onset	2.3	2	2.5
Types of major life events (stressors) in the year prior to onset	Surgery, illness, moving to new residence or area, relationship problems, loss of someone close	Loss of someone close, moving to new residence or area, career change, relationship problems, surgery	Career change, moving, relationship problems, loss of someone close, illness
Sudden onset of illness	36%	20%	29%
Gradual onset of illness	27%	10%	17%
Symptoms present for many years prior to developing full-blown illness	36%	70%	63%
The four most troublesome symptoms at onset	Fatigue (86%), neurocognitive symptoms (38%), pain (28%), headache (28%)	Pain (78%), fatigue (48%), sleep disorder (15%), neurocognitive symptoms (15%)	Fatigue (80%), pain (69%), headache (23%), neurocognitive symptoms (23%)
Work status before onset of illness (percentages may not add to 100% due to rounding)	Full time (80%), part time (20%), did not work (0%)	Full time (86%), part time (10%), did not work (5%)	Full time (90%), part time (6%), did not work (3%)

CFS/FMS Questionnaire Responses

Symptom	CFS	FMS	CFS and FMS
Present work status (percentages may not add to 100% due to rounding)	Full time (20%), part time (16%), do not work (64%)	Full time (40%), part time (11%), do not work (40%)	Full time (22%), part time (18%), do not work (60%)
Number and severity of symptoms at the present time (from a list of 103 symptoms)	Mild (11), moderate (23), severe (30)	Mild (9), moderate (19), severe (22)	Mild (11), moderate (23), severe (34)
Therapies that reduce symptoms, in order of helpfulness	Sleep and rest, diet/nutrition, decreased stress, pacing and moderation	Sleep and rest, mild exercise, decreased stress, warmth and heat	Sleep and rest, decreased stress, diet/nutrition, warmth and heat
Factors that worsen symptoms, in order of severity of effects	Overexertion, stress, lack of sleep	Stress, lack of sleep, overexertion	Stress, overexertion, poor diet
Present illness status (percentages may not add to 100% due to rounding)	Partially recovered (21%), not recovered but stable (18%), steadily improving (7%), sick all the time (29%), steadily worse (18%)	Partially recovered (11%), not recovered but stable (22%), steadily improving (7%), sick all the time (33%), steadily worse (28%)	Partially recovered (14%), not recovered but stable (11%), steadily improving (3%), sick all the time (46%), steadily worse (20%)

Note: Limitations of this study are small sample size, reliance on self-report, response at only one point in time, and representation of only one geographical area. The seminar fee of forty dollars may have prohibited attendance in some cases, although fee waivers and payment plans were arranged. Those who are most severely ill were excluded by their inability to attend a full-day seminar.

who meet the criteria may have other illnesses. Criteria are often inadequate, in need of revision in part because they do not take into account the variability of the disorders among patients.

‣ **Complicating factors** include groups without access to good medical care, those told they aren't ill, those misdiagnosed with psychiatric disorders or "atypical" something (such as atypical multiple sclerosis), and those diagnosed with FMS based on pain but whose CFS symptoms aren't addressed in the diagnostic process.

‣ **Individuals vary** in symptom prevalence and severity over time.

‣ **No objective tests** exist to measure such symptoms as fatigue.

‣ **Large-scale comparative studies have not been funded.** Preliminary studies show conflicting results.

‣ **All studies have inherent limitations, and criteria lack uniformity.** Studies are usually performed with small numbers of patients who are not necessarily representative of general patient populations. Patients may be chosen by various methods, representing only one geographical area or from one clinic or specialist's practice. Different diagnostic criteria may be applied. The experimental design may be flawed. Many cases are undiagnosed and therefore not included. Both illnesses may contain various subtypes who will show differing test results.

‣ **Underdiagnosis.** For each person diagnosed with CFS and/or FMS, we do not know how many others have fallen through the cracks: some misdiagnosed, others dismissed, and some never having seen a physician.

‣ **Overdiagnosis.** Those whose symptoms suggest CFS or FMS may have other undiagnosed disorders causing their symptoms.

‣ **Patient reports are subjective, and no universal standards exist.** Since such symptoms as pain and fatigue cannot be measured, we rely on patient information, but what is described as severe by one patient may be moderate to another.

‣ **There are many ways to conduct studies, apply criteria, and interpret data.** Numbers and data do not represent ultimate truth. Medical news changes from day to day, and it has been said that 50 percent of current medical knowledge will prove incorrect in the future. Weighing the results of various studies, their methodologies, and unwarranted cause-and-effect associations tells us that it makes no sense to react to any individual study as if a definitive answer has been found.

Chronic fatigue syndrome and fibromyalgia syndrome are clearly interconnected, although the nature and extent of this link remain unclear. Both are invisible illnesses with profound life-altering effects. Neither a cause nor a cure is known for either syndrome. Although treatment is available for both, results vary among patients. In America alone, millions of people are afflicted with CFS and/or FMS, and numbers of new cases and newly diagnosed cases seem to be rising. The true prevalence of CFS/FMS is unknown.

Case definitions and criteria vary a good deal more than the symptoms, abnormalities, and experience of being ill with CFS and/or FMS. Perhaps the most striking similarity is "irritable everything"—abnormal sensory processing causing sensitization to all stimuli: pain, noise, light, heat, cold, medicines, chemicals, foods, odors, and so on.

Whether we all have the same illness, subtypes of one illness, or different illnesses, the bottom line is the same: More funding and larger, better-designed studies are needed. Government agencies have been less than eager to devote attention and dollars to illnesses that are not really taken seriously, regardless of rhetoric to the contrary. Complicated illnesses are more convenient to ignore than to tackle. Additional funding for fruit fly reproduction studies is unwarranted when millions of Americans suffer, perhaps needlessly, from poorly understood disorders. Having established that CFS and FMS and additional overlapping disorders affect significant numbers of people nationally and globally, we need to turn our attention from counting cases to problem solving.

5

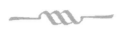

Symptoms

The symptoms of CFS/FMS vary among patients and in individual patients over time. As new symptoms crop up, we may find it hard to determine whether or not they are related to the syndrome. Symptoms at onset often determine the type of medical specialist one sees and the diagnosis. Pain, fatigue, and cognitive dysfunction are often the most prevalent and life-disrupting symptoms.

Betty describes the onset of her illness: "I had laryngitis for a month, and my throat hurt all the time. Later, I noticed difficulty walking. I felt as if I had run a marathon when all I had done was sit at my desk. I ached constantly."

"I hurt from head to toe and felt like a wimp," says Martin. "My muscles ached; my joints hurt. I was tired and brain-dead, and some days I could hardly move. I was a mess. I'm still sick, but now I'm getting medical care and I'm handling it better."

My illness began with a bout of what I thought was the flu: fatigue, malaise, aching, and lethargy. Within a few months I developed tinnitus (ringing in the ears), sore throat, equilibrium problems, irritability, morning nausea, weight gain, and shortness of breath. Additional symptoms then cropped up: unusual headaches, a tendency to become "overloaded" easily by activity or sensory stimulation, brief periods of severe depression, a periodic inability to find the right words as I spoke, slowed speech and thinking, photosensitivity, transient facial numbness, night sweats, "broken thermostat" (random sensitivity to heat and/or cold), heart palpitations, and general weakness. I popped vitamins and continued the hectic pace of my life as mother, psychologist, lecturer, college instructor, and jogger. I did what I had always done when something got in the way: I pushed hard and fought aggressively.

In retrospect, my "strategy" was misguided and inappropriate. Dogs have the good sense to rest an injured paw by walking on three legs until it has healed. I used to think symptoms were a signal to do *more* of what I was already doing. Early on, I didn't tell many people about my symptoms because I felt wimpy, vulnerable, and a bit crazy—and didn't want to risk being judged. Since I am not a weakling, hypochondriac, or hysteric, I tried to ignore my symptoms, certain they'd disappear. Sometimes they did, temporarily.

Others relate similar stories of the occurrence, disappearance, and reappearance of an array of unusual, bewildering symptoms. In the past, many had experienced allergies, colds, aches, and viral illnesses from which they had typically recovered within weeks. They assumed that their new symptoms would follow a similar course. But all of us have been astonished by the variety, unpredictability, and duration of the symptoms we have experienced. Toni Jeffreys describes the cycling of multiple symptoms as a "cafeteria in a nightmare" with a "horrendous array of horrors" (1982).

FATIGUE

To the healthy, fatigue means feeling tired or worn out and needing sleep or rest. CFS/FMS fatigue is of a different nature, defying description and measurement. It is described as debilitation, exhaustion, or feeling drained, washed out, weak, and unable to function mentally or physically. As David Bell, M.D., has pointed out, the term "fatigue" is used incorrectly in this context. Fatigue is defined as a state brought about by activity or exertion that is relieved by rest. In CFS and FMS, fatigue may be present without recent exertion or activity and is unrelieved by rest.

Some patients are literally too exhausted and weak to get out of bed. Many describe the experience of waking up, showering and dressing, and returning to bed, having depleted the day's energy supply. Even the simple act of brushing one's teeth can become a monumental chore, as unbelievable as this may seem.

Fatigue is often accompanied by a sense of general malaise, or feeling sick all over. It is worsened by physical, cognitive, and emotional exertion. Sleep does not necessarily relieve the fatigue. Although the perceived need for sleep may be great, sleep is often unrefreshing and nonrestorative; we may awaken just as tired as we were at bedtime.

SLEEP DISORDER

Sleep is often characterized as nonrestorative and unrefreshing, the feeling that one has barely slept, probably due to decreased deep (slow-wave or delta) sleep. Difficulty falling asleep and maintaining sleep are common. Sleep may be disrupted by pain, frequent need to urinate, sleep apnea (a breathing disorder), and nightmares or disturbing dreams. Early in the course of the illness, many experience hypersomnia, sleeping many hours, while hyposomnia, or lack of sleep, is more prevalent later. One may feel "tired and wired," exhausted but too "hyped" to sleep. Poor quality of sleep contributes to many other symptoms associated with CFS and FMS. Over time, circadian rhythms become disrupted, and the body's internal clock ceases to follow a normal sleep-wake cycle.

Fatigue is exacerbated by such sleep disorders as lack of deep sleep, difficulty falling asleep, and frequent awakenings. Many patients feel tired all the time but are unable to sleep more than a few hours per night. The quality of sleep may be poor and is often characterized by alpha-delta intrusion, a near-waking state that intrudes upon deep sleep. Lack of deep (stages 3 and 4) sleep may leave us feeling that we have just "skimmed the surface" of sleep. Nightmares and vivid dreams, often caused by medications, may disturb sleep, leaving a "haunted" feeling upon awakening.

◆◆ Restless Leg Syndrome and Periodic Limb Movement Disorder ◆◆

Restless leg syndrome (RLS) is characterized by sensory and motor abnormalities, felt particularly in the legs. RLS is characterized by paresthesias, or abnormal sensations such as numbness, tingling, restlessness, or a crawling feeling. Its severity ranges from infrequent, minor annoyance or discomfort to daily pain, accompanied by a crawling sensation, particularly at night when lying down. RLS may be relieved by moving the legs, particularly by walking around. Most patients with RLS also have PLMD (periodic limb movement disorder), the jerking or twitching of the legs or arms during sleep. Both disorders interfere with sleep and are treatable.

PAIN

Joint pain and muscle pain may be constant or intermittent. Pain may be bodywide or localized, often migrating from one site to another. It may be experienced as aching, burning, piercing, radiating, or stabbing, often varying in nature. Lymph nodes may be tender, although not necessarily swollen, particularly in early stages for those with infectious-type onset. Pain in the shoulders, neck, and back is common and may be accompanied by headache, sinus pain, or eye pain. Tender points are common in those diagnosed with FMS and CFS. Feelings of muscle weakness, sometimes to the point of near-paralysis, may be exacerbated by routine activity. Muscle spasms and twitching may occur. Allodynia, a pain response to stimuli that are not normally painful, is common.

Several chest pain syndromes may accompany CFS and FMS. Chest pain often provokes the fear that symptoms are due to cardiac problems, and all chest pain should be investigated to rule out this possibility. Thoracic pain and dysfunction is associated with continuous forward body posture (such as working at a desk), shallow breathing, and postural problems. Costochondralgia is a type of muscle pain in the area where the ribs meet the chest bone.

Body stiffness may be particularly apparent upon awakening and after prolonged periods of maintaining a fixed position. Changes in temperature or humidity may also cause stiffness. Paresthesia—numbness, tingling, or burning sensations, particularly in the hands or feet—may accompany CFS and FMS.

Unexplained dental pain, sometimes compared to the sensation that accompanies a dying nerve, may be experienced and often migrates to different areas. Dental decay and gum disease are more common in CFS/FMS patients than the general population. Chronic sinusitis, sometimes felt as "dental" pain, may result from bacterial or fungal infection.

HEADACHE

The types of headaches experienced by people with CFS and FMS vary and are different from pre-illness headaches. Some are migraine-like, accompanied by nausea and sensitivity to light and noise. Others are experienced as severe pain behind the eyes, pressure at the base of the skull, sinus pain, or a sensation of brain swelling. Headaches may last for several hours or several days and may migrate to different areas of the head.

Migraine is often described as intense, throbbing head pain on one or both sides of the head, sometimes accompanied by light and sound sensitivity, nausea, and vomiting. Pain sensations vary. Duration varies from hours to days. Frequently preceded by dizziness or visual disturbances, classic migraine is often unilateral and of shorter duration. The cause of migraine, once believed to be solely vascular, is now associated with epilepsy-like brain disturbance, and it is not always distinct from muscle tension headache.

Temporomandibular joint dysfunction (TMD) occurs at the hinge of the jaw joint near the ear, producing pain at that site and sometimes in the neck, temples, face, and ears.

Sinus pain may be caused by inflammation or by a bacterial or yeast infection. The pain may vary with positional changes of the head.

SENSITIVITIES AND ALLERGIES

Allergies are common in CFS and FMS—both allergies of new onset and worsening of long-term allergies. In an allergic response, the immune system recognizes a foreign body as "not self" and mounts what is intended to be a protective response, even if the perceived invader is a harmless bit of pollen.

Allergies are distinct from sensitivities. Sensitivity, or intolerance with symptom development, occurs with exposure to environmental chemicals including perfumes, exhaust fumes, cleaning products, and pesticides. Reactions usually intensify with additional exposures and generalize to other offending substances, causing increased symptoms over time. Foods may be poorly tolerated, with sensitivities to such food additives as preservatives and coloring or flavoring agents; for example, sulfites, sodium benzoate, monosodium glutamate (MSG), and aspartame. Symptoms include odd neurological sensations, headache, nasal congestion, and general worsening of symptoms. Exquisite sensitivity to medications and alcohol, and alterations in taste, smell, and hearing are common. Alcohol is typically poorly tolerated.

Hypersensitivity to light, noise, odors, and weather patterns is common. Some patients can tolerate only a very limited temperature range, becoming unusually uncomfortable with small variations. Dysregulation of metabolism and body temperature mechanisms may cause one to feel unusually hot or cold when healthy counterparts are comfortable. Temperature changes may cause symptom exacerbation, with cold intensifying fibromyalgia pain.

INFECTIONS AND FLULIKE ILLNESS

Onset of CFS/FMS may follow another illness. It may begin with recurring flulike symptoms include sore throat; hoarseness; cough; and tender or swollen lymph nodes (glands), especially in neck or underarms; fever and chills; malaise; and swelling of nasal passages.

WEIGHT GAIN AND LOSS

In our society, overweight connotes weakness (lack of willpower) rather than a physiological or psychophysiological problem. Although weight gain in CFS and FMS is partly attributable to inactivity and carbohydrate and other food cravings, weight gain often occurs without any significant change in eating habits, perhaps attributable to alterations in brain chemistry and the body's ability to convert calories into energy. This trend is a leading cause of "high school reunion syndrome" ("I don't want them to see me like this"). Others, particularly those with severe food sensitivities and irritable bowel, may lose weight, sometimes to dangerous extremes. Excessive weight loss, although problematic, is unlikely to elicit understanding and sympathy, given our society's inordinately high value of thinness. Many patients report food cravings, particularly for carbohydrates.

DERMATOLOGIC SYMPTOMS: SKIN PROBLEMS

CFS/FMS patients may experience skin rashes or sores, eczema, psoriasis, hair loss, fungal infections, dry skin, and easy bruising. A butterfly rash may appear on the face. Dryness of the eyes and mouth is partially attributed to certain medications.

THERMOREGULATION PROBLEMS

Persons with fibromyalgia tend to be highly sensitive to ambient temperature. Some often feel abnormally cold compared to others around them; others feel abnormally warm. Their hands and feet may be generally cold, in some cases associated with Raynaud's phenomenon, an unusual sensitivity to cold in the hands or feet accompanied by skin color changes.

◆◆ Low Body Temperature, Fever, and Sweats ◆◆

Subnormal body temperature often occurs in CFS and FMS, with or without thyroid dysfunction. Low-grade fevers may occur either intermittently or constantly. Night sweats resemble hot flashes: an abrupt rush of heat and sweating, especially in the upper portion of the body.

UROGENITAL SYMPTOMS

Many CFS/FMS patients experience increased urinary frequency and urgency and bladder pain or pain on voiding, often accompanied by increased thirst, although fluid retention is common. Some may develop a chronic, painful inflammatory condition of the bladder wall known as interstitial cystitis (IC).

Women may have more painful menstrual periods or worsening of CFS/FMS symptoms premenstrually. Conditions such as vulvar vestibulitis and vulvodynia, characterized by a painful vulvar region and painful sexual intercourse, may also develop in women. Endometriosis may be more common than in the general population. Males may experience prostatitis, inflammation of the prostate gland, with symptoms of pain in the prostate area, painful urination, and impotence. Libido (sex drive) is decreased in men and women.

Treatment of these genital-pain disorders with antibiotics is usually unsuccessful, since they are typically characterized by inflammation rather than infection.

GASTROINTESTINAL SYMPTOMS

Irritable bowel symptoms, such as nausea, gassiness and bloating, abdominal cramps, vomiting, esophageal reflux (heartburn), diarrhea, and constipation may be constant or intermittent, mild or severe.

◆◆ Candidiasis: Yeast Overgrowth ◆◆

The incidence of yeast overgrowth in CFS and FMS remains controversial. *Candida albicans* is normally present in the body, particularly in the intestinal tract. Under certain conditions, yeast cells proliferate out of control in the intestines and elsewhere in the body, causing rectal or vaginal itching, gas and bloating, and feelings of spaciness or disorientation. Some patients feel better on an "antiyeast" diet that eliminates alcohol, sugars, other refined carbohydrates, and sometimes yeast and dairy products if the patient is sensitive to them.

NEUROLOGICAL SYMPTOMS

Neurological problems include visual disturbances; vestibular (balance) problems; disorientation; dizziness; vertigo (a sense that the environment is moving or spinning); light-headedness; abnormal movements; tremors or trembling; seizures or seizure-like episodes; numbness or tingling; visual sensitivity and distortions; speech disturbance; confusion; tinnitus; shortness of breath or air hunger; frequent sighing; heart palpitations; "not quite seeing what you are looking at"; low blood pressure; and, most common and troublesome of all, "brain fog" or "fibrofog"—the inability to think clearly or to focus or maintain attention.

Abnormal gait, walking into things (often the result of altered spatial perception), clumsiness, and dropping things are not uncommon. Syncope (fainting) or, more commonly, faintness may occur when dysequilibrium is associated with orthostatic intolerance, an abnormal drop in blood pressure when standing (explained further in Chapter 9). Although seizures are reported in only a small number of cases, subclinical seizures or seizure-like events may occur. Driving is often difficult or impossible as a result of fatigue, spatial disorientation that affects the ability to judge distances or stay within a lane, concentration impairment, and poor judgment.

Such symptoms may appear at onset but usually emerge or intensify months later. Neurological deficits range from mild to acute, varying in severity over time.

COGNITIVE SYMPTOMS

Unusual cognitive complaints are, increasingly to me, the
single most important symptom.
— *Paul Cheney, M.D., Ph.D.*

Our brains aren't working right or functioning as they did prior to
becoming ill, leading to frustration and fear. Although native intelligence remains constant, the ability to apply it is compromised. We
may be painfully aware of "brain glitches" either as they occur or
afterward, when we discover misplaced objects or find ourselves sitting in the passenger seat, unable to start the car.

Cognitive difficulties include the following:

- impaired short-term memory, involving learning and retaining
  new information: difficulty understanding, acquiring, and
  encoding new information, with new memories being fragile
  and easily forgotten; difficulty integrating new information
  with existing memories; new memories disrupted by attention
  to additional information; inability to benefit from cues; and
  greater difficulty with auditory than visual memory

- use of simplistic and ineffective memory strategies

- slowed retrieval of long-term memories

- impaired visual discrimination; for example, looking at something but not quite seeing it

- spatial/perceptual and directional difficulties, such as misjudg-
  ing distances when driving, getting lost in familiar territory,
  and being unable to follow directions

- disorders of color perception—recognizing colors but forgetting what they mean, as with traffic lights

- altered time perception; "losing" periods of time while driving
  and in other settings

- impaired concentration and attention deficit

- easy distractibility

- difficulty processing simultaneous input (competing stimuli),
  such as following a conversation when background noise is
  present

- confusing left and right

- impaired auditory-verbal information processing
- expressive aphasia: word-finding difficulty, an inability to retrieve the name of an object
- paraphasia: incorrect word selection, such as using the wrong word from the right category or using a word that sounds similar to the desired word but has a different meaning
- transposition: reversal of letters, words, or numbers when speaking or writing
- nonrecognition of a visual stimulus
- prosopagnosia: inability to recognize faces; difficulty associating faces with names
- slurred speech
- difficulty expressing ideas
- dysarthria: difficulty producing speech, as in moving one's mouth to speak
- slowed rate of speech; stammering or stuttering
- losing one's train of thought in midsentence or midtask
- dyscalculia: difficulties with math and using numbers
- difficulty with problem solving and decision making
- difficulty following oral or written directions
- cognitive slowing: slowed performance speed and motor function, often varying with fatigue level
- forgetting how to perform routine tasks
- comprehension deficit
- impaired abstract reasoning and concept formation
- sequencing problems: inability to follow directions (as in recipes, series of errands, or assignments with multiple steps)
- poor judgment
- difficulty organizing, integrating, and evaluating information to form conclusions or make decisions
- volitional problems: difficulty starting or stopping tasks
- difficulty adapting behavior to current context
- difficulty getting organized

In addition to cognitive impairments, patients often experience fine and gross motor skill difficulties, slowed coordination, clumsiness, and decreased ability to perform work tasks.

In a 1987 *Rolling Stone* article, Hillary Johnson wrote about her inability to concentrate, hold a conversation in a group, use appropriate and often simple words, sustain a train of thought, and recall such familiar things as names of her friends and schools she had attended. Her behavioral errors included picking up the wrong object (a comb instead of a pen), trying to replace a drawer in a space that was actually a shelf, and being unable to fasten her seat belt on an airplane.

Betty describes her deficits and fears: "I used to do research and write for professional journals, but now I have to read and reread; I kept forgetting. I had the telltale signs of presenile dementia. At meetings it was almost impossible to concentrate, and I didn't know how to express my ideas, to find the right words, so I was quiet." She became reclusive, afraid others would find out. "It became hard to remember where my office was, and once I got there, what I was supposed to be doing. I was useless and finally stopped working." She also has problems driving. "I have to force myself to focus so I won't do something dangerous or stupid. I forget where I am, where I'm supposed to be going, and why."

Many patients report problems with common, routine tasks such as turning on the car headlights, making coffee, finding something that is right in front of them, and ascertaining their whereabouts in familiar territory. Susan became lost while driving in her neighborhood and asked her five-year-old son to direct her home, pretending it was a game. Many can no longer drive due to poor judgment, driving errors, and spatial disorientation.

Many react slowly and speak slowly. "My brain is broken," laments Kyle. "I depended on this wonderful tool that I have, my brain, and it just doesn't work very well any more. I get spacey and lose pieces of information."

Ron says, "When I can't recall something, I'm devastated. When my once-excellent memory failed me, I felt frightened; I was losing myself. I was a rising star at work before this struck. I became hopelessly lost; I couldn't think."

Forgetting is a common problem: Where did I put my keys? How did I lose the pen that was right in front of me? What did I come into the bedroom for? What is the name of the person to whom I was just introduced? Have I already told you what I am about to say? What is that word on the tip of my tongue? What are my shoes doing in the freezer?

Many describe this confused state as "brain spin" or "brain storm," a trancelike state of altered perception, or as a feeling of being drugged or poisoned. Others say:

I feel like there's an infection in my brain. It just isn't working right.

I've got cotton in my synapses.

This feels like Alzheimer's, or maybe just "Halfheimer's."

I feel disoriented, like being in a different dimension.

My mind is like a camera lens that can't focus.

I've been short-circuited.

Of all the things I've lost, I miss my mind the most.

Memory is a complex process of transforming a stimulus into meaning, of making updates to previously acquired memories. Difficulty understanding stimuli and absorbing new information and distortions in how stimuli are processed are problematic, with short-term memory particularly affected. Difficulty understanding or "registering" stimuli short-circuits one's ability to make new memories, and once made, memories are fragile and easily perturbed.

Findings on brain scans are often consistent with neurocognitive dysfunction.

OCULAR SYMPTOMS: EYES AND VISION

Light sensitivity is common in those with CFS/FMS. Many avoid bright sunlight, wear dark sunglasses outdoors, and keep indoor lighting dim. Fluorescent lighting may seem harsh and disturbing. Exposure to bright light may cause equilibrium problems, dizziness, headache, nausea, and "blinding."

Other eye problems include impaired depth perception, bouncing images, transient blurred vision, blind spots, transient diplopia (double vision), dryness, burning, and pain. Difficulty switching focus from one point to another is called accommodation difficulty. Changes in visual acuity (the ability to see well) often do not show up on eye tests and have been attributed to muscle fatigue or neu-rological dysfunction.

VESTIBULAR (BALANCE) PROBLEMS

Vestibular symptoms include dizziness, vertigo, spatial disorienta-tion, difficulty navigating (loss of balance, frequently bumping into things, or listing to one side), and nausea. These problems may be constant or intermittent. Patients also report a variety of unusual sensations: a sense of trancelike unreality; feeling "foggy," "spacey," or light-headed; inability to orient themselves in space; increased disorientation in the dark; and a need to restrict motion. These sen-sations may be produced or heightened by certain types of motion (including escalators, elevators, and some forms of transportation), noise, odors, and bright light.

Harold Levinson, M.D., suggests these symptoms are caused by abnormalities of the cerebellar-vestibular system (CVS), which is responsible for processing and making sense of external sensory input to maintain orientation and balance. When this "filter" mal-functions, incoming messages become scrambled or blurred, result-ing in distorted signals and odd sensations.

Overload, the result of too much conflicting sensory input, causes an exaggerated response to even small amounts of additional input. In high-level sensory situations, such as shopping in crowded stores or malls, one is bombarded with motion, lights, colors, shapes, odors, conversations, music, and other noise. Large amounts of visual, auditory, and motion-related stimulation result in confusion, disorientation, chaotic perceptions and reactions, dizziness, slurred speech, fatigue, tripping, stumbling, and impaired coordination.

PSYCHIATRIC AND EMOTIONAL SYMPTOMS

Historically, illnesses are attributed to temperament when sci-ence lacks, or refuses to seek, answers.

— *B. E. Synhorst, M.S.W.*

The medical profession often views depression or inability to cope productively with stress as the cause of any symptom for which a physiological cause is not evident. Psychiatry becomes a convenient dumping ground for those with unexplained illness. However, indiscriminate attribution of symptoms to psychological factors is inappropriate.

When a "physical" cause of symptoms cannot be found, we may be told that it is an "emotional" problem, that it is "all in our heads." In the sense that CFS and FMS are disorders of central processing and sensitization, the problems *are* in our heads. The notion that we cannot handle life, fabricate symptoms, or develop illnesses in order to receive special attention is ludicrous. Attribution of illness to such conscious or unconscious motivation is inaccurate, unfair, and insulting. Phrases such as "can't manage stress" and "mind over matter" add insult to illness. Emotional symptoms are no less real than physical ones, with no line of demarcation between the two. Illness-related emotions—depression, anxiety, anger, frustration, and disappointment—are part of and appropriate to the situation. *Any* illness is an emotional event.

Depression, anxiety, panic disorder, mood swings, irritability, and angry outbursts may accompany CFS and FMS as a result of neurohormonal abnormalities and the stress of being ill. Abrupt mood swings may be triggered by minor events or occur without apparent cause. When we're sickest, even minor sensory input is intolerable. Music or conversation becomes grating. Touch becomes painful. With a lowered tolerance threshold, our reactions are extreme, out of proportion to events, and atypical of past responses. We react very strongly to any sort of demand, frustration, or problem. We are often aware of our overreactions but powerless to change them.

Rage attacks are sudden, intense anger outbursts that are inappropriate to the situation and often surprising not only to others but to the individual as well. Personality changes, often worsening of previous tendencies, may also occur.

◆◆ Anxiety and Panic Disorder ◆◆

Anxiety may occur in response to an identified source or apparently at random. "In response to almost nothing… my heart pounds, my skin burns, my anxiety level skyrockets," remarks Yolanda. "I just can't handle stress."

Other patients comment:

I always feel nervous now. I'm nervous when I awaken. I'm nervous right now. My nerves are whacked out.

My heart starts to pound, and I feel as if I'm going to pass out—for no reason! I can't figure out what causes this; I really don't feel anxious about anything in particular.

I've gotten uptight about tests or interviews, but always for a reason. Now I get all worked up about nothing, or something really minor.

The cause of panic disorder is a misfired signal in the brain occurring at an inappropriate time, that is, when a protective fear response is elicited by a stimulus that would ordinarily be considered nonthreatening. Symptoms include feelings of fear or dread, light-headedness, dizziness, pounding heart, chest pain, cold hands and feet, shortness of breath, a sense of unreality, distorted perceptions, and fear of losing control or dying. Harold Levinson, M.D., links anxiety, panic, and phobias to the "internal state of alarm" that "results when the brain receives scrambled information." The fight-or-flight response is a normal reaction to stressful stimuli. In the absence of dangerous stimuli, the unexplained sensations exacerbate anxiety and discomfort.

Panic disorder is diagnosed when one or more panic attacks have occurred, with continuing fear of having another. It may become difficult to go places where panic attacks have occurred, such as supermarkets, restaurants, and malls, since those locations become associated with panicky feelings. Such avoidance may develop into agoraphobia—the fear of being out in public, around people, or away from home. Panic attacks are involuntary and can happen to anyone. There is no cure, but panic disorder is treatable.

◆◆ Depression ◆◆

Depression almost invariably accompanies chronic illness on a chronic or intermittent basis. Depression has traditionally been separated into endogenous and exogenous types but is probably more often a combination of the two. Endogenous depression, or depression from within, is thought to have a physical origin—an imbalance in brain chemistry—with a genetic basis. The onset of endogenous depression may be abrupt or gradual. Exogenous depression (also called reactive depression) is depression from without, attributable to an external event, such as loss or chronic illness. Disturbed body chemistry combined with deprivations, losses, changes in lifestyle, and a lack of understanding and empathy of others can produce profound depression. The incidence and severity of the depression may vary, sometimes in rhythm with other symptoms. Some CFS/FMS patients experience little or no depression.

Symptoms of depression include the following:

▶ fatigue and loss of energy

▶ feelings of hopelessness, helplessness, emptiness, and loss of control over one's own life

▶ anhedonia: loss of pleasure in life, especially in activities once enjoyed

▶ feelings of worthlessness, self-deprecation, and guilt

▶ inability to concentrate; memory problems

▶ changes in weight and appetite

▶ frequent tearfulness

▶ sleep disturbance

▶ loss of interest in the outside world

▶ loss of interest in sex

▶ thoughts of or plans for suicide, or suicide attempts

Some patients describe their feelings of depression:

Out of nowhere, a black cloud envelops me. I hole up in my room. I have no interest in other people or in anything, least of all myself. Nothing is right with the world; it hurts more than I can stand. The depression lasts a day or two, lifting as suddenly as it hit.

I've been situationally depressed in the past. This is different. I feel crazy and out of control. Life just seems pointless.

I have reached the point of planning suicide but I don't have the energy. I can't work, can't pay my bills, or keep my personal life going. This is unacceptable for someone who has always done everything, graduated summa cum laude, and excelled.

Others may react strangely to our depression, often not understanding that it is beyond voluntary control, that we cannot think positively or snap ourselves out of it. Their attempts to cheer us up often backfire, causing us to feel misunderstood.

Depression is not a sign of unworthiness, incompetence, or weakness. It is more profound than the sense of discouragement that accompanies exacerbation of symptoms. Depression is a serious matter; its severity and debilitating effects must not be minimized. If depression is prolonged, severe, or accompanied by suicidal thoughts, seek treatment immediately. It is not your fault, and help is available.

OTHER ILLNESSES

Other illnesses and infections commonly appear early on, usually becoming less frequent over time. Some patients report continuation of frequent infections and illnesses, with a tendency to catch "whatever is going around," while others find they are less prone to catching other illnesses, possibly due to the immune system being turned on, in constant fighting mode. Additionally, CFS and FMS may occur simultaneously with other chronic illnesses.

6

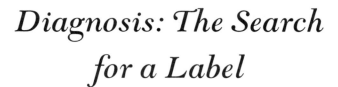

Diagnosis: The Search for a Label

As I talked to these patients, I began to hear a recurrent theme. It was as though I was listening to the first four notes of Beethoven's "Fifth Symphony." Once you've heard those notes, you know the rest of the music.
— *Harvey Moldofsky, M.D.*

Attitude as much as data determine diagnosis.
— *Frank Albrecht, Ph.D.*

People treat you nice once you're "officially" sick. [If] you don't feel good, you're just a pain in the ass.
— *George Carlin*

We know what it's like to feel well and what it's like to feel sick, but the distinction is difficult to verbalize. For no apparent reason our bodies and minds are not behaving right. We want—*need*—some sort of explanation. We want to know why and what to do about it. In the beginning, we'll settle for a label, anything that validates our experience and reassures us we're not crazy.

Many symptoms are invisible, not observable or measurable. And the symptoms come and go on their own schedule without permission or warning. Other people have difficulty understanding how absolutely rotten we feel, in part because our numerous symptoms are invisible. "You look fine," they tell us. One patient wears a button proclaiming, "I look better than I feel."

Our society has many unwritten rules about sickness, including the expectation that someone who is ill will either recover or die. It's okay to break a limb—as long as it heals in a timely manner and one does not complain excessively. To have symptoms that cannot be seen or understood by others is not okay. Anything that cannot be fixed, diagnosed, or neatly categorized is likely to be disbelieved.

Patients must often solicit numerous opinions before obtaining an accurate diagnosis. Some give up along the way for a number of reasons. The energy expenditure involved in seeking one opinion after another may simply be too much. The financial expense may be too great. Dismissive physicians may cause patients to turn away from the medical profession. Patients labeled somatizers, hypochondriacs, or malingerers may cave in, adopting the attitudes of their accusers and regarding their litany of complaints—unrelenting pain, fatigue, shortness of breath, ringing in the ears, headache, inability to think clearly or to do simple math—as evidence that no sane individual could possibly experience such a variety of crazy symptoms. Poorly understood syndromes involving multiple symptoms are culturally and medically delegitimized.

We do not enjoy being ill and have nothing to gain by manufacturing a list of crazy symptoms, a living hell on earth. The supposed secondary gains are nonexistent. We may not be well enough to go to work but may not be ill enough to spend all our time in bed. Some days we can accomplish a lot; other days mere survival needs require all of our limited energy. We slip through the cracks.

Step one in the diagnostic process is to schedule an appointment with a doctor. The receptionist may ask the nature of your illness but prefers not to hear your symptom soliloquy. The appointment may be granted as if it were a special favor rather than a two-way business transaction, and the preparation begins. "What can I say to convey the seriousness of this to the doctor; how can I describe what is happening to me? If I bring a list, the doc will think I'm neurotic. If I don't, I'll forget important information. How healthy should I look? If I look okay, I won't be taken seriously. I know I'm sick; why should I have to convince anyone?" In Sefra Pitzele's words, we are in a "well until proven sick" situation.

Feeling increasingly helpless and lost, we begin to wonder whether our symptoms are imaginary. Self-confidence plummets; doubts flourish. We doubt our doctors; we doubt ourselves. With self-esteem at low ebb, we are surrounded by others who cannot possibly understand how we feel. Armchair advice and diagnoses from concerned others may do more harm than good, and the same is true of the reactions of many of the doctors we approach with desperation and fear. Still we pursue a diagnosis: proof of legitimacy.

DOCTORS AND DIAGNOSES

Diagnosis is both an art and a science. The diagnostician's expertise and intuition are supplemented with diagnostic tests— not the other way around. Diagnosing an elusive illness can be exceptionally difficult, in this case because cause is unknown and no specific diagnostic tests have been developed. The process is perplexing for medical professionals as well as patients and their families.

One may see several doctors before a correct diagnosis is made. The search requires determination, and many give up along the way. Although awareness within the medical profession has improved, too many doctors still don't "believe in" CFS and FMS, as if such disorders were akin to the tooth fairy.

The anxiety of waiting for test results is often more traumatic than the tests themselves. Like a teenager awaiting a prom invitation, I sat near the telephone waiting to hear whether I had a brain tumor, hypoglycemia, heart problems, multiple sclerosis, or an ulcer. Initial relief at knowing what I *didn't* have was quickly replaced with fear of not knowing what I *did* have. I assumed that if the right test were run, I'd be diagnosed, treated, and cured. With each negative test result, I became more rather than less concerned; perhaps it would be concluded that I didn't "have" anything at all. I had been taught to believe in the wisdom of doctors and medical tests, but instead felt misunderstood and mistreated. Two incredibly long years passed before my illness was properly diagnosed.

No definitive test to diagnose CFS or FMS exists at this time. Specialized tests may indicate abnormalities, but these findings are not diagnostic. Depending on one's symptoms, some of the following may need to be ruled out:

- viral illnesses, including cytomegalovirus (CMV), chronic mononucleosis (Epstein-Barr virus infection), toxoplasmosis, herpesviruses (simplex I and II, herpes zoster, HHV-6), mycoplasmal pneumonia, coxsackie B, hepatitis A and B, chronic active hepatitis, rubella, and HIV disease

- other infectious diseases, such as localized infections and bacterial infections (e.g., tuberculosis, brucellosis, endocarditis, and Lyme disease)
- collagen vascular diseases (e.g., systemic lupus erythematosus)
- rheumatoid arthritis
- immune deficiency state (e.g., low immunoglobin A, or IgA, which helps fight infection)
- chronic inflammatory diseases (e.g., sarcoidosis and Wegener's granulomatosis)
- toxic agents (e.g., chemical solvents, heavy metals, and pesticides)
- allergies
- malignancies, especially lymphoma
- chronic psychiatric diseases (e.g., depression, anxiety, and/or panic disorder) as the sole cause of symptoms
- chronic systemic diseases (e.g., pulmonary, renal [kidney], cardiac, hepatic [liver], and hematologic [blood] diseases)
- anemia
- neuromuscular diseases (e.g., multiple sclerosis and myasthenia gravis)
- fungal diseases, including candidiasis (which may be a separate illness or part of the CFS cluster)
- endocrine diseases (e.g., hypothyroidism, Addison's disease, Cushing's syndrome, and diabetes mellitus)
- parasitic infection (e.g., giardiasis, amebiasis, or helminthic infection)
- drug side effects, dependency, or abuse (including alcohol); drug interactions

Routine laboratory tests sometimes reveal abnormalities, often subtle:

- CBC: elevated hematocrit (red blood cell count)
- macrocytosis with elevated MCV (large red blood cells with elevated volume)

‣ mild leukocytosis, modest leukopenia, moderate monocytosis, and atypical lymphocytes

‣ liver function tests: mildly elevated SGOT and SGPT

‣ thyroid values: T_4 and thyroid stimulating hormone (TSH) usually normal; T_3 uptake subnormal or at the low end of normal; elevated blood levels of antithyroid antibodies

‣ elevated antinuclear antibodies (ANAs), usually a speckled pattern

‣ low sedimentation rate (although in some cases slightly elevated)

‣ lipid panel: elevated lipids, including LDL; decreased HDL

‣ electrolytes: decreased potassium, sodium

‣ urine: increased pH (alkaline)

Doctors often become annoyed and skeptical when confronted with illnesses with which they are not well-acquainted. The symptoms are often diverse and vague, the clues subtle, and the search frustrating. Unfortunately, psychiatry and psychology become dumping grounds for those with elusive illnesses. Would a cancer patient be told, "You can't possibly have cancer because you are depressed"? How does one negate the other? To assume that the psychological factors associated with CFS and FMS are causal is to confuse correlation with causation. When nothing "turns up" on lab tests, the patient is often presumed physically healthy but psychologically suspect. To be told "I can't find anything, so it must be a psychological problem; go see a shrink" is neither constructive nor logical.

THE OFFICE EXAM

Findings present in a physical examination of a CFS/FMS patient may include the following:

‣ tender points consistent with fibromyalgia

‣ abnormal neurological functioning

‣ excessive titubation (staggering or stumbling) or inability to maintain Romberg or tandem stance and tandem walk (standing or walking with eyes closed)

‣ end-gaze nystagmus (involuntary eye movements)

- intermittent aniscoria (unequal pupil size) in dim light
- photophobia (light sensitivity)
- difficulty with cognitive functioning: serial 7s (counting backward from 100 by 7s), recalling the names of three items following intervening stimuli, mathematical calculations, spelling words backward (neurocognitive test performance may not accurately reflect the extent of these difficulties)
- fever or subnormal body temperature
- low blood pressure
- intermittent tachycardia (increased heartbeat)
- abnormal oral pharynx (throat) exam, including buccal mucosal ulcerations (sores in the mouth), posterior cobblestoning or erythema (swelling or redness), blisters on tongue or coated tongue (sometimes thrush), and crimson crescents (purplish-red discoloration of both anterior pharyngeal pillars)
- anterior and/or posterior cervical or axillary adenopathy or lymphadenia (swollen or inflamed glands), usually asymmetric
- rashes or sores
- brittle or thinning hair
- sallow complexion
- hyperreflexia (increased reflex reactions)
- intention tremor (quivering hand movements when attempting a task)
- mild tremor on drift testing (attempting to hold one's arm out in a stable position)
- mitral valve prolapse (an abnormality that causes a failure of this heart valve to close properly)
- diffuse abdominal tenderness
- mild to severe skin atrophy of distal finger tips; loss of fingerprints

(Paul Cheney, M.D., Ph.D., and Charles Lapp, M.D., March/April 1993)

The diagnosing physician will often ask about unreported symptoms that the patient may not have associated with the illness or that are difficult to describe without specific questioning, such as sensitivity to light, noise, and odors; food intolerances; feeling unusually hot or cold; specific cognitive problems (getting lost while driving, losing one's train of thought, quickly forgetting new information, difficulty with word finding, easy distractability, calculation difficulty, forgetting how to do routine things, "brain fog"); balance problems; presyncope (the sensation of impending faint); difficulty remaining standing; difficulty processing multiple sensory input; sensory overload phenomenon; and shortness of breath.

A daily log of symptoms, medications, and symptom fluctuations can be immensely helpful for the physician. A completed symptom list and other rating scales provide useful medical documentation and are especially important in disability determination.

LABORATORY TESTS

The practice of medicine relies upon laboratory tests for diagnosis. The emphasis on lab tests has been praised ("Incredible technology!") as well as damned ("Doctors treat test results instead of patients"). Sophisticated lab tests can be of great value but may be dangerously misused; they cannot replace the art of medicine, the practice of listening to the patient carefully and with an open mind. We should not value "scientific data" above good judgment. Reliable labwork should serve as an adjunct to rather than the basis of good medical practice.

Undergoing tests is emotionally and financially draining for patients, even when the procedures themselves are relatively innocuous. Although tests are routine for those who order and perform them, they are journeys into the unknown for sick patients, who may feel confused and diminished by the process. The equipment and procedures can be intimidating; technology can cause panic in the uninitiated—as it probably should.

The cost of a test may present greater discomfort than the test itself. Waiting for test results is nerve-wracking; the prospect of coming up with nothing is frustrating, and the possibility of finding serious disorder is frightening. The hours or days spent waiting for test results may seem like months or years, and although no one wants a diagnosis of cancer or lupus, we are nonetheless disappointed to have gone through blood tests and brain scans only to be told we have "nothing."

Although no specific diagnostic tests for CFS or FMS exist, certain tests should be performed to rule out other illnesses with similar symptoms or to identify concurrent illnesses:

- complete blood count
- SMA-20 (blood chemistry panel)
- erythrocyte sedimentation rate (ESR)
- tuberculin skin test and/or chest X-ray
- urinalysis (qualitative and microscopic)
- thyroid profile, including free thyroxine index (thyroxine and T3 uptake) and thyroid stimulating hormone (TSH)
- antinuclear antibody (ANA) blood levels
- syphilis test (RPR or VDRL)
- electrocardiogram (ECG)

Additional tests should be considered on a case-by-case basis, based upon individual symptomatology, sometimes to document abnormalities for disability determination and to help determine treatment:

- allergy testing
- skin test for anergy (lack of immune response)
- antithyroid antibodies
- tests to rule out cancer, hepatitis, HIV, Lyme disease, lupus, myasthenia gravis, multiple sclerosis, or parasites
- tilt table testing (to evaluate patients with episodes of light-headedness or fainting)
- viral PCR (polymerase chain reaction) or antibody tests for HHV-6 (a herpes virus), cytomegalovirus (CMV), Epstein-Barr virus (EBV), and the like; PCR for mycoplasma, chlamydia, and so on
- polysomnography (sleep study)
- fecal occult blood
- exercise testing with oxygen-consumption measurements
- toxic chemical analysis
- brain scans: CT, MRI, topographic computer EEG, NeuroSPECT, and PET scans

- neuropsychological testing
- vestibular (balance) testing
- immune tests: circulating immune complexes; IgA levels and IgG subclasses and so on
- lumbar puncture (spinal tap)
- upper and lower gastrointestinal (GI) series
- liver and spleen scan
- bone marrow aspirate
- lymph node biopsy
- perturbations of the 2-5A synthetase/RNaseL antiviral pathway
- hypoglycemia and/or insulin resistance testing
- functional capacity evaluation
- neuropsychological examination

FINALLY, A LABEL

It is well-established that the mere fact of knowing what hurts you has an inherent curative value.

— *Hans Selye, M.D.*

Obtaining a diagnosis is a good news–bad news proposition. The good news: this is a physical, organic illness. "I'm not crazy. There's a name for this miserable condition, and I'm not the only one who has it. I was right to listen to my body's signals that something is wrong. I have some control now that I know what I'm dealing with." One patient said, "I was so relieved to know I *had* something." A diagnosis gives us permission to be sick and lends validation of our complaints. The postdiagnostic double may be summarized: "Oh good, I'm really sick. Damn, I'm really sick."

The "honeymoon period," or the initial relief of having been diagnosed, is short-lived, leaving us to deal with the symptoms, the losses, the puzzlement of those around us. We wonder, "Knowing is good—but how do I recover?" and realize that the answer to this question is not included in the diagnosis. We are labeled, put into a cubbyhole. And the aftershock: the illness is real. It isn't going to go away overnight, if at all. Having obtained a diagnosis becomes a mixed blessing, initial relief followed by acknowledgment of the forthcoming journey into the unknown.

Acknowledging CFS and FMS means losing a large degree of perceived control over one's life. The illness continues to be unpredictable and unwelcome. The diagnosis brings with it a sense of betrayal, anger at one's body, feelings of fear and insecurity. And the inevitable question: *Why me?* We ride the emotional roller coaster of diagnosis like that of grieving: denial, shock, truth, disbelief, numbness, anger, relief. Since the illness is chronic, emotional effects are continuous and variable.

COMMUNICATING THE DIAGNOSIS
TO THE PATIENT

The way a doctor communicates a diagnosis has a profound influence on the patient. Many physicians say such things as, "Just accept this and go on with your life," or "You have a chronic illness. There's nothing I can do for you. It will probably never go away." This is incomplete information, delivered insensitively.

A CFS/FMS diagnosis is not a death sentence but may be a life sentence. Once a diagnosis has been made, it is time to discuss options, various treatment modalities and coping mechanisms, and the hope for a cure in the future. Physicians should try to motivate their patients, working together toward symptom alleviation. A dose of hope delivered along with the diagnosis is vital. The newly diagnosed need to hear such statements as, "You have quite a struggle ahead of you, but there is hope. We will try different treatments to see what works for you. You will probably improve over time and you may or may not fully recover, but many resources are available."

Despite the lack of a cure or even a reliable or specific treatment program, patients should consult only competent, open-minded, CFS/FMS-educated physicians and stay well informed about current theories and therapies. Patients who remain actively involved in treatment are more likely to do well than those who crawl back under the covers.

7

Overlapping Disorders:
Variations on a Theme?

Syndromal diagnoses are common . . . where there is a strong reliance on patient self-report rather than clinical signs or laboratory markers. Many clinical specialties identify syndromes closely related to CFS, but with varied emphasis on a particular symptom feature, such as musculoskeletal pain in fibromyalgia and gastrointestinal disturbance in irritable bowel syndrome.
— *Andrew R. Lloyd, Ian B. Hickie, and Robert H. Loblay*

Numerous chronic disorders share common features, including symptoms and abnormalities. The similarities are remarkable, yet the relationships among them are unclear. Skeptics who dismiss CFS, FMS, irritable bowel syndrome (IBS), and the like as "wastebasket" syndromes—that is, those that do not fit neatly into established categories of physical disease—imply that poorly understood conditions do not deserve the respect afforded "testable" illnesses. This practices lifts a burden from disinterested physicians and blames—even traumatizes—sufferers.

Double standards allow medical doctors to diagnose psychiatric illness in patients in the absence of a known physiological cause, but do not typically allow the psychiatrist or psychologist who rules out emotional causes to rule in physiologic illness. That is, acceptable practice allows a physician to say, "It is all in your head," but how often does a psychiatrist or psychologist say, "Nothing wrong with your head; the illness is all in your body"? Depression is diagnosed in large part on the patient's self-reported symptoms, but such reporting is criticized as too subjective in diagnosing "real" illness. Although psychiatric symptoms often accompany chronic illnesses, they do not cause them, and studies of a large group of chronic disorders differentiate them from major depression.

Overlap with so-called psychiatric disorders creates an artificial distinction between illnesses of the mind and those of the body. A "psychiatric" label is used pejoratively to characterize poorly understood disorders, implying emotional weakness, personal failure, and the inability to cope effectively with life. Illnesses such as multiple sclerosis (MS), rheumatoid arthritis, polio, HIV/AIDS, stomach ulcers, and diabetes were once considered to be of psychiatric origin. When markers or diagnostic tests were developed, the diagnoses shifted to "real" illnesses, those of the body. History repeats itself.

Overlap among medical disorders is common. Statistically, irritable bowel syndrome (IBS), CFS, restless leg syndrome, headache, and menstrual pain problems are more common in FMS patients than in the general population; this occurrence is far greater than it would be by mere chance. Restless leg syndrome occurs in 30 percent of people with FMS, 15 percent of those with rheumatoid arthritis, and 2 percent of the general population. IBS is common in FMS, and FMS is found in about 65 percent of people with IBS. Coincidence?

Several studies of such disorders as CFS, FMS, IBS, temporomandibular joint dysfunction (TMD), multiple chemical sensitivity disorder, myofascial pain syndrome, and Gulf War syndrome (GWS) reveal similar characteristics and findings, showing that several of these disorders commonly occur in the same patient. Because illnesses are compartmentalized and labeled, spanning a number of medical specialties, each is studied as a discrete disorder. As common factors become more apparent, the boundaries between illnesses tend to blur. Daniel Clauw, M.D., a rheumatologist at Georgetown University Medical Center, takes a broad perspective on such illnesses that share similar characteristics, conceptualizing them as components of a large spectrum of illnesses having similar characteristics with more commonalities than distinctions.

Muhammad Yunus, M.D., calls this spectrum of similar conditions with overlapping features and characteristics "central sensitivity syndrome," or CSS. He views CSS as a "paradigm of central sensitivity and neurohormonal dysfunction," citing central sensitization and neurohormonal, neuroendocrine, and brain imaging abnormalities as common factors (2000). The abnormalities differ from those found in psychiatric conditions, and routine lab tests and X-rays are normal. Shared symptoms include pain, hyperalgesia, poor sleep, and fatigue. Leslie Aaron, Ph.D., and Dedra Buchwald, M.D., describe a similar group of overlapping disorders in which the most consistent objective findings are tender points, along with decreased pain threshold and tolerance (2001). Yunus states that as a group, CSS syndromes are the most common reason for medical visits and "the number one cause of human suffering anywhere in the world."

Researcher Andrew Lloyd, M.D., notes the difficulty of establishing diagnostic boundaries among similar disorders, particularly those sharing fatigue as a major symptom. Because symptoms overlap, Lloyd speculates that all may be manifestations of the same disease state with similar or identical etiologic factors including pathogens, genetic predisposition, lifestyle, history of toxic exposure or emotional or physical trauma, and central nervous system (CNS) and hypothalamic-pituitary-adrenal (HPA) axis disturbances.

The consensus is clear: A large spectrum of overlapping disorders share common symptoms and abnormalities, each characterized somewhat differently, with no clear boundaries among them. A group of overlapping disorders is presented here. Numerous others have been excluded due to space constraints.

ALLERGY

Allergies occur when one's immune system mounts a specific response to an antigen.

Several tests measure allergies, including the scratch test (in which drops of antigens are applied to scratches made on the skin) and blood tests: the IgE RAST test that helps identify substances causing immediate reactions and the ELISA/ACT lymphocyte response assay that determines immunoreactive effects on the lymphocytes and delayed reactivity. Since test results are not absolute, personal experience must be used as a guide.

The degree of an allergic reaction varies with the amount of exposure to an allergen, simultaneous exposure to multiple allergens, and the general state of the immune system at the time of exposure. Allergies are known to change over time. They are not regarded as causal but may predispose one to become ill with other disorders.

AUTOIMMUNE DISEASE

Autoimmune disorders are those in which one's immune system attacks the body's own joints, tissues, and organs. Like CFS and FMS, autoimmune diseases are more common in women than men.

Rheumatoid arthritis (RA) is most apt to mimic fibromyalgia syndrome and includes morning stiffness, fatigue, and tender points. Pressing such points, however, does not produce the intense pain that occurs with fibromyalgia, and laboratory tests for abnormality can usually differentiate RA from FMS. Hashimoto's thyroiditis is an autoimmune type of hypothyroidism (low thyroid level) that, if undetected and untreated, can cause widespread muscle aches, depression, and fatigue. Other autoimmune disorders with similar symptoms and a higher prevalence in women are systemic lupus erythematosus (SLE) and multiple sclerosis. Fibromyalgia symptoms, in fact, are very common in SLE patients, although the two conditions are thought to be distinct. Autoimmune diseases evolve slowly, and even when physicians diagnose FMS, they should keep track of any changes in symptoms over time in order to rule out these other illnesses, which require different treatments.

The cause of autoimmune disease is unknown, probably involving several factors: pathogens, environmental factors, chemicals, and drugs, all of which may damage or alter body cells. Sex hormones and heredity are probably involved. Whether pathogens are causal agents, cofactors, or secondary superinfections remains speculative. For example, mycoplasmal infections have been reported in patients with various inflammatory diseases, such as endocarditis, pericarditis, and encephalomyelitis.

Treatment may involve nonsteroidal anti-inflammatory drugs (NSAIDs), such as ibuprofen and naproxen; glucocorticoids, such as cortisone and prednisone; and disease-modifying antirheumatic drugs (DMARDs), such as methotrexate.

COMPRESSED SPINAL CANAL: CHIARI, SYRINGOMYELIA, AND CERVICAL STENOSIS

Chiari type I is a relatively rare malformation at the juncture of the brain and spinal cord, with protrusion of the cerebellar tonsils (two appendages extending from the cerebellum) into the spinal canal. Chiari is associated with numerous symptoms, most commonly severe headache and neck pain, but many people with the disorder are asymptomatic. Syringomyelia, an associated disorder, is characterized by an abnormal collection of fluid in the spine in the form of a cyst, or "syrinx." Cervical stenosis (CS), a congenital narrowing of the spine in the neck area, is not relieved by surgery.

The most common intervention for Chiari is a lengthy, invasive surgery to achieve craniocervical decompression. Results vary, with some patients showing improvement and others becoming more symptomatic. Surgery has been performed on unsuitable candidates with poor results. A tiny subgroup of CFS/FMS patients may have concurrent or undiagnosed Chiari malformation or CS, but desperation should not drive one toward unnecessary surgery.

ENDOMETRIOSIS

Endometriosis, or overgrowth of cells from the uterine lining into the abdominal cavity, is characterized by menstrual pain, fatigue, bloating, heavy and/or irregular bleeding, and bowel disturbances. Some studies indicate a statistically significant overlap with CFS/FMS, while others do not. The two conditions may exist simultaneously but there is no known causal relationship, and it remains unclear whether the incidence of endometriosis is higher in the CFS/FMS population as compared to healthy individuals.

GENERALIZED ANXIETY DISORDER

Shared symptoms among generalized anxiety disorder (GAD) and CFS/FMS include fatigue, concentration difficulty, sleep disturbance, irritability, restlessness, and rapid heartbeat. However, the most prominent symptom in GAD is excessive, persistent worry, whereas the most prominent symptoms in CFS and FMS are fatigue, pain, and neurocognitive dysfunction.

Other primary misdiagnoses of CFS and FMS include conversion disorder (emotional illness manifesting as physical symptoms), panic disorder with agoraphobia, separation anxiety, parental over-protection of ill child, and Munchausen syndrome by proxy (MSBP), a rare disorder in which a parent purposefully creates symptoms in a child to gain attention for her/himself.

GULF WAR SYNDROME

The U.S. government has alternately acknowledged and denied the existence of a group of symptoms experienced by at least 100,000 of the 700,000 U.S. troops deployed to the Persian Gulf in 1990. Although no case definition for Gulf War syndrome (GWS), aka Gulf War illness (GWI), exists, its symptoms strongly resemble those of CFS, FMS, and rheumatoid arthritis. More than half of GWS patients meet criteria for CFS.

Symptoms occurring in Gulf War veterans include debilitating fatigue, postexertional fatigue, widespread muscle and joint pain, sleep disorders, temperature dysregulation, night sweats, pain and stiffness, headaches, numbness, swelling in joints and extremities, diarrhea, cramps, anxiety, irritability, depression, malaise, and neurological symptoms: blurred vision, irregular heartbeat, balance problems, dizziness, speech difficulty, weakness, tremors and shaking, seizures and other movement problems, and cognitive impairment (concentration deficit, memory problems, and confusion). Many Gulf War veterans have suffered long-term health problems, and their significant others have become ill as well.

Likely cofactors in the development of GWS include multiple exposures to chemical, biological, and emotional stressors. In addition to multiple vaccines (including anthrax and botulism), deployed veterans were exposed to high doses of at least eight pesticides (including organophosphate pesticides, high-concentration DEET (N,N-diethyl-2,5-dimethylbenzamide) insect repellant, and those in the acetylcholinesterase inhibitor class, such as carbamates), sarin nerve gas, mustard agents, pyridostigmine bromide (PB) tablets (an experimental drug used as protection against nerve gas but known to have side effects), disinfectants, chemical and biological warfare agents, smoke from oil fires, chemical warfare antidotes, depleted uranium and depleted uranium dust, special paints, heavy metals, jet fuel, decontamination solution, and petrochemicals (including kerosene used in heaters inside tents and diesel fumes from fuel sprayed on sand to harden it in making parking lots). In many cases, protective measures were not taken. The synergistic and long-term effects of many of these agents are unknown.

Several studies indicate that oil-well fires, combat stress, antibiotics to prevent anthrax, and antimalaria pills are unrelated to development of GWS. Infectious disease and posttraumatic stress disorder (PTSD) have been ruled out as causes. The factors that appear to be related are exposure to sarin gas, use of PB tablets, wearing of flea collars to repel insects (containing the pesticide chlorpyrifos, then called Dursban, now removed from the consumer market), applying copious amounts of the military-issue insect repellant containing DEET, and exposure to ethyl alcohol. Use of experimental vaccines and hazardous chemical exposure was greater for Gulf War veterans than any other known deployed military group.

Documented abnormalities includes loss of brain cells, with neuronal damage in the brainstem and basal gangli; functional MRI data abnormalities; and neurotransmitter derangement, particularly dopamine levels. Immune abnormalities include upregulation (overreaction) of cytokines and T-cells and diminished numbers of natural killer (NK) cells, abnormal CD4/CD8 ratios (related to cells that help control the immune response), NK cell abnormalities, reactivation of Epstein-Barr virus (EBV) and herpesvirus HHV-6, and changes in antinuclear antibodies (ANAs) with progression of the disease. Medical tests have evidenced neurotoxic effects and damage to deep brain structures. GWS symptoms and findings resemble those of diseases affecting these structures, such as Parkinson's disease, Huntington's disease, and amyotrophic lateral sclerosis (ALS). ALS, typically found in older people, has been diagnosed in some GWS veterans in their 30s and 40s. Correlations have been found between number of inoculations and musculoskeletal complaints, and between symptoms of toxic neuropathy and number of days spent handling pesticides.

A high rate of concurrent infections has been found: mycoplasma (particularly *M. fermentans*), chlamydia, brucella, borrelia, rickettsia, and possibly other transmittable, chronic bacterial and viral infections. Evidence exists for increased risk of leukemia and other cancers and symptoms of advanced acute toxicity after taking pyridostigmine bromide. Cardiovascular dysregulation has been evidenced by decreasing blood pressure during mental arithmetic tasks and speech. GWS-associated disorders suggest additional risk of developing respiratory ailments, rheumatoid arthritis, cardiac diseases, autoimmune diseases, and immunosuppressive diseases.

The U.S. government has been accused of shortchanging Gulf War veterans who have developed debilitating symptoms. Suspected risk for developing Parkinson's disease, ALS, and other neurological disorders in aging Gulf War veterans are cause for concern.

INFLAMMATORY BOWEL DISEASE AND IRRITABLE BOWEL SYNDROME

Gastrointestinal symptoms are common in CFS and FMS, more typically irritable bowel syndrome (IBS) than inflammatory bowel disease (IBD). IBD is a serious, chronic condition, often accompanied by arthritis-like pain and occurring in a waxing-and-waning pattern, that significantly impacts one's lifestyle. Two serious types are Crohn's disease, a severe inflammation of a part of the gastrointestinal (GI) tract, and ulcerative colitis, an inflammatory process of the large intestine. Crohn's disease is characterized by abdominal pain, diarrhea, fever, and weight loss, sometimes with serious complications. Symptoms of ulcerative colitis include abdominal cramps, blood and mucus in the stool, and increased urgency to defecate. Attacks may be severe and sudden, with the possibility of serious complications.

Pathogenesis of IBD may be related to immune dysregulation, with Crohn's disease a manifestation of an exaggerated Th1 response and ulcerative colitis an exaggerated Th2 response (Th1 and Th2 cells are involved in the body's immune response). Treatments include antibiotics, probiotics, anti-inflammatories, steroids, and immune system modulators.

IBS, a disorder of bowel function rather than structure, is estimated to affect 20 percent of adults in the Western world. A distressing disorder that greatly affects one's quality of life, IBS was once dismissed as a mild, psychogenic disorder of gut motility. It is now regarded as the result of brain-gut dysfunction with dysregulation of the autonomic nervous system. Autonomic dysfunction may account for the presence of IBS in CFS and FMS. Neuromodulators such as norepinephrine, dopamine, acetylcholine, and neuropeptides (including substance P) occur in both brain and gut, affecting bowel function and perhaps causing cytokine production that leads to inflammation. Serotonin plays a significant role and is often used in treatment.

This often-lifelong condition commonly begins in childhood or young adulthood, afflicting more women than men. Incidence is estimated at 15 to 20 percent of the general adult population, although many do not seek medical attention. Screening tests include blood tests; stool hemoccult; flexible sigmoidoscopy; lactose tolerance evaluation; and X-rays, colonoscopy, or biopsy if indicated. Diagnosis is based on the Rome II criteria: abdominal discomfort associated with additional symptoms. Patients typically experience abdominal pain, straining or urgency, increased colonic motility after eating, bloating, and mucus in the stool. Many doctors are unfamiliar with diagnostic guidelines and underestimate the seriousness of IBS, attributing symptoms to psychiatric factors. Treatment is often challenging. A recent study found bacteria in the GI tract of IBS patients, and antibiotic treatment has shown promise in treatment.

LYME DISEASE

Lyme disease is a multisystem inflammatory disorder that may affect the skin, joints, heart, eyes, and nervous system. The most common tick-transmitted disease in the United States, it is caused by the bite of a tick infected with the spirochete *Borrelia burgdorferi* or related species. Since blood tests are often unreliable, diagnosis is also based on clinical signs and symptoms and ruling out other disorders, particularly those with neurological symptoms. The CDC-recommended standard approach to diagnosis is based on two tests, the western blot and ELISA, which are only somewhat reliable. PCR (polymerase chain reaction) testing is more reliable, although more expensive. A potential marker for Lyme disease is being studied, and a vaccine has been developed. The CDC estimates 50,000 cases of Lyme disease in the United States, while the Lyme Disease Foundation's study suggests 1.5 to 2 million cases.

Lyme disease often begins with a telltale bull's-eye-shaped rash and flulike symptoms (fatigue, fever, headache, stiff neck, and joint and muscle pain), although many patients are unaware of receiving a tick bite, and the rash may escape detection. Antibiotic treatment is most successful in the early stages. Multiple antibiotics may be given sequentially (on an alternating basis) or simultaneously. Some respond well to treatment, others recover over a long period of time, and some fail to recover fully, with a lingering postinfectious syndrome or development of other serious illnesses such as Lyme arthritis.

Months to years after the initial infection, later symptoms include arthritis pain and swelling, sleep disorder, generalized achiness, stiffness, weakness, heart palpitations, headache, fever, shortness of breath, swollen lymph glands, weight gain, tingling or numbness in the extremities, abnormal pulse, sore throat, sexual dysfunction, irritable bladder, GI symptoms, vision problems, alcohol intolerance, multiple chemical sensitivities, balance problems, light-headedness, disorientation, confusion, dizziness or vertigo, photophobia, anxiety, depression, mood swings, and cognitive problems (concentration deficit, anomia, and memory deficits).

The possibility that Lyme disease is related to CFS and FMS has been explored, with no clear consensus. Some physicians find that patients diagnosed with CFS and FMS actually have undiagnosed Lyme disease.

MAJOR DEPRESSIVE DISORDER

Major depressive disorder (MDD) is characterized by feelings of hopelessness and helplessness, decreased libido, anhedonia (decreased ability to experience pleasure), frequent tearfulness, changes in appetite and weight, hypersomnia or hyposomnia, decreased energy, feelings of guilt and worthlessness, and cognitive dysfunction.

The history of psychiatric disorders in the CFS/FMS population is similar to that in the general population. Depression and CFS/FMS may coexist due to changes in brain chemistry and as a normal reaction to debilitating chronic illness. Depression does not cause these syndromes and it is not present in all cases; however, many patients are given a psychiatric diagnosis when a physiological diagnosis is not apparent. Overlapping symptoms, presence of depressed mood in some patients, lack of a known cause or marker, and simple ignorance causes confusion between CFS/FMS and depression.

Depressive symptoms in physically ill patients may be a result of immune activation and cytokine secretion, in addition to a psychological reaction to illness-related distress and incapacitation. Complex interactions among the immune system, the HPA axis, and other neurological factors affect stress levels, emotions, and vulnerability to illness. Illness, in turn, affects these body systems. Specific cytokines have been associated with depressed mood, anxiety, and memory impairment. Studies show that immune activation may precede the development of depression, with increased levels of certain cytokines, in addition to a psychological reaction to the effects of illness (Yirmiya 2000).

The rate of depression is not necessarily higher in patients with the most severe symptoms. Low doses of antidepressants do help with sleep disorder, pain, energy levels, and cognitive dysfunction, and standard doses are used to treat symptomatic depression if present. Nonantidepressant medications common in CFS/FMS treatment are not effective in treating MDD.

Psychological tests are frequently used to "rule in" depression and other psychiatric disorders; however, they cannot distinguish between a test-taker's medical and psychological disorders. One who endorses numerous physical complaints is likely to be labeled depressed. "Results in ill populations may be falsely elevated for psychological disorders" (Jason, Richman, et al. 1997).

The table on pages 102–103 compares CFS/FMS with MDD in terms of patient and illness characteristics, symptoms, and typical test results.

MULTIPLE CHEMICAL SENSITIVITY DISORDER

Multiple chemical sensitivity (MCS) disorder, also known as environmental illness (EI), is characterized by immediate or delayed reactions to various environmental chemicals. Chemical intolerance (CI) is a symptom of MCS, although the terms are often used interchangeably. Sick building syndrome (SBS), a subset of MCS, is characterized by fatigue, upper respiratory infections, and difficulty concentrating.

Toxins are ubiquitous in our environment. Offending chemicals are found in food additives, drugs, perfumes and other scented products, pesticides, herbicides, fuel and engine exhaust, environmental tobacco smoke, disinfectants and room deodorizers, natural gas, building materials (e.g., paint and particleboard), solvents, new carpets, and household furnishings. Some offending substances that

Comparison of CFS/FMS and MDD

Symptom	CFS/FMS	MDD
Onset	often but not always abrupt	gradual
Pain	strongly associated	weakly associated, if present
Age	most prevalent in middle years	occurs increasingly with age
History	incidence of mood disorder same as in general population	often history of mood disorder in patient and family
Pattern	no characteristic pattern	likely to awaken depressed and improve as the day progresses
Duration	usually persists for years or indefinitely	average duration six months
Motivation	interested but unable to engage in activities	lack of interest in previous activities
Social	lacks energy to be "social"	reclusive, loss of social interest
Treatment	symptomatic only; does not resolve	usually resolves with treatment
Response to antidepressants	some symptom relief: pain, allergy, mood, cognition; many unable to tolerate regular dose	significant relief; cure or remission likely; able to tolerate typical dose
Symptoms	(see Chapter 5)	most symptoms of CFS and FMS are absent
Attribution	views illness as being caused by external factors	views illness as being caused by inadequacy, personal failing
Fatigue	severe, debilitating, or disabling	less severe
Exercise	exacerbates symptoms	improves symptoms
Exertion	decreased brain perfusion (blood flow) and brain activity	increased brain perfusion and brain activity
Cognition	often varies with fatigue and pain levels	deficits proportional to degree of depression

Comparison of CFS/FMS and MDD

Symptom	CFS/FMS	MDD
Sleep disorder	abnormal brain waves during sleep; does not correlate with depression; increased REM latency; alpha-delta intrusion; abnormal breathing; involuntary limb movements	normal brain waves during sleep; usually improves when depression is treated; reduced REM latency
Immune abnormalities	Numerous, e.g., decreased NK activity and altered levels of certain interleukins	few immune abnormalities noted
Antibody production	common	uncommon
Cortisol level	decreased	increased
CRH	decreased	elevated
Tender points	common	absent
MRI brain scan	punctate lesions	few or no lesions
SPECT brain scan	hypoperfusion to localized areas of the brain	hypoperfusion has different pattern; more diffuse
Metabolic defects	common	uncommon
Alcohol use	poorly tolerated	use is common
Test performance	overestimate test performance	underestimate test performance
MMPI-2	Unique profile: elevated 1, 2, 3, 7, and 8. Elevation of subscales 1, 2, and 3, typical of chronic illness.	elevated 2; 2 and 7; or 2, 4, and 7
Other neuropsychiatric tests:	Differing findings for CFS and FMS vs. depression on WAIS-R IQ test, memory tests, and neurological test battery subscales	

The Minnesota Multiphasic Personality Inventory-2 (MMPI, Version 2), widely used to diagnose psychopathology, shows distinct scale elevations ("profiles") for MDD and CFS/FMS.
When "neurological" items were removed from the test and the tests were rescored, all scores dropped to within the normal range; that is, no elevations remained. This finding provides evidence that neurological dysfunction rather than psychopathology accounts for the typical CFS profile.

are inhaled, eaten, or drunk are able to cross the blood-brain barrier, causing neurological damage.

Several definitions of MCS have been proposed. MCS may start with either acute or chronic toxic exposure, with the response increasing over time, even to small amounts of the substance, and generalizing to other substances generally regarded as nontoxic, neutral, or mildly unpleasant in a process called cross-sensitization. Reactions may be abrupt or delayed and are exacerbated by multiple exposures, stressors, and neuroimmune factors.

The mechanism by which sensitization occurs is unclear. Chemical, biologic, and psychological stimuli can initiate sensitization. The site of the amplification may be the limbic system, which receives input from the olfactory pathways, leading in turn to behavioral, autonomic, endocrine, and immune system dysfunction. Chemical intolerance may be a measurable indicator of the brain's ability to amplify symptoms and sensations, including pain. High levels of body chemicals such as substance P (known to be elevated in FMS patients) may cause brain sensitization and malfunctioning, producing amplified symptoms. Iris Bell, M.D., suspects that temporal lobe epilepsy may be present.

Symptoms of MCS span multiple organ systems: dizziness, headache or migraine, nausea, spaciness and other neurological sensations, breathing difficulty, cognitive deficits (impaired concentration and memory), weakness, irritation (of the eyes, mouth, throat, and ears), balance difficulties, skin rash, musculoskeletal pain, abdominal pain, and affective symptoms (irritability, depression, and anxiety).

The disorder is not new, but its prevalence is increasing as new chemicals are developed and introduced. Environmental toxicologists report increased incidence of cancer, brain disorders, asthma, autoimmune disease, and other health problems directly related to the recent proliferation of synthetic chemicals. This multitude of toxins includes arsenic, chlordane, polychlorinated biphenyls, trichloroethylene, and toluene.

The true incidence of MCS is unknown because diagnostic criteria vary and many physicians regard the problem as psychogenic. An estimated 15 to 34 percent of Americans experience some symptoms of chemical sensitivity, with 4 to 6 percent severely affected. (Bell 1998). Various studies suggest that MCS is present in

40 to 80 percent of people with CFS, FMS, and GWS, and the majority of people with a primary diagnosis of MCS have concurrent CFS, FMS, GWS, and allergies. MCS is more prevalent in women than men (except in older populations), with age of onset typically in the thirties and forties. Although there is no specific test for MCS, abnormalities have been detected on immune and brain imaging tests.

MULTIPLE SCLEROSIS

A chronic, progressive, and often disabling disease of the central nervous system, multiple sclerosis (MS) is characterized by the destruction of myelin, the insulating fatty sheath surrounding nerves that helps to transmit nerve signals to and from the central nervous system. Twice as common in women than men, MS is usually diagnosed between the ages of twenty and forty, most often in the early thirties, and is believed to be most prevalent among Caucasian women. The estimated prevalence in the United States is 100 cases per 100,000, with about 350,000 afflicted, and more than 1 million cases worldwide. MS is more common in certain geographic areas, particularly higher latitudes.

MS may be caused by multiple factors: genetic, viral, immune, and environmental. An autoimmune response may be triggered by one or more infectious agents in those who are genetically susceptible. Suspected agents include *Chlamydia pneumoniae*; human herpesvirus 6 (HHV-6), canine distemper virus, measles virus, rubella (German measles) virus, human T-cell leukemia virus type 1 (HTLV-1), an unidentified pathogen, or co-infection with several pathogens. Increased antibodies to numerous viruses have been found in the blood and spinal fluid of MS patients. Although believed to cause demyelinating disease in humans and animals, viruses may not play a direct causal role in MS but may trigger relapses. MS may be the result of genetic predisposition coupled with an environmental agent that triggers an autoimmune response directed against myelin.

Abnormalities include serotonin, acetylcholine, and dopamine deficiencies; damaged cellular ion channels; cellular metabolic defects; disordered brain functioning; and immune dysfunction. Symptoms range from mild to severe, determined by the location of the plaques (lesions) in the central nervous system: fatigue, weakness, sensory disturbance (numbness, tingling, pain), visual impairment, muscle function problems (tremors, incontinence, spasticity), dysequilibrium (dizziness, vertigo, incoordination, balance and gait problems, paralysis), and cognitive impairment.

There is no evidence that MS is contagious or directly heritable. Diagnosis is based on patient history and symptoms, evidence of demyelinization, nature and severity of attacks, and ruling out other illnesses, such as collagen vascular diseases, Lyme disease, and HIV. MRI is not a definitive diagnostic tool, since lesions may not be present early on, other diseases cause similar lesions, and healthy people may have similar findings.

Treatment is aimed at symptom improvement, alteration of abnormal immune and neurotransmitter dysfunction, combating infectious agents, and restoring myelin. Standard treatment includes tricyclics, antiepileptics, immune mediators, corticosteroids, and stimulants. Cannabis has been helpful in clinical trials.

The course of MS is individual and unpredictable; exacerbations may be triggered by infection or trauma. Various clinical courses of the disorder have been identified based on frequency of relapses and degree of recovery.

POSTPOLIO SYNDROME

Many survivors of paralytic and nonparalytic polio have developed symptoms years after the initial infection, possibly caused by neuron damage. Symptoms of postpolio syndrome (PPS) include new-onset chronic fatigue triggered or exacerbated by physical exertion and emotional stress; joint and muscle pain; cold intolerance; sleep disorder; cognitive impairment (problems with attention, concentration, memory, word finding, information processing speed, and difficulty thinking clearly); headache; neck pain; myalgia (muscle pain); low-grade fever; irritability and anxiety; hypersomnolence; and weakness, often in muscles unaffected by the initial infection. (Hugh Moldofsky, M.D., notes that PPS is not associated with tender points, morning stiffness, or alpha EEG sleep anomaly.) Severity of the initial illness does not correlate with severity of PPS symptoms.

Outbreaks of "abortive" or "atypical" polio cases occurred in numerous locations. In the 1940s, an illness dubbed the "summer grippe" (or "Iceland disease") was characterized by abrupt onset, duration of less than a week, and flulike symptoms: headache, aching, fever, stomach pain, nausea, and sore throat. Since the syndrome went unrecognized at the time, most cases of nonparalytic polio (NPP) were unreported. NPP outbreaks commonly occurred during or immediately following polio outbreaks, often among hospital personnel. The causative agent was later identified as a milder, low-virulence Type II poliovirus. None of those with summer grippe developed Type I polio; apparently the milder illness conferred immunity against Type I polio. However, even mild polioviruses may have damaged the central nervous system without causing weakness or paralysis. "Potentially half of those diagnosed today with CFS may in fact have had Summer Grippe or undiagnosed nonparalytic polio as children in the years before the polio vaccine became available," reports Richard Bruno, M.D.

Paralytic and nonparalytic polio (NPP) are now recognized as varying severities of the same disorder. Dr. Bruno now associates NPP with myalgic encephalomyelitis (ME), otherwise known as CFS.

Abnormalities in PPS include brain lesions on MRI; impaired HPA and cortical activity; slowed brain waves; and decreased levels of ACTH, cortisol, peptides, and growth hormone. Brain stem centers are involved even in milder polio cases. Dopamine deficiency may underlie symptoms. Bruno states, "We believe that brain activating system damage causes fatigue in both polio survivors and those with CFS."

RHEUMATOID ARTHRITIS

Rheumatoid arthritis (RA) is a systemic autoimmune disorder in which the immune system attacks the body's healthy tissues: the synovium, or joint linings, and/or internal organs. Inflammation may be chronic or periodic, with flares and remissions. RA afflicts approximately two million Americans, most commonly middle-aged women, although it may begin at any age.

Usually beginning in the hands and feet, RA may also affect knees, ankles, hips, wrists, elbows, shoulders, neck, and jaw, usually on both sides of the body. Symptoms include joint pain, stiffness, warmth, swelling, and redness; fatigue and decreased energy; presence of tender points; loss of appetite; and fever. Inflammation may damage bone and cartilage, resulting in pain and loss in range of movement.

The cause is unknown and no definitive test exists. Diagnosis is based on symptom patterns, physical exam, lab tests for rheumatoid factor, X-rays, and ruling out other disorders. Early diagnosis and treatment allow symptom reduction and modification of the disease course before damage occurs. Adjunctive therapies include rest, exercise, and physical and occupational therapy.

Viruses are suspected to play a role in susceptible individuals; one genetic marker has been tentatively identified. Certain cytokines (chemical messengers between cells) such as tumor necrosis factor (TNF) and interleukin-1 (IL-1) are involved in the inflammatory response and disease progression. In RA these proinflammatory forces outweigh the mechanisms attempting to keep the inflammation in check. The resulting inflammation contributes to cartilage damage and bone erosion.

SJÖGREN'S SYNDROME

Sjögren's syndrome (SS) is an autoimmune disorder characterized by xerostomia (dry mouth) and keratoconjunctivitis sicca (dry eyes, often described as a feeling of sand or gravel in eye). Primary Sjögren's syndrome occurs alone, while secondary SS co-occurs with connective tissue disease such as rheumatoid arthritis, systemic lupus erythematosus, polymyositis, or systemic sclerosis.

SS is most common in females in their forties and fifties but occurs in either sex at any age. Prevalence has been estimated at 1 to 3 percent of the population. Although the illness has a genetic component, with a slightly increased incidence of autoimmune diseases in siblings and children, it is not believed to be contagious. The cause of SS is unknown, but it may be virally triggered in genetically susceptible individuals. SS is associated with characteristic abnormalities in blood tests and salivary gland biopsies.

Eye infections are common due to decreased production of tears that normally lubricate and protect the eye. Mouth and eye dryness may be caused by destruction of salivary glands or from interruption of nerve signals that control secretion. Onset is usually gradual, with patients noticing increasing dryness of eyes and mouth and difficulty swallowing dry foods. As the syndrome progresses, the dryness leads to increased swallowing difficulty, peri-odontal disease, and oral *Candida* infections. The gastrointestinal system, spleen, liver, pancreas, kidney, and lung may also be affected. Other common symptoms include fatigue, joint and musculoskeletal pain, depression, photophobia, hypothyroidism, anemia, sleep disorder, memory and concentration problems, skin rashes, lung inflammation, swollen lymph nodes, sinusitis, dental decay and chronic oral candidiasis, atrophic rhinitis (chronic inflammation of the lining of the nose), hoarseness, dryness of skin and hair, dryness of mucous membranes (genital and rectal), and increased incidence of Raynaud's phenomenon.

In the absence of uniform criteria, diagnosis is symptom-based, confirmed by evidence of keratoconjunctivitis sicca (eye inflamma-tion and dryness), with abnormal findings on the Shirmer test (a measure of eye dryness), salivary gland biopsy, and the presence of autoantibodies. Treatments include artificial tears and lubricating ointments, antifungals for candidiasis, NSAIDs and steroids for inflammation, and various disease-modifying agents. Although there is no cure, significant symptomatic improvement can be achieved and serious complications may be avoided by early recog-nition and treatment.

SOMATOFORM DISORDERS AND FUNCTIONAL SOMATIC SYNDROMES

The *DSM-IV*, the handbook of psychiatric diagnoses, characterizes somatoform disorders by the presence of physical symptoms that suggest but are not explained by a medical illness, direct effects of a substance, or another mental disorder. Symptoms are involuntary, causing significant distress and impairment of social and occupa-tional functioning.

Somatization disorder, formerly referred to as hysteria, is a type of somatoform disorder that begins before age thirty, lasts for years, and is characterized by multiple, unexplained somatic complaints (a combination of pain and gastrointestinal, sexual, and pseudoneuro-logical symptoms). Fatigue is not necessarily a prominent symptom.

Somatizers often seek treatment from several physicians con-currently, describing their symptoms in colorful, exaggerated, and inconsistent terms, although laboratory findings are unremarkable.

They are likely to exhibit impulsive and antisocial behavior and to be anxious or depressed, sometimes with suicidal threats and attempts and a tendency to form unstable relationships. Prevalence of certain personality disorders is high, and the disorder occurs with greater frequency in women. The disorder may fluctuate over time but rarely resolves completely. Several other variants of somatoform disorder exist, with medically unexplained symptoms and prominent psychological factors.

CFS and FMS share common factors with somatoform disorders—multiple symptoms, lack of consistent lab test findings, presence of psychiatric disorders, and functional impairment—but are excluded from this category by symptom prevalence, age, suddenness of onset, lack of prevalent personality disorders, and exercise and alcohol intolerance.

The term functional somatic syndromes (FSS) refers to suffering in the absence of specific medical findings. This term is often inappropriately applied to poorly understood illnesses such as CFS, FMS, GWS, IBS, and MCS. FSS patients are said to self-diagnose exaggerated symptoms and distress, embrace the sick role, amplify their degree of impairment and disability, expect their illnesses to become worse over time, be nonresponsive to treatment and reassurance, and have a continuing history of psychiatric disorders. Such individuals have a "strong sense of assertiveness and embattled advocacy with respect to their etiologic suppositions, and they may devalue and dismiss medical authority . . . that conflicts with their beliefs," with "very explicit disease attributions for their symptoms," resistance to "information that contradicts these attributions," and a suspicion of physicians, whose authority they undermine (Barsky and Borus 1999). FSS disorders are framed with circular reasoning: "You think you have a serious illness but you don't because we have no specific test for it." The alleged secondary gains of illness are typically absent, yet patients are accused of being entrenched in the sick role and embracing their symptoms, which are said to become more pronounced in the absence of medical or societal validation.

Functional somatic syndromes do exist, with desperation and certain personality traits amplifying symptom perception. However, a diagnosis of FSS more often provides a convenient way to dismiss patients' symptomatic complaints whose cause is unknown. The absence of diagnostic tests for many known disorders creates fertile ground for physicians who view any difficult-to-diagnose disorder as imagined illness. However, an illness that defies current scientific knowledge is still an illness.

SYSTEMIC LUPUS ERYTHEMATOSUS (LUPUS)

Systemic lupus erythematosus (SLE), a complex autoimmune, multisystemic, autoinflammatory disease, is believed to affect 40 to 50 people per 100,000, with variability among racial and ethnic groups. Most common in females aged eighteen to forty, the female-to-male ratio in this age group is about 8:1, decreasing to a ratio of 2:1 or 3:1 in later years. Of unknown cause, SLE may be triggered in genetically predisposed individuals by infectious agents, stress, environmental toxins, diet, sun exposure, or certain medications. Overproduction of autoantibodies leads to inflammation of the skin, tissues, and internal organs, causing pain, redness, heat, and swelling.

Symptoms include the classic butterfly-shaped rash on the cheeks and bridge of the nose; sun sensitivity; rashes and skin lesions; fatigue; generalized arthralgias; inflammation of the kidneys, heart, and skin; swollen, tender joints; transient lymphadenopathy; dry eyes and mouth; and arthritis-like problems in the hands, wrists, ankles, and knees. Abnormalities include low white cell count, increased rates of spontaneous abortion and premature birth, multiple autoantibodies, hypercoagulable state (an increased tendency to form blood clots), and nonspecific spinal fluid abnormalities. Central nervous system symptoms include headaches, cognitive deficits, neuropathies, seizures, and depression. SLE may coexist with other connective tissue disorders.

Diagnosis is based on history and symptoms, physical exam, ruling out similar disorders, and laboratory tests. Abnormalities on blood tests for antinuclear antibodies and CT and MRI scans may be present but are not diagnostic. Treatment, including lifestyle modification, is aimed at reducing inflammation and modulating immune activity. SLE is a chronic disease with flares and remissions. The survival rate is 90 percent at five years and 80 to 90 percent at ten years, with older patients having more benign courses of the illness.

CONCLUSION

The illnesses profiled in this chapter overlap in terms of symptoms (notably pain, fatigue, and sleep disorder); complexity; chronicity; poorly understood pathophysiology; variability among cases; trial-and-error treatment; prevalence in women; primarily clinical diagnoses; possible involvement of infectious agents; dysfunction of the immune and central nervous systems, including autonomic and neuroendocrine dysfunction; known or suspected autoimmune component; characterization by exacerbation and partial remission; and dismissal or lack of "real" illness status unless a marker or test has been identified. However, their relationships to one another remain unclear.

Many conditions characterized by overlapping symptoms and characteristics breed speculation that they are either related or are different manifestations of the same illness, perhaps caused by similar factors. Similarities of symptoms and multiple dysregulations suggest a common mechanism in several conditions, possibly hypothalamic-pituitary-adrenal (HPA) axis dysfunction. Neuroendocrine mechanisms of the HPA axis are complex and delicate, and minor variations in dysfunction might account for similarities among these disorders.

8

Cause: In Search of a Unified Theory

A simple cause-and-effect answer to the question of causation eludes us, since we do not understand CFS and FMS well enough to develop a neat, inclusive explanation for illness manifestations and abnormalities. Most findings are considered speculative, and none fully explains all cases of CFS or FMS.

The essential question is not simply, "What causative agent or abnormality makes us sick?" but the more complex question, "What factors interact to cause CFS and FMS?"

In the movie *Outbreak,* the virus causing a terrible disease is isolated quickly, rapidly followed by development of a curative and preventative vaccine. The likelihood of such a simplistic scenario as identification of agent x that causes disease y, followed by drug/vaccine z (the cure!), has not been known to occur in real life, where few medical puzzles are easily solved.

A tentative causal consensus points to the involvement of a combination of factors including genetic predisposition, central nervous system abnormalities, endocrine factors, a dysregulated immune system, trauma and stress, environmental toxins, and infectious agents. Although these elements appear in many cases, the sequence of events is unknown. CFS/FMS populations may represent a heterogeneous group of variations on a theme associated with a variety of causal agents and triggering factors.

Hypotheses are numerous and overlapping; some are more widely accepted than others. Concepts wax and wane in popularity in the scientific community, depending on the weight of the current evidence for particular causal models. The many hypotheses are not mutually exclusive; many of them fit together well. Several factors may be involved: one to set the stage, one to ignite the fuse, and others to perpetuate the process. Some of the possibilities (both popular and unpopular) are explored in this chapter.

SINGLE AGENT THEORIES

A single causal agent is a ubiquitous (common) pathogen to which only some people are susceptible due to constitutional or environmental factors, which may affect how the illness manifests. The causal agent is an uncommon, possibly contagious pathogen.

Despite evidence of viral and bacterial infections, no particular agent has been linked to CFS or FMS. Wide speculation exists regarding the role of pathogens. If a pathogen does play a causal role, is the agent new to the host or a reactivation of a previously dormant organism? Is the pathogen known or as yet undiscovered?

MULTIPLE CAUSAL AGENT THEORIES

In theories proposing multiple causal agents, several causal agents of CFS and FMS, along with host factors, account for the variability among cases.

Infection with one or more agents triggers disease by dysregulating various body systems, while the agents themselves do not cause any symptoms.

The "two-hit event" theory proposes that one must be infected with two agents, such as herpesviruses HHV-6 plus a retrovirus or bacterium.

◆◆ A Spectrum of Disorders ◆◆

CFS and FMS lie on a continuum of neurological, neuroimmune, and neuroendocrine illnesses caused by one or more pathological agents. Manifestation of the disease is related to the location and severity of the presumed brain infection.

◆◆ The Hit-and-Run Theory ◆◆

The hit-and-run theory contends that an agent infects the host, causing immune dysregulation and symptoms, and then disappears while its effects continue. One theory holds that virally caused DNA damage persists after the virus has left, altering DNA transcription to new cells.

IMMUNE DYSREGULATION THEORIES

FMS, and especially CFS, have been viewed as disorders of the immune system, with underlying viral or bacterial infections suspected as cofactors. No specific pathogen or immune abnormality has been consistently or uniquely associated with either illness.

In theories pointing to immune dysregulation, an agent causes an initial infection, dysregulating the immune system and thus allowing previously dormant viruses to emerge from latency and actively reproduce. Cytokines, produced in response to reactivated viruses, continue to cause symptoms.

A vulnerable immune system allows opportunistic infections to develop, further dysregulating the immune system and affecting other body systems, notably the central nervous system.

Activation of certain cytokines may cause disruption of the hypothalamic-pituitary-adrenal (HPA) axis, with abnormal levels of HPA-related chemicals creating a vicious cycle and persistent symptoms.

GENETICS

CFS and FMS tend to run in families, particularly among first-degree blood relatives. In previous generations, the disorders may have remained undiagnosed or misdiagnosed as "atypical" forms of other illnesses. Those most prone to become ill have had periodic illnesses and infections throughout their lives, alternating with periods of feeling well. Many patients report medical histories of long-term, low-level pain, frequent infections, low body temperature, and other symptoms suggestive of subclinical disorders. Some who had regarded themselves as healthy and active do recall in retrospect unusually high numbers of illness episodes over the years from which they recovered uneventfully. Some recall that their energy level has always been low but that they learned to compensate. However, others report having been healthy until the onset of CFS and FMS.

Genetic predisposition may be a cofactor that, along with other factors, plays a causal role. Cofactors may include the following:

▶ Central nervous system (CNS) disruption is caused by the interplay of a combination of factors—genetics, stress, trauma, infection, and so on—causing further disruption of the CNS and every organ system, resulting in such phenomena as altered metabolism and cardiac functioning. Jay Goldstein, M.D., regards CFS and FMS as psychoneuroimmunological phenomena, characterized by limbic encephalopathy in a dys-regulated neuroimmune network.

‣ Neuroendocrine factors: Impairment of the hypothalamic-pituitary-adrenal (HPA) axis characterizes CFS/FMS. The pre-cise role of neuroendocrine disturbance in these illnesses is not clear.

‣ Neuroendocrine interaction with immune activation causes autonomic changes and alterations in the HPA axis. Immune abnormalities dysregulate the autonomic nervous system and the HPA axis, often following exposure to an antigen or a toxin.

‣ Immunizations: Routine immunization has obliterated several life-threatening illnesses but may also have negative effects on the immune systems of susceptible individuals. Vaccines con-tain attenuated (weakened) viruses to stimulate the produc-tion of antibodies so that the individual will not get an active infection if exposed to the virus at a later time. However, the injected viruses may be transmitted from those vaccinated (usually children) to others who are sufficiently sensitive to react to the virus and become ill. In some cases, live virus is included in vaccines, often by accident, or vaccines are con-taminated with other viruses; this has been cause for investiga-tion. For example, evidence indicates that polio vaccines in the 1950s and 1960s may have been contaminated with a simian virus, which has been hypothesized as a cause of later illness.

CFS AND FMS AS PSYCHOLOGICAL OR PSYCHIATRIC DISORDERS

Historically, illnesses are attributed to temperament when sci-ence lacks, or refuses to seek, answers.

— *B. E. Synhorst, M.S.W.*

Depression and anxiety are symptoms often associated with chronic illness, both endogenously, due to internal chemical changes, and exogenously, as reactions to the difficulties of living with chronic illness. Not all individuals with CFS/FMS are depressed or anxious. The pre-illness incidence of major depressive disorder (MDD) and other psychiatric disorders is roughly equal to that in the general population.

Depression is associated with chronic illness, but it is considered a secondary symptom rather than a causal factor. Although symptoms of depression and anxiety are present in some CFS/FMS patients, most symptoms associated with CFS are not characteristic of so-called psychiatric disorders (see Chapter 7).

CFS AND FMS AS SOMATOFORM DISORDERS OR FUNCTIONAL SOMATIC SYNDROMES

Under the guise of adopting an integrative model of mind and body, or medicine and psychiatry, a small number of physicians classify unexplained chronic illnesses as somatoform disorders. This rationale is based in part on decreasing medical costs rather than serving the needs of the patient (Reid and Wessely 1999).

> *While proponents of this theory address the need to get away from simple medical vs. psychological models, they reinforce the 'all in your head' philosophy of unexplained illness, emphasizing the role of psychiatric morbidity. (Hickie, Scott, et al. 1998).*

In their "subjective suffering from non-verifiable symptoms," patients are said to suffer from symptoms that are falsely attributed to "real" (objectively proven) illness (Barsky and Borus 1999). Some medical researchers and practitioners equate poorly understood disorders with somatization (a somatoform disorder) or functional somatic syndrome (FSS). Although multiple symptoms are seen in somatization disorder, symptom clusters typical of CFS and FMS are not found in this group, nor is sudden onset, which often characterizes CFS/FMS (see Chapter 7).

SELF-RESPONSIBILITY FOR ILLNESS

Humans are unwilling to believe that great suffering and disaster can be inflicted without moral justification.
— *Rita Mae Brown,* **High Hearts**

Many of us are told that we have brought illness upon ourselves as a result of character deficiencies or weak moral fiber, flaws we could voluntarily correct if we were properly motivated. Illness has been viewed as a punishment for improper living, the result of an inadequate spiritual belief system, or a self-created opporunity to grapple with certain life lessons. Remaining ill connotes that we have failed to learn the right lessons or to conquer our imperfections. Such beliefs inappropriately blame the patient for the illness

Susan Sontag (1977) views the punitive notion of disease causation as long-standing and counterproductive, encouraging the patient to engage in self-blame for having become ill and for not getting well. Blaming ourselves for being ill is self-defeating and injurious. We do not have a choice about being ill.

PERSONALITY TYPE AND ILLNESS

Many of us were once energetic, driven, aggressive, intelligent, perfectionistic, goal-oriented people with busy lifestyles. Phillip Rubin, M.D., said at a Phoenix support group meeting, "Most of you do in your impaired state more than most people do in their normal state." Many of us were overextended caretakers in our personal and professional lives. We felt most comfortable when giving or providing, had difficulty requesting and receiving, and prided ourselves by being available and reliable at all times. Hardworking and even sacrificial, we have been described as driven, Type A overachievers, caretakers, and stress addicts with a tendency to overwork and overexert.

However, many with CFS/FMS never led this type of lifestyle, and most so-called overachievers have not become ill, so we cannot assume causation. Perhaps the driven, Type A group is more inclined to persist in the pursuit of a diagnosis and more likely to become active in support and advocacy groups, and is therefore overrepresented in the literature.

Research has shown that CFS/FMS is an equal-opportunity illness. Psychosocial factors and traits play a role in all illnesses, although not typically a causal one. For example, stress or depression may be both predisposing and perpetuating factors in illness. Emphasizing the role of psychiatric factors is often an attempt to dismiss patients with poorly understood disorders that are difficult-to-treat.

LIFESTYLE AND LIFE EVENTS

◆◆ Stress and Trauma ◆◆

Stress, the continual adaptation to changes and demands from without and within, is natural and necessary. Stress urges us forward, allowing growth and progress. All change, whether positive, negative, or neutral, is stressful. Sources of stress are everywhere in our lives, for example, too much or too little activity, demands of families and employers, responsibilities, time schedules, and exposure to noise and environmental pollution.

Acute and chronic stressors tax even the strong and hardy. When stressors are numerous, severe, and constant, or when we fail to adapt successfully, the result is physiological and emotional change. Stressful events—individual or family difficulties or crises, death of loved ones, breakup of significant relationships or other losses, illness, surgery, childbirth, career or job changes, financial problems, geographic relocation, highly active lifestyles, changing roles, rapid technological change, spiritual and existential concerns, life dissatisfactions, time pressure, and lack of social structure—often precede the onset of illness. Stress activates a protective fight-or-flight response, causing bodily changes that include the release of various chemicals, some of which inhibit immune system functioning. As the body continually taps its resources, certain body chemicals become depleted and exhaustion may set in, rendering us susceptible to illness.

Too often we neglect our restorative needs because we're programmed to do more, better, faster, living in a state of tension and anxiety. Societal, familial, and self-induced pressure to push and achieve, while neglecting self-care, takes a negative toll on health.

The stress of chronic illness is heightened by physical or mental activity, travel, chemical exposure, hormonal fluctuations, family problems, and personal issues, rendering the body exquisitely sensitive even to minor assaults. Trauma—acute physical or emotional stress—triggers dysregulation of body systems leading to symptoms that further disrupt the body's ability to function normally. Stress and trauma are often cofactors in the onset and perpetuation of illness.

ENVIRONMENTAL THEORIES

While the leaders of government everywhere are worrying
about the Big Bomb, mankind everywhere is poisoning the
ground and the waters we depend on for life.

—*Andy Rooney,* The Dead Land

Many theorize that a massive environmental assault (toxins, stressors, and the like) allows an already damaged immune system to
succumb to an agent it cannot fight off.

Pesticides, hormones, drugs, and other chemicals pollute our
air, water, soil, vegetables and fruits, meat and poultry (see Chapter
9). Substances banned in the United States are used in countries
from which we import foods. New chemicals are being added to our
environment at an alarming rate, increasing the overall risk. We
suffer both major toxic events and long-term, low-level exposure.

Neurological, cognitive, and behavioral disturbances have been
found in those exposed to solvents and other chemicals in the
workplace. Sick building syndrome occurs in poorly ventilated or
sealed buildings, where endlessly recirculating air increases exposure to chemicals and pathogens. Daniel Peterson, M.D., observed
in the early-1980s CFS outbreak in Lake Tahoe that local schools
with poor air exchange had a significantly higher rate of illness than
did schools with better air circulation (1991).

The synergistic effects of radiation and other environmental
factors increase susceptibility to disease. In the 1940s, low-level
ionizing radiation began to be released into the environment with
nuclear weapons plants, bombings, and aboveground bomb tests.
Underground tests started in the 1960s; later, nuclear power plants
were built. Radioactive fallout, resulting from aboveground tests
and leakage from nuclear energy plants, is released locally and may
be carried widely by winds and precipitation. A general disregard for
public safety is also evidenced by such phenomena as groundwater
contamination and governmental approval of chemicals that have
not been thoroughly tested.

Much of the damage could not be undone even with an aggressive national cleanup program, since many substances are stored
indefinitely in adipose tissue (fat), cumulative and synergistic
effects are unknown, and irreversible genetic changes may have
already taken place. A comprehensive program to make dramatic

changes in our use of these chemicals would be politically unpopular because of its astronomical cost and because it would anger political contributors who manufacture these substances.

The toll on human life is gradual, subtle, and alarming. Many toxins remain in the body for years, and pesticide residues or metabolites are believed to be present in all American adults. Long-term bodily damage cannot be assessed, but neurological and immunological damage and increased disease rates appear over time. Concern about elevated incidence of cancer and other illnesses in response to environmental pollution continues, but little formal testing has been done.

THE JURY IS STILL OUT

The single-cause approach is tantalizingly simple. All we have to do is identify the culprit, kill that rotten germ, and be well again. But as in any war, the problem is not as simple as merely obliterating the immediate enemy. There will always be other enemies. Interaction among such factors as environment, heredity, behavior, infectious agents, immune functioning, central nervous system functioning, coping strategies, self-expectations, and stress are likely determinants of who will get ill and who will not. Other determinants of disease resistance include such psychosocial factors as lifestyle, job, place of residence, cultural background, personality type, race, sex, and social status.

CFS and FMS defy the standard medical concept of separate disorders, each with a known cause and consistent abnormalities. Doctors and patients remain puzzled and frustrated in the face of unexplained suffering with no identified cause. Studies continue, abnormalities are found, and hypotheses multiply with no conclusive findings. We've learned a lot, but we don't know much yet. It is of some comfort that the plethora of documented abnormalities challenges the "nonbelievers," many of whom are finally recognizing the legitimacy and seriousness of these disorders.

The lack of a unified hypothesis indicates the need for divergent research in which many possible etiologies are explored. We need to learn more not only about pathogens but about interconnections among body systems and between organism and environment. Multifaceted, multidisciplinary research will contribute to our understanding of the pathophysiology of baffling disorders.

RESEARCH FUNDING AND GOALS

Research funds are difficult to obtain, especially to study invisible illnesses whose names are inaccurate and trivializing. Inadequate funding has resulted in little progress over the years. Funding has been allocated to numerous epidemiological studies, each indicating a higher number of cases than the last. CFS and FMS are debilitating and often disabling illnesses that exist in a substantial portion of the world's population. Numerous studies have negated the antiquated concept that these are nonexistent, imagined, or psychiatric illnesses, yet these images continue to prevail in many circles. Polio, syphilis, arthritis, multiple sclerosis, and pernicious anemia were similarly dismissed, but as tests or causative agents were identified, each gained legitimacy. Have we not learned from these experiences? When will those afflicted be able to shed the defensive posture of justifying, attempting to prove their illnesses real and their credibility intact?

The Centers for Disease Control and Prevention (CDC) has admitted that a large portion of the small allocation of funds for CFS research was spent on other projects instead. Having appropriated this funding, why is Congress not outraged at the misspending and cover-up? We have already lost years of potentially helpful research—years stolen from patients' lives. Why do we not have more advocates? Why has most research been funded by private contributions rather than government dollars? Why aren't these insidious, debilitating, costly illnesses a national and international priority? The neglect and outright refusal of the government to allocate adequate funds to the study of illnesses affecting millions of Americans is a national disgrace.

PART TWO

What These Illnesses Do

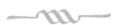

9

Psychoneuroimmunology

Psychoneuroimmunology (PNI) is an age-old but newly em-
braced interdisciplinary approach to understanding the interconnectedness of the central nervous system (CNS, the brain and
spinal cord), the immune system, thought, mood, and behavior.
Growing evidence suggests that "psychiatric" and "somatic" disorders overlap and should be granted equal credibility, withdrawing
the judgmental bias that so often prevails in our attempts to make
artificial distinctions between illnesses of the mind and the body,
inextricable parts of a whole. In efforts to create a simplistic model
that distinguishes the "somatic" from the "psychiatric" (the body
from the mind) and to explain each disorder individually, we over-
look their commonalities and connections, unable to see the forest
for the trees. Many diseases are labeled psychiatric or "stress" disorders until causal agents or illness markers are identified, at which
time they graduate to the status of legitimized, genuine illness. (A
"marker" is a distinct abnormality found in those with an illness,
with little or no known incidence in other disorders or in healthy
populations.)

Psychoneuroimmunology is a phenomenon at once amazingly
simple and incomprehensibly complex. The simple part is acknowledgment that the mind, brain, and immune system are interactive
components of one integrated system. The complex part is how this
works. Countless electrochemical signals occur constantly and
simultaneously, integrating all the cells in the body. The chemical
messengers dashing about madly inside us are influenced no less by
emotions than by medications and other "physiological" events.
This intricate process explains who we are and how we function.

Together, these functions create a state of balance, or equilibrium, in which body systems are in constant communication with
each other. A change in any part of the system affects the entire

organism, just as tapping any one part of a delicately balanced mobile sets all other parts into motion. Once this occurs, the mobile naturally seeks to restore equilibrium, or homeostasis. The body is an infinitely more elaborate version of the mobile, with an ongoing basic need to restore homeostasis following any disruption, whether labeled physical or emotional. Symptoms are indicators that home-ostasis has gone awry.

Western thought is steeped in dualism, the notion that the mind is one thing, the body another. We underestimate the role of emotions in "physiological" illness and the role of physiology in "emotional" illness. However, all illness is psychosomatic, involving both mind and body (the mindbody), for they are inseparable. The term "psychosomatic" is often misused to mean "psychogenic," that is, caused by psychological factors or "all in one's head," or to refer to illnesses more imagined than real. In fact, "psychosomatic" refers to the interactions of psyche (mind) and soma (body), without implying exclusive causation in either realm.

Western thought is based on specifics, finding diagnostic cubby-holes into which our diagnoses fit neatly and breaking things apart to isolate and examine their smallest components. Eastern thought is more highly focused on connections and unity, in which viewing individual components matter insofar as they contribute to the whole. An integrated approach points to commonalities shared by overlapping disorders. The so-called functional syndromes (e.g., CFS, FMS, IBS, and MCS) share common symptoms and possibly common or overlapping etiologies. The more specialized and sub-specialized we become, assigning illnesses to increasing numbers of diagnostic cubbyholes, the greater our failure to see the big picture. Accepting the interconnectedness, the mindbody, is a sticking point in an era of increasing specialization and compartmentaliza-tion. Combining Eastern and Western thought, we see the forest *and* the trees. Thus, illness is much more than a simple interaction between a germ and a body.

CFS and FMS serve as models to help us recognize and respect the importance of the integration of mind, spirit, and soma (body), to see them as inextricably interconnected. Malfunction in one sys-tem creates imbalance, causing malfunctions in other areas. CFS and FMS may thus be seen as a model of neuro-endocrine-immune interactions.

Various studies illustrate the factors that influence health. Hospital patients who see trees and grass outside their windows heal faster than those facing a brick wall. The response rate to placebos (pills without active ingredients) is often dramatic. Asthmatics exposed to the scent of vanilla when using their inhalers later improved in response to the aroma of vanilla. Symptoms improve when our doctors provide an infusion of hope. The inner pharmacy is wise and helpful.

Breast cancer patients with high levels of anxiety about their disease experienced a significant reduction in the effectiveness of their natural killer (NK) cells compared to those with low levels of stress. Breast cancer patients with good emotional support had higher levels of NK cells. When a partner, close friend, or physician provided that support, the increase was even greater. A group receiving both support and medical care was less anxious, less depressed, and less bothered by pain, living eighteen months longer than control patients. Those with malignant melanoma who underwent a program of group therapy and education experienced less psychological distress, coped more effectively, and had increased numbers and activity of NK cells and better survival rates.

If you are skeptical, try this quick exercise: Imagine cutting into a large, ripe lemon. As you slice into it, lemon juice trickles onto your hand, onto the counter. Having cut a juicy wedge, bring it to your mouth and take a bite of the sour juice. Are you salivating? This simple exercise can convert even the most stalwart dualist.

Norman Cousins wrote in 1979:

Illness is always an interaction among both [mind and body]. It can begin in the mind and affect the body, or it can begin in the body and affect the mind, both of which are served by the same bloodstream. Attempts to treat most mental diseases as though they were completely free of physical causes and attempts to treat most bodily diseases as though the mind were in no way involved must be considered archaic in the light of new evidence about the way the human body functions.

The way we conceptualize a problem is reflected in the ways we attempt to solve it, and we are often guilty of oversimplifying and applying faulty logic. There is no clear distinction between physiological and psychiatric disorders; no disorder in either category excludes the other. Every physiological event has psychological correlates, and vice versa. We continue to seek distinctions although connections are more illuminating.

Although the practice of holism has come to imply quackery, multilevel sales, and sci-fi medicine, its true meaning is the treatment of body and mind as an integrated system in which all parts communicate with each other to maintain balance and health, with the whole greater than the sum of its parts. What the mind believes is what the body believes.

The process of disease is not merely physical, nor is the process of mood only emotional. When we stop viewing these separately, we begin to understand how we work. Genetics, stressors, environmental pollution and illness, brain and immune dysfunction, and pathogens are inextricably related in the development of chronic illness.

Psychosocial and environmental events take their toll on the immune system, but the way in which this occurs is not fully understood. In *The Healer Within*, Locke and Colligan discuss the tendrils of nerve tissue from the brain that run through the most important parts of the immune system: the thymus gland, bone marrow, lymph nodes, and spleen. Hormones and neurotransmitters secreted by the brain have an affinity for immune cells. Active lines of communication connect the brain and the immune system; brain chemicals have both positive and negative influences on immune functioning. The brain-immune system link works both ways; changes in either entity affect the other because they are inextricably bound, each influencing the other. Links among all body systems present the opportunity for our emotions to influence how well the body is able to defend itself.

THE ENVIRONMENT

Too many major American industries dig up the good things
out of the earth, spit out what they can't use and produce
poisonous waste by-products that are eventually going to kill
the land and then us.

— *Andy Rooney,* The Dead Land

Science moves at a dazzling pace, with both positive and negative consequences. Hippocrates stressed the importance of viewing the human body within its context—its geography, climate, diet, and so on. Our environment is hazardous; we breathe pollutants, eat additives, and drink contaminants, ingesting startling amounts of harmful chemicals daily. We poison ourselves slowly with substances whose potential damage we can only estimate. So-called safe amounts of many chemicals are mere guesses; their long-term and synergistic effects are unknown. Government regulations are inadequate and poorly enforced, and industry, aware of many harmful properties of chemicals, regularly withholds information from workers and consumers for the twin aphrodisiacs of profit and power.

Highly advanced yet absolutely stupid, we tamper with biology without fully understanding the consequences. We send a rocket to the moon and invent microchips that outperform the human brain. But on a daily basis, we ingest multiple chemicals whose consequences and synergistic properties we cannot assess. We know some of them make us sick but pay the price for the sake of progress and convenience.

In recent years the number of new chemicals introduced into our bodies has increased dramatically; our bodies are heavily and unreasonably taxed chemical-processing plants. In the name of progress, we have created compounds both helpful and harmful and bear the brunt of their assault. Just a few of the culprits are pesticides (insecticides and herbicides such as chlordane), food additives (such as preservatives; flavoring and coloring agents; steroids, veterinary medicines, and antibiotics in meat and poultry; waxes; thickening agents; and emulsifiers), and air pollutants (such as sulfur dioxide).

Kat Duff, author of *The Alchemy of Illness,* views us as "canaries in the coal mine." Some of us are sick, some are dying, and others remain blissfully asymptomatic and unaware. Our heightened sensitivity, susceptibility due to genetics, lifestyle, and other factors should serve as a warning to others, especially since it is yesterday's news that pollution and other chemical assaults fell the vulnerable first. As a society, we would apparently prefer to expose ourselves to toxins and then use our vast but inadequate technology to treat resulting illnesses. Health is too big a price to pay for what passes as success or progress.

In a game called "what I can't see won't hurt me," we expose ourselves to arsenic, aldicarb (a pesticide), vinyl chloride (used in making plastic), polychlorinated biphenyls (PCBs), hazardous industrial solvents, radioactive wastes, and heavy metals (such as chromium, lead, and cadmium). Emerging illnesses over the coming years will bear out the inestimable damage to neuroimmune functioning. To allow ourselves to be reassured by information provided by industry and government is foolish. We know better. The very things intended to enhance our lives are killing us... gradually, so perhaps we won't notice.

THE IMMUNE SYSTEM

Pathogens are tiny, talented, elusive creatures that are capable of infecting, hiding, mutating, and combining. Viruses and slow-growing infections can make us miserable while eluding detection. When weakened by physical and emotional factors, we create an opportunity for pathogens to flourish.

Immunology is a relatively new field of medicine, far more complex and important than previously imagined. Once believed to be a self-contained system that operated independently of other body systems, the immune system is now known to be integrated with all other bodily systems. It has no central regulating organ, as do other body systems (e.g., the heart in the circulatory system, the lungs in the respiratory system). Its components are located throughout the body. Communication takes place among immune cells and between them and other organs.

The function of the immune system is to be sensitive to invaders, to distinguish between "self" and "nonself." Anything foreign to the body is "nonself": a potential enemy, called an *antigen.* Once an enemy is recognized, a complex process is set in motion. In response to an antigen, or invader, phagocytes (scavengers that gobble up invaders) go to work, attempting to destroy the offending pathogens or substances. If unsuccessful, T- and B-cells, lymphocytes that flow through lymph channels throughout the body, are called into play: helper T-cells join the battle, in turn summoning killer T-cells to kill invaded cells, and B-cells, the equivalent of munitions factories, to produce antibodies specific to the invader. After a successful battle, suppressor T-cells call off the attack, shutting off the immune response, and peace is restored. Memory cells guard against a subsequent attack by the same agent.

When the complex functioning of the immune system is disrupted, its components and functions can be upregulated (over-
reactive) or downregulated (underreactive). When upregulated,
components of the immune system are switched on and left on, and
the host becomes reactive to all types of substances perceived as
"nonself." Symptoms associated with battle and illness are produced. The ratio of helper to suppressor T-cells functions as the on-
off switch of the immune system, with a normal ratio of 2:1 or 3:1.
The balance between them is critical to proper immune response
and functioning. During and following illness, this ratio varies.

Autoimmune disorders are characterized by an immune system
that has lost its ability to distinguish between "self" and "nonself,"
leading the body to attack its own tissue as if it were an antigen
(enemy). In the process, healthy cells are attacked and destroyed.

When the immune system is generally downregulated, a state of
immunosuppression allows enemy cells, such as viruses, to reproduce actively, because the immune system is unable to rid the body
of invaders. The result is an ongoing battle with no victor and
increased symptoms for the host.

Immune dysfunction is caused by a variety of factors. Primary
immune deficiencies (those that are congenital, or present from
birth) may not become apparent until later in life when exposure to
certain antigens creates symptoms. Secondary immune deficiencies
are acquired; they develop as a result of such factors as nutrition,
age, sleep, surgery and general anesthesia, infections, injury, certain
drugs, emotional state, hormonal imbalance, stress level, and environmental exposures.

Negative emotional states, such as loneliness and depression,
can impair immunity to a significant degree because of alterations
in neuroendocrine function. Intense or prolonged stress adversely
affects immune, neurological, and endocrine function. Conversely,
the positive emotions are believed to enhance immune functioning.

When the immune system is out of balance, some parts become
overactive and others underactive, resulting in inappropriate reactions. Signals within the immune system or between the immune
system and other body systems are distorted, creating widespread
malfunctioning. The immune system may mount an exaggerated
response to benign invaders, such as pollen, wreaking havoc on the
body in the process.

STRESS AND THE HYPOTHALAMIC-PITUITARY-ADRENAL AXIS

Keeping up with the fast pace of life and barrages of sensory input can be overwhelming. We live a crazy lifestyle in which denial of personal needs is considered heroic. We travel widely, diet frequently, intersperse dieting with junk food pig-outs, try to force rapid recovery after surgery or illness, ignore the problems and symptoms that are trying to give us messages about our needs, and spend so much time "taking care of business" that we neglect to take care of our bodies. Neglecting self-care (sufficient sleep, moderate exercise, relaxation, and adequate diet) and constantly pushing to get ahead are valued in society but detrimental to health. Many of us live in a state of constant tension and anxiety.

Stress is inescapable and continuous: the acute stress of a traumatic event, such as the death or illness of a loved one or the loss of a job, or the chronic day-to-day wear and tear of traffic jams, isolation, and worries about work, finances, and personal problems. Stress is the natural and continual adaptation process that both motivates and taxes the body. All change, good or bad, is stress producing. When stressors are numerous, severe, and constant, or when we fail to adapt successfully, the result is bodily damage. Our bodies do not differentiate physical, emotional, and cognitive stressors, which impact us in the same ways.

The total stress load on an individual consists of stress from within and without. Unrelenting stress or a series of highly stressful events is taxing even to the strong and hardy, often resulting in illness. Although acute and chronic stressors contribute strongly to the development of illnesses, stress alone does not cause illness. In turn, illness causes stress, creating a loop. Stress is associated not only with increased risk for illness but with slower healing time as well.

Stressful events that precede the onset of illness may include death of a loved one; divorce or breakup of a significant relationship; other illnesses and health problems, including infections and surgery; childbirth; job change; a highly active and busy lifestyle; financial difficulties; changing roles; life dissatisfaction; time pressure; relocation; and other individual or family crises.

Stress activates the fight-or-flight response, a protective process in which bodily changes take place and numerous chemicals are released. In response, blood platelets aggregate, immune cells activate, blood sugar rushes to muscles to give them energy, the heart and breathing rates quicken, and blood pressure rises. Cortisol, a steroid hormone, initially sustains the stress response and later slows it down so the body can return to normal functioning. Sometimes this feedback loop goes awry. If stress is chronic, or if hormones fail to turn off once the challenge has passed, cortisol and other hormones become dysregulated. Instead of providing protection, they may suppress the immune system by interfering with the regular repair and maintenance functions of the body, leaving us open to infections and disease. The price our bodies pay for accommodating to stressful changes may be high; some people develop a hyperactivity or hypoactivity—too much or too little—of the normal stress response.

As the body continually taps its resources for coping with stress, certain chemicals become depleted and exhaustion may set in, rendering us susceptible to illness. In the face of continuing challenges, we push rather than rest, compounding the problem. Essentially, we are drawing from a depleted account that has dipped deeply into credit reserve. Long-term stress leads to immune dysfunction, such as reduced CD8 cells (involved in the cellular immune response) and decreased natural killer cell function. Stress-related immune system changes contribute to the development of many types of illness, as varied as depression, heart attacks, cancer, and chronic disorders. Many illnesses are stress driven but not stress caused.

The body's response to stress is regulated by the hypothalamic-pituitary-adrenal (HPA) axis, composed of the hypothalamus, the pituitary gland, and the adrenal glands. This complex system releases hormones, triggers other glands to release hormones, and influences physiology, psychology, and behavior. The HPA axis interacts with other central nervous system (CNS) functions including mood, pain perception, and cognition.

The hypothalamus controls appetite, body temperature, and hormones and secretes corticotropin releasing hormone (CRH) to stimulate the pituitary gland.

The pituitary gland, located beneath the hypothalamus, is called the "master gland" since it produces and secretes a wide range of hormones. In response to CRH, it releases adrenocorticotropin releasing hormone (ACTH). ACTH signals the adrenal glands to produce and release cortisol.

The two adrenal glands, located next to the kidneys, release a group of hormones that affect the body's metabolism and fluid balance, producing adrenaline (or epinephrine) and certain steroid hormones including cortisol. Cortisol, the major stress hormone, plays a primary role in the body's response to stress and recovery from stress. An immune suppressor, cortisol regulates liver enzymes, glucose levels, and metabolism.

In managing the body's response to stress, the HPA axis produces stress hormones to alert the body and create adaptive physiologic and behavioral changes to restore homeostasis. The hypothalamus secretes CRH, which causes the pituitary gland to release ACTH, which signals the adrenals to produce cortisol. This adaptive response creates the fight-or-flight response, causing increased arousal, alertness, and vigilance. Long-lasting stress or multiple stressors can cause damage to the HPA axis, dysregulating this delicately balanced system. Chronic activation of the HPA axis is a factor in the development of illnesses, including depression.

In CFS and FMS, HPA axis functioning may be disrupted by CNS and immune abnormalities, including elevated levels of certain cytokines, causing a vicious cycle and persistent symptoms. CFS and FMS are stress-related syndromes, since stress plays a key role in triggering both onset and exacerbations. These syndromes are characterized by low cortisol levels and an exaggerated stress response. The stress response, and hence cortisol, may be chronically activated at the onset of CFS and FMS, in conjunction with overresponse of the immune system; over time, inadequate stress responses occur as cortisol production decreases.

Inadequate production of stress hormones can be just as harmful as too much, because it may trigger the secretion of other substances that compensate for the loss. For example, if cortisol does not increase in response to stress, inflammatory cytokines (peptides that mediate brain-immune system communication) rise. For unknown reasons, stress hormones sometimes do not decline once a stressful event has passed, and some individuals lose the ability to produce stress hormones when they are needed.

THE CENTRAL NERVOUS SYSTEM

Every cell in our body is controlled by the central nervous system (CNS), consisting of the brain and spinal cord. The chief organ of the CNS is the brain, a miracle of complexity in a hard shell. Despite all we have learned about how the CNS functions, we know very little. The process of learning about the CNS is essentially the brain's attempt to understand itself, but we are incapable of comprehending its multitude of intricate interconnections. We still do not understand consciousness, know where the mind is, or understand what feelings are.

Although we study the brain's function and structure, we see only a small piece of what goes on. We cannot perform invasive procedures for study, and animal models are inadequate for understanding language, creativity, feelings, or higher mental functions.

The sciences of neurology and psychology are merging into one: the study of the brain. Chronic disorders of the brain occur just as they do in other body systems. As a diabetic depends on insulin, someone with depression or obsessive-compulsive disorder may depend on serotonergic chemicals to live normally. Such disparate problems as learning disorders, balance problems, and depression indicate abnormalities in brain function.

CFS and FMS are considered neurosomatic disorders since the CNS plays a prime role in the illness, one that is not yet well understood. (Perhaps we should no longer feel insulted when told the illness is "in our heads"!) Many symptoms associated with CFS and FMS and similar disorders are of central (brain) origin, rather than peripheral (local) origin. Interconnected parts of the brain are involved in pain, fatigue, sleep, thermoregulation, cognitive dysfunction, vision and the other senses, emotions such as depression and anxiety, rage, balance, chemical sensitivities, metabolism, respiration, hormones, hunger and thirst, libido, and cardiac functioning.

The limbic system in the brain, for example, helps to maintain internal homeostasis by integrating internal and external events, coordinating input from our inside and outside worlds. A complex neural network, the limbic system is a rim of cortical structures above and highly interconnected with the hypothalamus, the area of the brain that controls the endocrine system and the autonomic nervous system, which generates the drives and instincts that promote survival of the self and the species. The limbic system affects most aspects of bodily functioning, including emotion and mood (and their connection with behavior), respiration, memory, appetite and weight, fatigue, sleep, libido, and the immune and endocrine systems.

THE EMOTIONS

I shouldn't precisely have chosen madness if there had been any choice. What consoles me is that I am beginning to consider madness as an illness like any other and that I accept it as such.

— *Vincent van Gogh*

Darkness, however terrible, never fully extinguishes the spark of light.

— *Depak Chopra*, The Path to Love

The mind remains a mystery. Where does it reside: in the brain, or in every cell? What we think affects body functioning, but what causes us to think as we do? How do our thoughts affect our feelings, and how do our thoughts and feelings affect our health?

The idea that emotions and health are connected originated centuries ago, when doctors believed that "the passions" played a role in causing disease. Having gained a better understanding of cellular functioning, researchers have more recently found that illnesses characterized by chronic immune system activation are associated with depression, a problem that is underreported and often untreated. Thus, depression may be the result of increased cytokine levels as well as a response to the losses and limitations associated with medical conditions.

Numerous researchers have written about the role of the positive emotions in determining psychophysiological responses to illness—the powers of hope and positive expectations versus remaining stuck in anger, prolonged depression, despair, blame, hatred, and bitterness. Studies demonstrate the negative effects of stress and other negative moods on immunity and well-being.

Why are these scientists writing about hope rather than microbes and medication? In ways that seem mysterious, love, positive beliefs, and spirituality contribute to healing in a remarkably complex process in which thoughts and beliefs play a vital part.

"I have learned never to underestimate the capacity of the human mind and body to regenerate—even when the prospects seem most wretched," wrote Norman Cousins in 1979. "The life-force may be the least understood force on earth." Cousins stressed the importance of the "human apothecary"—hope, positive beliefs, a positive patient–doctor relationship, reassurance, purpose, faith, love, determination, and playfulness, all "powerful biochemical pre-scriptions." Our life philosophies affect the ways we think and feel and how our bodies behave. What the mind believes is what the body believes.

The positive emotions include hope, love, determination, faith, optimism, humor, spirituality, connectedness, and pleasure. Hope is what keeps us alive when we wish we were dead, what allows us to hang on for one more day just in case things get better. It allows us to give even when we thought we had nothing left and allows us to delight in the mundane. Hope is putting one foot in front of the other, even when we're not sure why we bother: It is the triumph of the human spirit over adversity.

The positive emotions have important physiological benefits. The importance of humor, hope, and the other positive emotions are underemphasized in our concepts of illness and wellness, per-haps because they are not sufficiently "scientific." However, I don't need a lab test to tell me that my sense of humor, enjoyment of music, and creativity are excellent barometers of how ill or well I feel. When I laugh, I feel better, and when I feel better, I laugh. It's that simple—and that complex.

Realistically, we cannot always maintain hope, singing and laughing our way through life. The human condition is a lifelong struggle between positive and negative forces. Lacking predictabil-ity, security, and a sense of control, we have ample reason to feel hopeless and helpless. At times we feel isolated, invisible, burden-some, misunderstood, and diminished by illness and other prob-lems. We sustain injuries, losses, and fears. We especially fear that which we do not understand and cannot predict.

Hope, although not a cure-all, enables our bodies to mobilize toward healing and helps to improve our quality of life. Although elusive at times, the presence of hope is like a pilot light that con-tinues to burn through feelings of desolation and helplessness. The resiliency of the human spirit is greater than we had ever imagined. Is there any better medicine?

10

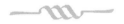

Abnormalities

Once scarce, CFS/FMS research literature is now abundant—in medical journals, newsletters, and Internet postings—but findings are contradictory and inconclusive. Various causal hypotheses gain and lose popularity in the CFS/FMS scientific community.

CFS and FMS are associated with numerous, often conflicting, abnormalities. We are unable to determine what these findings mean in terms of cause, contributing factor, or result of the illness. Data regarding the presence of similar abnormalities in the healthy population are not always available, and we lack specific guidelines to distinguish between "normal" and "abnormal."

RESEARCH

The plural of anecdote is data.

— *Mark Bekoff, University of Colorado biologist*

Abnormalities in CFS and FMS are inconsistent, and causal attributions are uncertain. Variations among symptoms and findings obscure the big picture. We cannot tell whether a particular finding identifies a causal, contributing, or perpetuating factor; a secondary effect resulting from multisystem dysregulations; or an epiphenomenon (an abnormal finding that may or may not be related to the primary illness).

Most studies focus on only one factor because limiting variables makes results clearer. However, this method does not allow study of combined effects, which may differ significantly from the myopic, one-factor-at-a-time approach. Combinations of factors often yield more useful results, particularly when the subject under scrutiny is complex.

Lack of collaboration among researchers who work in isolation prevents them from integrating their findings. Looking at one area at a time leaves us in a situation like that of the blind men and the elephant, with each "seeing" (touching) one part of the elephant—the trunk, a tusk, a foot—and drawing erroneous conclusions about the entire beast. In order to develop a more accurate concept of "elephant," they would need to pool their ideas. Accomplishing this in medical research is a complex undertaking, requiring the coordination of multidisciplinary research efforts.

Findings and theories pile up like hundreds of puzzle pieces. Some will prove central to the big picture, some are part of smaller pictures, and others do not belong. Identifying the relevance of information and assembling pieces to see the whole picture may take more than a village.

Before the causative agent of HIV disease was identified, the medical community was baffled by patients with such various disorders as Kaposi's sarcoma, wasting syndrome, and PCP pneumonia, which were not initially recognized as presentations of the same underlying illness. The shift came only when a causative agent was identified and the variability of the illness was better understood. Similarly, CFS and FMS vary in their manifestations, with symptoms and abnormalities that overlap between them and with other disorders. We lack a clear understanding of the various presentations of each disorder and their relationships to each other.

The abnormalities and suspected causal agents of CFS and FMS have been implicated in other illnesses, blurring boundaries. Some identified abnormalities are found in healthy populations and in spouses and family members of patients.

Systemic vulnerabilities of different patient groups may create variability in findings. Each of us has a "weak link," a heightened vulnerability in a certain organ system, that predisposes us to particular clusters of symptoms, even if the primary causal factor is the same.

Research yields tentative conclusions rather than hard answers. Findings "lead us to believe" or "may indicate" or "could point to." Conclusive findings may be one study away or may not emerge for years. Lack of funding hinders research. The trivializing names, invisibility of the disorders, and controversies surrounding CFS and FMS do not attract research dollars.

In attempting to identify causal or contributing factors and markers (abnormal findings that distinguish those with an illness from those without the illness), we encounter pitfalls and difficulties:

▶ The interrelationships among CFS, FMS, and similar illnesses are unclear: Are they distinct disorders, overlapping syndromes, or variations on a theme with numerous subgroups? CFS and FMS remain poorly defined by inadequate and varying criteria. One's diagnosis may depend on primary symptoms and/or on the specialty of the diagnosing physician. We are unable to differentiate CFS and FMS accurately, and the majority of patients seem to have elements of both. Many FMS patients find that initial pain is joined by debilitating fatigue and impaired cognition; CFS patients often find that flulike symptoms and neurological complaints are accompanied by increasing pain and the presence of FMS tender points. If we choose to study subgroups, we must select a method of identifying them; for example, on the basis of the most prevalent symptoms, abnormalities, type of onset, onset triggers, length of time ill, gender, and/or geographic area.

▶ Lack of uniform laboratory criteria render us unable to compare findings at different labs, with laboratory error compounding the problem.

▶ Studies are limited by lack of funding, poor design, inclusion criteria, studying only small numbers of patients, variations in testing techniques, timing of examinations or blood collection, and prohibitively expensive testing costs.

▶ Most tests are performed at one point in time, not necessarily presenting a true picture due to variability of symptoms and abnormalities. Few longitudinal studies have been done, so we have little information about what occurs over time.

▶ We are limited to testing for known pathogens and abnormalities, and only those for which tests are available.

▶ Many aspects of the illnesses are unquantifiable on standard measures. For example, there is no reliable test of fatigue or pain. Some tests lack adequate standardization.

▶ In scientifically valid, double-blind placebo studies, anecdotal information is ignored. Informal, nonstandardized studies or clinician observations may also yield useful findings. Although typically dismissed, anecdotal information frequently provides a foundation for future research.

Clues abound in the minds of those who explore this murky and uncertain territory. As research progresses, the interplay among factors will become clearer. Some of the more promising theories may turn out to be irrelevant, and some unlikely factors may play pivotal roles in the development and continuation of CFS and FMS studies.

The bottom line: Although promising theories and findings are abundant, the experts don't have the answers. At this time, our collective feet are firmly planted in midair.

Some of the findings in this chapter apply only to those diagnosed with CFS or FMS studied as individual disorders, while others apply to both disorders. Many abnormalities found in one disorder have not been tested in the other. Findings are not uniform, varying among research studies. In the future, some findings will prove valid and relevant, some will serve as springboards for future research, and others will be proven untrue and discarded. The information presented in this chapter is complex and technical, but space limitations preclude full explanations.

The temptation is great to seize upon the latest research "breakthrough," attribute one's illness to the newly uncovered factor or agent, and seek treatment with expectations of a cure. However, the reader is urged to exercise caution in drawing hasty conclusions regarding possible abnormalities and causal or triggering factors.

The categorization of abnormalities for the sake of convenience belies the complex interaction of body systems and interrelation of findings.

IMMUNE SYSTEM ABNORMALITIES

In an important sense, the immune system is far greater than
the sum of its parts.

— *Mizel and Jaret,* **The Human Immune System: The New
Frontier in Medicine**

Immune abnormalities have been documented in CFS and FMS, but research findings are inconsistent among patient groups. Although many aspects of immune functioning are overactive, the immune system is not wholly overactivated; some functions are underactive or in the normal range. The immune system interacts with the autonomic nervous system and the hypothalamic-pituitary-adrenal (HPA) axis, as well as with all other body systems. FMS and CFS are associated with various immunologic abnormalities, as evidenced by laboratory test findings and symptoms. However, limitations of these findings include inaccurate measurements of immune parameters at commercial labs, inconsistencies among results from different labs and from patient to patient, and lack of correlation between immune dysfunctions and illness severity.

Dysregulation or imbalance of the immune system affects other body systems. When the immune system is constantly turned on, it becomes aware of all types of substances perceived as "nonself" and reacts, producing symptoms that are caused by the body's *reactions* to particular agents rather than by the agents themselves.

Immune dysfunction is a contributory factor in many currently unexplained illnesses. Immune dysfunction occurs when the immune system underreacts, overreacts, or reacts inappropriately to an invader. When the immune system reacts appropriately, we are able to fight off infection. When its attempts are inadequate, illness results. We are constantly exposed to many antigens but become ill only when the antigens "win."

A state of *immunosuppression* allows enemy cells, such as viruses, to reproduce actively. When the immune system rallies, symptoms subside. When the disruptive agent becomes stronger, symptoms increase; neither side is able to sustain a victory and end the war. As the war continues, the infectious agent retains a degree of control. If the agent "loses," it is killed. If the agent "wins," it kills its host, thus destroying itself. So it is to the invader's advantage to stay in control by using the host but not killing it. In the process, it disrupts the host's functioning in ways that cause symptoms. When the situation is a "standoff," the immune system is unable to rid the body of invaders, which remain in the body.

A variety of factors impact immune functioning. Primary immune deficiencies (those that are congenital, or present from birth) may become apparent later in life with exposure to certain antigens. Secondary immune deficiencies are acquired, resulting from nongenetic factors such as nutrition, age, sleep disorders, surgery and general anesthesia, infections, injury, certain drugs, emotional state, hormonal imbalance, stress level, environmental toxins, and allergens. Such deficiencies are either transient or persistent.

Although we can measure aspects of immunity, we are unable to measure the strength of an individual's immune system. Inconsistent immune abnormalities in CFS and FMS have been identified. Some abnormalities correlate with symptom presence and severity, while others do not. Some immune parameters fluctuate over time, making it difficult to establish a typical CFS/FMS immune profile. Abnormalities in various body systems, including the immune, neuroendocrine, and central nervous systems, may represent causes or effects of the illness.

Immune abnormalities in CFS and/or FMS include the following:

- recurrent illnesses and infections, especially early in the disease (acute phase);
- allergies; skin test atopy (hypersensitivity) or anergy (lack of immune response);
- abnormal CD4 and CD8 (cells that turn the immune response on or off) numbers and ratios—particularly low suppressor cells, which keep the immune system active and cause production of symptom-producing cytokines;
- low natural killer cell cytotoxicity (NKCC);
- autoantibody production: elevated blood levels of antithyroid antibodies and antinuclear antibodies (ANAs), usually a speckled pattern;
- low sedimentation rate (although in some cases it is slightly elevated);
- changes in white blood cells: mild leukocytosis; mild leukopenia; moderate monocytosis; atypical lymphocytes; abnormal macrophage, B-cell, and neutrophil functions;
- frequent immunoglobulin deficiencies (most often IgG1 and IgG3);
- altered levels of cytokines (immune messengers between cells): elevated proinflammatory cytokines (e.g., IL-1, IL-6, and tumor necrosis factors); and alterations in interleukin levels and activity;
- abnormal interferon levels (e.g., elevated alpha interferon, decreased gamma interferon);

› abnormalities in the complement cascade as demonstrated by C_3, C_4, CH_{50}, and immune complex levels;

› Th2 shift: Two key types of immune pathways are categorized as Th1 and Th2. A healthy immune system is able to switch between the two as needed to maintain a balance. Dysregulation by viruses and other factors shifts this mechanism, "fooling" the immune system into responding inappropriately. Th1, or cell-mediated immunity, involves activation of macrophages, interleukin-2, gamma interferon, and NK cells that attack invading pathogens such as viruses, mycoplasma, chlamydia, yeast, and cancer cells, normalizing once the pathogen is eliminated. When the Th1 response is deficient and unable to conquer invaders, they persist, overburdening the RNaseL antiviral system. The Th2 system, or humoral immunity, involves the production of white cells such as eosinophils, antibodies, and certain interleukins (IL-4, IL-5, and IL-10). When Th2 is dominant, the immune system can mount a response to reactivated pathogens, including allergens, bacteria, toxins, and parasites. When either system is overactive, the other is underactive. In overly activated Th2 illnesses, antibodies are overproduced and NK function decreases;

› Perturbations of the 2-5A synthetase/RNaseL pathway (the intracellular antiviral cellular defense mechanism, an enzymatic pathway that is activated when defending against a virus) and an abnormal, low molecular weight (LMW) form of RNaseL have been identified in CFS. REDD, or RNaseL enzyme dysfunction disorder, occurs with overproduction of the abnormal LMW (low molecular weight) RNaseL, which damages the body by consuming ATP, the energy source within cells (those with FMS are believed to have a much smaller percentage of defective RNaseL than those with CFS);

› Autoimmunity is increased in many patients, raising the possibility that CFS and FMS are autoimmune illnesses. CFS and FMS are often present in those with autoimmune disorders, and those with CFS and FMS may go on to develop autoimmune disorders;

‣ Leaky gut syndrome is a somewhat controversial condition in which intestinal-wall permeability allows potentially allergenic substances (proteins) to cross the intestinal wall and enter the bloodstream, causing allergic reactions and numerous other symptoms;

‣ Increased sensitivity (not allergy) to chemical exposure can trigger acute or chronic reactions. Sensitization and consequent exposure can lead to dysregulation of autonomic, endocrine, and immune system functioning, possibly mediated by the limbic system. Hypersensitivities to environmental metals, pesticides, chemical spills, and chemical residues in foods cause neurological, immunological, gastrointestinal, and respiratory problems. The issue of dental metals remains controversial;

‣ Comorbid conditions and symptoms are believed to include nasal allergies, hives, fatigue, arthralgias, sinusitis, rhinitis, bronchitis, migraine, irritable bowel, peptic ulcers, food sensitivities, arthritis, ovarian cysts, breast cysts, menstrual dysfunctions including PMS, hypothyroidism, depression, anxiety, and panic disorders;

‣ Silicone gel breast implant rupture and certain vaccines (such as hepatitis B and early polio vaccines) are hypothesized to cause or trigger CFS and FMS.

INFECTIOUS AGENTS

The microbe is nothing; terrain is everything.

— *Louis Pasteur*

In many instances, CFS and FMS begin suddenly with a flulike condition. Because most of the features of these disorders resemble those of a lingering viral illness, many researchers view infectious agents as causes or results of immune abnormalities. However, not all cases are preceded by infection, and most cases occur sporadically (not as part of a cluster), so contagion is believed unlikely. Certain infections common in patients are found in the general population as well. If an infectious agent is involved, it may be a mutated form of typically harmless pathogens, or a hit-and-run agent that infects and disappears, leaving immune dysfunction and resulting symptoms in its wake.

Other theories hold that immune or neurologic abnormalities cause reactivation of a viral or bacterial infection that had presumably resolved. Previous infections may predispose one to new, chronic infection. Alternatively, the illness may be caused by a low-level viral infection that provokes an immune response, leading to chronic symptoms.

◆◆ Viruses ◆◆

"Virus" is a word used by doctors a great deal. It means,
"Your guess is as good as mine."

— *Bob Hope*

Viruses are submicroscopic, protein-covered bundles of genetic material containing blueprints for self-reproduction. Incapable of reproducing on their own, these nonmalicious organisms seek a place to replicate, searching for host cells to invade to accomplish this purpose. They invade cells (like checking into a motel), give genetic orders, and turn invaded cells into virus factories. Their offspring burst forth, destroying the previously invaded cell and seeking out new, healthy cells for their continued reproduction. A successful virus coexists with its host in order to survive and serve its needs, whereas a virus that is too successful sabotages its own life by killing its host. Unlike bacteria, which are living organisms, viruses are neither alive nor dead.

There are probably millions of different viruses, only a small number of which have been identified. Because viruses are adept at escaping detection, viral illnesses are often diagnosed on the basis of antiviral antibodies and symptoms, and by exclusion of other possible illnesses. Viral presence can be tested by polymerase chain reaction (PCR), a sophisticated technique that allows amplification of DNA or RNA sequences and that has detected new viruses associated with known illnesses (e.g., Kaposi's sarcoma, associated with HIV disease).

Notoriously elusive, viruses are capable of hiding, mutating, and combining; their versatility allows them to exist in an active, dormant, or low-level state, producing various immune reactions. Some remain in a latent (inactive, nonreproducing) state in our bodies for long periods of time without producing symptoms. Slow viruses have lengthy incubation periods and can cause persistent disease (often neurological) after being in the body for a long period of time. Viruses may cause chronic illnesses by alternating between dormant and active (replication) phases. Reactivation of latent viruses may follow trauma, such as infection, chemical exposure, or any physical or emotional stress. Certain viruses are linked with disruption and disorders of body systems (e.g., the immune, endocrine, and central nervous systems); these links are the subject of continued research. In the development of chronic illnesses, a weakened immune system may allow replication of previously dormant viruses.

A virus may be a causal or triggering agent. Nonviral triggering factors that interfere with immune functioning may allow viruses to move from dormant to active states so that viral activation is an effect, rather than a cause, of illness. The cause may turn out to be a newly discovered virus, a more virulent strain of a known virus, a recombinant virus, a faulty immune system reacting inappropriately to a "normal" virus, all of the above—or none of the above. CFS/FMS may be an umbrella term for a number of different but similar illnesses with various causative factors.

Among the viruses that possibly play a role in CFS and FMS are adenoviruses, herpesviruses, stealth viruses, enteroviruses, retroviruses, parvovirus, and Borna virus. Many viruses, particularly the herpesviruses, are ubiquitous; that is, most adults have been exposed to them and continue to harbor them in a dormant (inactive) state.

Adenoviruses, associated with respiratory and intestinal infections, can persist in body cells for long periods of time. They can reproduce slowly but consistently, producing low-grade infections and causing ongoing immune activation.

Herpesviruses include herpes simplex, herpes zoster, cytomegalovirus (CMV), and human herpesvirus type 6 (HHV-6). Infections include cold sores, herpes encephalitis, influenza-type illness, chicken pox and shingles (both caused by the varicella virus), cytomegalovirus-related illness (which occurs mainly in fetuses and babies, but which can also produce a mononucleosis-like illness), and Epstein-Barr (EBV, implicated in most cases of mononucleosis and, less frequently, certain cancers). Viruses in the herpes class demonstrate a particular ability to remain latent for long periods of time, often becoming more active when the human host is under increased stress. Persistent cardiomyopathy (disease of the heart muscle) resulting from EBV and/or CMV infection has been proposed to play a causal role in CFS.

The Epstein-Barr virus (EBV) is a herpes virus that infects virtually everyone; 90 to 95 percent of the adult population have been infected at some time during their lives (in many cases, without obvious symptoms). Once the virus has infected an individual, it persists for life, generally remaining inactive following the initial exposure, probably because we have developed enough antibodies to suppress the virus but not kill it. EBV infections in children are generally asymptomatic, while young adults initially exposed to it may develop mononucleosis. Once believed to play a causal role in CFS, EBV has proven to be one of many persistent dormant viruses.

Human herpesvirus type 6 (HHV-6), a central nervous system virus initially isolated in 1986, is a common virus, although infection is often asymptomatic. Like other herpesviruses, it may remain dormant for many years until reactivated by trauma, such as stress, infection with another agent, or changes in the immune system. A high frequency of HHV-6 reactivation may indicate a causal role or may be the result of immune dysfunction. Other herpesviruses that may play a role in causation and symptom production include cytomegalovirus (CMV, which causes EBV-like manifestations, notably neurological symptoms), herpes simplex I and II, herpes zoster (the cause of chicken pox and shingles, remaining dormant in the nerve cells thereafter), and gamma herpesviruses.

Stealth viruses infect the brain without causing inflammation, successfully evading the immune system, unchecked by normal antivirus defense mechanisms. These atypically-structured cytopathic viruses, possibly related to CMV, induce multisystem neurologic illnesses in both humans and animals. John Martin, M.D., suspects that stealth viruses commonly play a role in brain disorders of children and adults.

Enteroviruses include coxsackie A, coxsackie B, echovirus, and poliovirus. There is some speculation that CFS is another form of poliomyelitis or is caused by a nonpolio enterovirus—or that enteroviruses do not play a causal role but are reactivated by immune dysregulation, as are the herpesviruses.

Retroviruses contain an enzyme, reverse transcriptase, that allows them to reverse the order of genetic information processing. They carry genetic information that directs the construction of a protective envelope that allows them to infect new cells, and new individuals, to continue the replication process. Retroviruses are neurotropic, living in the brain and other parts of the central nervous system, and have been implicated in such illnesses as HIV/AIDS, a rare type of leukemia, and certain forms of cancer.

◆◆ Bacteria ◆◆

Enigmatic mycoplasmas, the smallest self-replicating bacteria, are capable of altering immune, metabolic, and biochemical functioning. They may enter cells and damage the mitochondria, the cells' energy-producing centers. Garth Nicolson, M.D., has detected mycoplasmas in the majority of CFS/FMS patients, as well as those with related autoimmune and inflammatory disorders. Strains of these slow-growing bacteria in CFS and FMS include M. *fermentans*, M. *incognitus*, M. *pneumoniae*, M. *penetrans*, and M. *hominis*.

Chlamydia is a chronic infection that disrupts the immune system and leads to a chronic inflammatory response. Of several strains, C. *pneumoniae* is a common cause of respiratory and coronary artery infection and has been implicated in CFS, FMS, GWS, and other chronic illnesses.

Rickettsia is a small, intracellular bacteria that may penetrate and persist in macrophages, disrupting their functioning and causing other immune aberrations.

Coxiella burneti, a rickettsia-like organism that fits between viruses and bacteria, is the causative agent of Q fever and other diseases in humans and animals. It is believed to be asymptomatic and therefore significantly underdiagnosed. Its prevalence in humans and possible role in CFS and FMS remain unknown.

Ehrlichia, a type of rickettsia, cause disease primarily in animals, although prevalence in humans may be underestimated. Capable of persisting in a dormant state for long periods of time, ehrlichia may cause neurological disorders in humans.

Toxin-producing **staphylococci** may produce damage to membranes and cause fatigue and pain, thus potentially playing a part in CFS and FMS.

❖❖ Systemic Yeast/Fungal Infection ❖❖

Whether systemic candidiasis is related to CFS and FMS is a controversial issue; many believe this condition is overdiagnosed. Yeast overgrowth may be a causal contributor or a secondary effect of the illness, or both may be attributable to immune dysfunction. Contributing factors to both conditions may include nutritional deficiencies, overuse of antibiotics, extended use of birth control pills, environmental toxins, and emotional stress, all of which are believed to have detrimental effects on immunity. That antiyeast medications and diet are often helpful does not prove a causal relationship but does indicate that further research is warranted.

CENTRAL NERVOUS SYSTEM ABNORMALITIES

Neurological dysfunction is considered the principal mechanism of both physical and mental fatigue in FMS and CFS. Many symptoms of CFS and FMS suggest central nervous system (CNS) involvement: sensations of unreality or "spaciness," cognitive abnormalities, headache, irritability, dizziness, light-headedness, visual disturbances, muscle aches, tingling in fingers or toes, profound fatigue, depressed feelings, chest discomfort, shortness of breath, digestive problems, loss of motivation, and disordered sleep. CFS/FMS symptoms resemble those found in closed head injury and limbic or temporal lobe epilepsy: sensory alterations (tingling, numbness, or a "crawling" feeling), stuttering or slurred speech (or speech arrest), and autonomic manifestations (flushing, dyspnea, a feeling of weight on the chest, air hunger, chest pain, palpitations, sinus tachycardia, nausea, or epigastric distress). Seizure disorders, including subclinical seizures, have been tentatively linked to CFS and FMS.

Neurotransmitters, the brain's electrical/chemical communicators, are key players in establishing two-way communication between the CNS and all other organs and cells. Altered neuro-transmitters in CFS/FMS patients include the following:

> Elevated substance P (SP) in the cerebrospinal fluid (CSF), related to the transmission of pain signals in FMS. SP facilitates pain messages to the brain by a sequence of chemical reactions known as nociception. Elevation can amplify pain perception, particularly in inflammatory states that increase both SP and its receptors. Elevated in rheumatoid arthritis and lupus, SP is increased more dramatically—twofold to four-fold—in the CSF of FMS patients, although blood levels are normal. Levels vacillate in some and remain constantly elevated in others. Levels of SP change in response to pain, which may be the reason for increased prevalence in those diagnosed with FMS or CFS/FMS, as opposed to CFS alone, which is less likely to be characterized by severe pain.

> Decreased neuropeptide Y in the blood.

> Decreased serotonin, associated with mood, sense of well-being, sleep disorders, gut functioning, and pain perception.

> Altered levels of 5-HIAA, a metabolite of serotonin, possibly resulting from impaired neuroendocrine stress responses mediated through a deficient dopaminergic system. This finding is considered a potential marker for CFS and FMS.

> Decreased dopamine levels, as found in postpolio syndrome.

CNS dysfunction may be a primary phenomenon related to CNS damage or it may be secondary to unidentified systemic factors. Jay Goldstein, M.D., views virtually all symptoms and abnormalities as stemming from "limbic system dysregulation in a neural network or an immunoneuroendocrine network that involves the brain and the entire body" (1993). Altered neurotransmitter levels may impair the processing of sensory input, according to Goldstein. The brain is equipped with the ability to separate important input from unimportant garbage, but when this mechanism malfunctions, the brain becomes unable to separate the signal (the stimulus one wants to pay attention to) from "noise" (extraneous input that should be in the background). Thus, competing sources of input (odors, sensations, noises, movements, pain, and other interfering factors) cannot be filtered appropriately. As competing stimuli bombard the brain, causing confusion and sensory overload, the result is a scrambled message or misinterpretation of what is occurring.

The autonomic nervous system (ANS), the "automatic" or self-controlling part of the nervous system, controls vital functions including blood pressure, pulse rate, breathing rate, digestion, bowel function, stress response, and body temperature regulation. Small studies have indicated ANS abnormalities in the majority of CFS/FMS patients. Both branches of the ANS, the sympathetic and parasympathetic, are dysregulated and unable to function in their normal, complementary fashion.

Dysautonomia is the inappropriate (delayed or exaggerated) ANS response to external or internal stimuli. It may be the cause of panic attacks, changes in blood flow, heart and blood pressure abnormalities, and breathing problems.

SLEEP ABNORMALITIES

The purpose of sleep is to repair and rejuvenate the body. Normal sleep patterns contain four stages, from light sleep to deep sleep. It is further divided into rapid eye movement (REM) sleep periods, which occur every 90 to 120 minutes during sleep, and non-REM sleep. Most dreams occur during REM sleep. Sleep typically begins with stages 1 and 2 sleep, followed by REM sleep, and progressing to deep sleep, cycling through the stages several times each night. Deep sleep is restorative, associated with respiration, blood pressure, growth hormone secretion, and other regulatory functions. Lack of deep sleep has been associated with altered immune functioning. The quality as well as the quantity of sleep is important. Sleep deprivation causes significant dysregulation of bodily functioning and is associated with pain, daytime drowsiness, cognitive dysfunction, decreased alertness, and irritability.

Prevalent sleep disorders in CFS/FMS patients include the following:

▸ hypersomnia: sleeping many hours, often present in early stage of illness, or in cycles, often alternating with periods of hyposomnia

▸ hyposomnia: need for sleep but inability to fall asleep or obtain restful sleep (a "tired and wired" feeling)

- increased sleep latency (delayed onset of sleep)
- shortened REM latency (delayed onset of rapid eye movement sleep) and increased REM activity and density
- increased sleep fragmentation: frequent awakenings
- reduced slow-wave (deep) sleep with alpha-delta intrusion: alpha wave (lighter) sleep intrusion into delta wave (deeper) sleep, causing unrefreshing, nonrestorative sleep
- abnormal night temperature variations
- night sweats (usually upper body)
- night headaches, which may cause awakening
- sleep paralysis, usually upon awakening: a state that may last for several minutes, in which voluntary movement is impossible despite clear consciousness, sometimes accompanied by vivid hallucinations
- vivid, disturbing dreams and violent, graphic nightmares
- "waking dreams" that continue from sleep into waking consciousness
- changes in breathing, including sleep apnea (frequent awakening due to breathing cessation)
- altered circadian rhythms: often difficulty falling asleep until early morning hours and sleeping late; energy often best in the late afternoon or evening
- restless leg syndrome (RLS; leg movements, restlessness, and/or tingling—often relieved by walking) and periodic limb movement disorder (PLMD)
- bruxism (grinding of the teeth)
- nocturnal panic attacks

Sleep disturbance and relapse are strongly associated, with sleep disruption causing increased pain, profound fatigue and lethargy, reduced sensory threshold for pain, disordered temperature regulation, cardiovascular abnormalities, disturbed higher cerebral function, and increased depression. Sleep studies (polysomnographs) may not reflect these abnormalities accurately.

VISION ABNORMALITIES

CFS/FMS patients may have the following visual abnormalities:

▶ intermittent blurred vision, close and distant

▶ photophobia (light sensitivity)

▶ oscillopsia (bouncing, jiggling vision)

▶ driving problems (impaired night vision, inability to concentrate, overload, and problems with spatial relations such as judging distances)

▶ latency in accommodation (slowed shifting focus from one place to another, e.g., near to far)

▶ nystagmus (abnormal eye movements), usually primary horizontal nystagmus

▶ eye sensitivity (dry, scratchy, gritty, or burning)

▶ discomfort looking at complex patterns (probably due to abnormal sensory processing)

▶ diplopia (double vision; less common)

NEUROPSYCHOLOGICAL ABNORMALITIES

Although the term dementia has been associated with CFS and FMS, cognitive problems are not progressive, as in Alzheimer's disease. Though cognitive dysfunction and other neurological symptoms may become more pronounced over time, they tend to follow a waxing-and-waning pattern. This multifocal pattern of impairment has been classified as an atypical brain syndrome, possibly due to encephalopathy of viral or other origin. Native intelligence is largely unharmed, but the ability to use or apply it suffers. Memory and concentration are most impaired. Cognitive deficits are described in Chapter 5.

◆◆ Neuropsychological Testing ◆◆

The findings on neuropsychological tests and brain scans often correlate with symptoms; however, the frequency, severity, and waxing-and-waning nature of cognitive symptoms are not always reflected adequately in test results. Many patients have learned to compensate well when cognitive glitches occur.

On the Wechsler Adult Intelligence Scale-Revised (WAIS-R), full-scale intelligence quotient (IQ) is lower than would be expected, given an individual's vocational and educational background, or as compared to pre-illness IQ scores. Verbal scores are usually higher than performance scores, which are often significantly impaired (e.g., digit span, especially repeating digits backward; arithmetic; digit symbol; block design; and picture completion subtests). Scores on subtests vary considerably, indicating organic brain deficits with attention-concentration, visual-perception, and visual–motor speed impairments; and problems with memory, sequencing, visual discrimination, abstract reasoning, and spatial organization. "IQ loss on repeated IQ measures over time . . . indicates definite shifts in intellectual functioning during the course of the illness" (Bastien and Peterson 1994).

The Minnesota Multiphasic Personality Inventory-2 (MMPI-2) reveals a profile of acute psychological disturbance related to illness. Linda Iger, Ph.D., found a unique profile of elevated scores on subscales 1, 2, 3, 7, and 8 in CFS. These scale elevations resemble those found in other chronic illnesses. When "neurological" items were eliminated, scores dropped to within normal limits. Valid profiles were obtained, reflecting depression, somatic concerns, social withdrawal, anxiety, pessimism, extreme concern for well-being, and awareness of somatic and sensory difficulties.

Scores on the Wechsler Memory Scale-Revised (WMS-R) demonstrate memory deficits described by patients on both immediate and delayed memory impairment, with verbal memory more impaired than visual memory. Subjects with CFS had a tendency to overestimate performance as opposed to depressed individuals, who underestimated performance. New memories were found to be fragile and easily perturbed, and when a memory task is followed by an irrelevant task, subsequent retesting indicates that the material learned in the original memory task is lost ("proactive inhibition").

The Halstead-Reitan Neuropsychological Test Battery reveals abnormalities on several subtests: category, tactual performance, finger oscillation, dynamometer, seashore rhythms, trailmaking A and B, speech sounds perception, and grip strength, indicating impaired nonverbal reasoning, poor visual sequencing, altered spatial perception, impaired motor functioning, and mildly impaired abstract reasoning.

◆◆ Brain Studies: Neuroimaging ◆◆

Brain scans are of two types, structural and functional. Although brain abnormalities are found in CFS/FMS patients, particularly on tests of function, the lack of consistent findings renders neuroimaging a research tool and technique for ruling out other disorders rather than a diagnostic measure. Brain scan abnormalities reinforce the possibility of an encephalomyelitic pathogenesis (defects in the myelin coating of nerve fibers in the brain).

The brain positron emission tomography (PET) scan measures brain metabolism. Hypometabolism (significantly reduced glucose metabolism) of the brain stem has been reported, particularly in the pons, a mass of nerve cells located on the brain stem. In FMS patients, bilateral activation is shown even when a pain stimulus is applied to only one side of the body.

Single photon emission computed tomography (SPECT) scans reveal significantly decreased blood flow, or hypoperfusion, to areas of the brain in CFS/FMS patients. Abnormalities are most marked in the frontal lobes and brain stem, and often in the temporal lobes. Lack of consistency across studies and overlap with other illness groups render SPECT results nondiagnostic. SPECT scan results often correlate with cognitive deficits reported by patients.

Magnetic resonance imaging (MRI) reveals small areas of high signal intensity (punctate lesions), seen as small, scattered dots in the cerebral white matter. Although these may be seen in healthy controls, their number is markedly increased in those with CFS and FMS. Abnormalities in brain activity during cognitive tasks are seen on functional MRI, as the brain appears to be working harder than that of a healthy person doing the same task. Other parts of the brain that would not normally be activated seem to be brought in to assist. Results of MRI and CT scans in CFS and FMS yield inconsistent and inconclusive results.

Electroencephalogram (EEG) results suggest the possibility of a distinct profile for CFS. Quantitative EEG (Q-EEG) reveals a pattern that differentiates CFS patients from controls and those with depression. These findings, along with patient symptoms, parallel those of temporal lobe epilepsy. The very high amplitudes in the occipital and temporal regions of CFS patients are also seen in persons suffering from head injury, drug abuse, extreme sleep deprivation, and encephalopathy.

ENDOCRINE AND NEUROENDOCRINE ABNORMALITIES

◆◆ Hypothalamic/Metabolic Dysregulation ◆◆

Dysregulation of the hypothalamic-pituitary-adrenal (HPA) axis with associated abnormal stress response (as discussed in Chapter 9) is characterized by decreased corticotropin releasing hormone (CRH), cortisol, epinephrine, norepinephrine, and DHEA. At onset, FMS and CFS may be chronically activated stress–cortisol states due to infection or other trauma, followed by an overresponse of the immune system. The ability to produce cortisol then decreases over time, resulting in an inadequate stress response.

Additional abnormalities include the following:

▶ Elevated liver enzymes (slightly elevated SGOT and SGPT).

▶ Abnormalities in the liver detoxification processes.

▶ Hypothyroid (often after the first few years of illness): decreased thyroid hormone related to metabolism, with deficiency causing slowing of the heart rate, sluggishness, fatigue, dry skin, insomnia, decrease in body temperature, cold intolerance, cognitive dysfunction, and depression. Common in CFS and FMS, hypothyroidism may be associated with abnormalities in the pituitary gland's release of thyroid stimulating hormone (TSH). Conversion of T_4 to T_3, the usable form of thyroid in the body, may be disrupted.

▶ Reduced TSH (thyroid stimulating hormone) and response to TRH (thyrotropin releasing hormone).

▶ Altered cycles of hormone production.

▶ Dehydroepiandrosterone sulfate (DHEA-S) and pregnenolone are produced by the adrenals and related to the production of the sex hormones estrogen and testosterone. Although their production typically declines with age, levels in CFS/FMS patients are lower than normal, possibly contributing to negative effects on memory, mood, and energy levels.

▶ Low levels of growth hormone (GH), vital to brain and immune function, metabolism, conversion of stored fat into energy, healing and tissue repair, and resistance to oxidative damage. GH secretion is regulated by the interaction between GH releasing hormone and somatostatin, or somatotropin release inhibiting hormone. This process is influenced by other neurotransmitters and hormones that may play a role in GH deficiency, probably due to HPA axis abnormalities. Insulin-like growth factor 1 (IGF-1), a stable marker that reflects pulses of growth hormone, is low, probably due to HPA axis abnormalities. GH promotes growth in the young and decreases steadily with age. Symptoms of deficient GH include reduced plasma volume, reduced exercise capacity, low blood pressure, low energy, dysphoria, decreased libido, impaired cognition, poor general health, muscle weakness, cold intolerance, and decreased lean body mass. Growth factor is short-lived and therefore difficult to measure.

▶ Elevated prolactin in a subset of FMS patients who report the most severe pain.

▶ Decreased relaxin, a hormone present in high levels during pregnancy. Relaxin is involved in the production of collagen and associated with relaxation and muscle elasticity; inability to properly use relaxin may be associated with the pain and muscle spasms of FMS.

▶ Increased cortisol response to 5-HT (serotonin).

▶ Mitochondrial impairment (abnormality in the cells' ability to produce energy).

▶ Krebs' cycle abnormalities: depleted adenosine triphosphate (ATP), the energy source within individual cells, resulting in mitochondrial damage; hypercitricemia, high citric acid levels in the urine, a potential cause of chronic tissue hypoxia; high blood levels of pyruvate; and low levels of carnitine, acylcarnitine, and acetylcarnitine.

▶ Low nicotinamide adenine dinucleotide phosphate (NADP), a cofactor in tryptophan metabolism.

▶ Decreased amino acids: L-Carnitine/Acylcarnitine, L-Alanine, L-Serine, L-Lysine, L-Histidine, L-Proline, L-Threonine, and L-Tryptophan.

▶ Elevated excitatory amino acids hypothesized to transmit pain: glutamine, asparagine, glycine, and taurine.

▶ Increased homocysteine, a naturally occurring amino acid, secondary to insufficient levels of B_6, B_{12}, and folate.

- Altered oxygen/energy mechanisms.
- Decreased glutathione.
- Decreased elaidic acid.
- Increased stearic acid.
- Elevated lipids, including LDL ("bad") cholesterol.
- Essential fatty acid (EFA) deficits.
- Alkaline urine.
- Presence of urinary metabolites associated with altered proteolysis.
- Albumin deficiency.
- Minerals: low potassium, calcium (high calcium has also been reported) and calcitonin; phospate, creating an energy-deficient state in muscle tissues; zinc; magnesium, critical for ATP production for the Krebs' cycle and for conduction of nerve and muscle impulses; and malate, believed to be an aluminum detoxifier. High levels of mercury and aluminum, purported to block ATP synthesis.
- Abnormal phosphate levels, reported in some studies to be low and in others to be high.
- High nitric oxide and peroxynitrite levels.
- Insulin resistance may be more common in CFS and FMS than in the normal population. Insulin resistance is a condition in which insulin is overproduced and unable to function properly in aiding the conversion of glucose and protein to fat. This condition may result from hereditary factors; age; physical activity; and overconsumption of refined carbohydrates, such as sugar and white flour, and saturated fats. Elevated insulin can result in obesity, diabetes, and cardiovascular abnormalities. Decreased insulin sensitivity may disrupt the action of serotonin in the hypothalamus, causing carbohydrate cravings and weight gain, and also impacting immune functioning.

ORAL HEALTH ABNORMALITIES

CFS/FMS patients may experience these abnormalities of the mouth:

- oral infections, including abscesses

- red, persistent sore throat
- papules (elevated red bumps) and vesicles (which resemble blisters) in the back of the throat and lining of the cheeks
- aphthous stomatitis: inflammation of the oral mucosae in the back of the throat and on the tongue, gum tissue, and buccal mucosae (inner cheeks and lips), similar in appearance to strep throat
- cobblestone appearance of reddened spots in the back of the throat
- crimson crescents
- herpetiform lesions
- candidiasis on tongue and cheeks (thrush)
- brown or black "hairy tongue"
- xerostomia (dry mouth)
- increased incidence of periodontal disease

ABNORMALITIES OF THE FINGERS

CFS/FMS patients may also experience these abnormalities of the fingers:

- fingertip abnormalities
- flattening of the dermal ridges, often resulting in loss of finger-prints (a phenomenon of aging that occurs at an accelerated rate)
- longitudinal creasing of the fingertips

ABNORMAL RESPONSE TO EXERCISE

Exercise is important to prevent deconditioning but is not always well tolerated. Any exercise regimen should be implemented gradually and carefully.

Abnormalities during and following exertion include the following:

- quickly reached anaerobic threshold (AT), the point at which one becomes completely fatigued and cannot exercise any longer
- decreased cortisol

- decreased growth hormone
- decreased catecholamine response
- endorphins increase less than in healthy individuals; decreased enhancement of dopamine release
- increased IL-1; IL-6 not increased
- temperature doesn't increase as much as in healthy individuals and might decrease
- exaggerated increases in blood pressure
- decreased cerebral perfusion (blood flow to brain)
- postexertional cognitive abnormalities
- abnormal aerobic threshold; impaired VO2 utilization and reduced VO2 max (a measurement of oxygen consumption)
- difficulty with regulation of breathing and erratic breathing patterns; irregular tidal volume rates (breathing patterns)
- abnormal lactic acid accumulation
- decreased functional capacity
- inefficient glucose usage
- muscle abnormalities
- oxidative muscle damage
- increased muscle fatigability
- slowed recovery phase after muscle use
- hyperalgesia (pain)
- selective muscle hypersensitivity
- histologic abnormalities: degenerative changes in muscle depending on chronicity and severity, including "moth eaten" filaments, swollen mitochondria, "rubber band morphology," bandlike compression of muscle fibers, and microspasm of muscle bundles
- skeletal muscle defects: degeneration of muscle fibers
- edema, increased mast cells and fluid content, and increased interstitial fluid
- difficulty with regulation of breathing and erratic breathing patterns

- abnormalities in muscle blood flow; compromised capillary microcirculation and ischemia with hypoxemia
- decreased intramuscular levels of ATP and phosphocreatine
- increased anaerobic metabolism with accumulation of metabolic products
- decreased muscle strength
- altered perception of muscle force

ABNORMAL PAIN LEVELS AND PERCEPTION

Evidence of alteration of pain-sensing mechanisms occurs in CFS and FMS, with increased sensitivity to pain:

- allodynia (pain sensitization to normally nonpainful stimuli)
- hypoperfusion to pain-processing centers in the limbic system
- altered cytokine and neurotransmitter levels, possibly related to continuous nociception
- downregulation or absence of certain opioid receptors in skin and muscles
- overproduction of nitric oxide in the CNS
- NMDA receptor activation secondary to pain, leading to central sensitization
- prostaglandins, cytokines, and growth factors released following tissue damage
- malfunction of the diffuse noxious inhibitory pain control (DNIC) system
- decreased serum sodium
- altered output of amino and organic acids
- increased ALT and AST (markers of tissue damage)
- increase in the tyrosine/leucine ratio

CARDIAC AND CIRCULATORY ABNORMALITIES

CFS and FMS are associated with these abnormalities of the heart and circulatory system:

- extremely low circulating blood volume

▶ elevated red blood cell count

▶ macrocytosis with elevated MCV (large red blood cells with elevated volume)

▶ below-average pumping action

▶ reduced stroke volume

▶ reduced cardiac output

▶ blood vessel constriction

▶ decreased potassium in heart muscle

▶ hypercoagulability

▶ abnormal red blood cell membranes

▶ elevated serum angiotensin-converting enzyme (ACE, a blood pressure regulating mechanism)

▶ microcirculation disturbances

▶ low blood pressure

The prevalence of low blood volume, particularly of red blood cell volume, results in less oxygen being carried to various parts of the body. This problem may contribute to the prevalence of orthostatic intolerance (OI), with blood pooling in the legs and feet and a diminished supply to the brain. OI is a type of dysautonomia, an abnormal autonomic nervous system response that may produce hypotension, presyncope (feeling of faintness), light-headedness, dizziness, nausea, tremors, breathing or swallowing difficulties, headache, visual disturbances, profuse sweating, and pallor when standing or sitting upright.

Neurally mediated hypotension (NMH) is a type of OI characterized by a dramatic drop in blood pressure and increased heart rate (pulse) when upright, even for a short time. An abnormality in the central nervous system (CNS) is believed to signal the heart to slow down and decrease blood pressure when a person stands up, causing blood to pool in the feet and legs. This causes further activation of the sympathetic nervous system, which inappropriately releases such chemicals as cortisol, dopamine, epinephrine (adrenaline), and norepinephrine, increasing vasoconstriction and producing symptoms of light-headedness, fainting or a sense of impending faint, increased pulse, panicky feelings, and exhaustion. This disorder seems to result from miscommunication between the brain and the heart. Tilt table testing, used to diagnose NMH, reveals an abnormal drop in blood pressure followed by lack of restoration of normal circulation.

Another type of OI known as positional (or postural) orthostatic tachycardia syndrome (POTS) is a rapid increase in heart rate when standing. Symptoms are similar to those of NMH, with the heart speeding up in response to upright posture.

Both conditions are associated with pooling of blood in the extremities and reduced blood flow to the brain. They may be triggered by physical exertion, hot showers, prolonged sitting or standing, warm environments, sodium depletion, mental or emotional stress, medications, pain, and exercise. Possible causes include decreased blood volume, autonomic dysregulation (overactivity of the sympathetic nervous system), infection-caused injury to the CNS, and neuroendocrine disturbances.

Tilt table testing is performed in a quiet room with minimum external stimuli. Strapped to a table that is tilted to a semi-upright position, the individual may experience an abnormal drop in blood pressure, syncope (fainting or a feeling of faintness), and/or a significantly increased heart rate compared to healthy individuals. Many of the same responses are evoked by prolonged standing during which the blood pressure is taken several times, often called the "poor man's tilt test," although results are not as specific or well documented.

The abnormalities found in CFS and FMS are numerous, and many are based on only small, preliminary, or inadequate studies. Findings may vary among subgroups, leading to conflicting results when large groups are studied. Some of these abnormalities result from illness, while others may be causal factors.

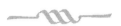

11

Overwhelmed and Uncertain: The Effects of CFS and FMS

Let me tell you that from a purely experiential, sensory perspective, CFIDS lives in the brain, and in the soul. It cripples
the mind and the spirit as much as it does the body.

— *Marc Iverson*, The CFIDS Chronicle

Incurable chronic illnesses fall into the category of incomprehensi-
ble things that happen to other people. Their onset is met with a
sense of disbelief and betrayal. As an illness lingers, it becomes more
difficult to deny its foothold on our lives. Careers and educational
plans must be modified or discontinued. Depression and anxiety are
frequent complications. We face financial issues, difficult decisions,
and the inability to function as before. Massive skepticism by the
medical community, general public, and significant others contribute to the problems. These difficulties both result from illness
and, like all stressors, perpetuate its severity.

Just as a senseless death is a tragedy, so is a senseless life.
Chronic illness can rob us of our former lifestyles, activities, hopes,
and dreams. Periodically we get some of it back, only to lose it
again. Unpredictability of symptoms presents a burdensome and
continuous challenge. Those most severely afflicted lead a day-to-
day existence and are capable of taking care of only their most
basic needs. Essentially bedridden, they must depend on others
financially and emotionally. For others, the illness is cyclical:
"Down" periods are interspersed with more productive days.

The devastation of CFS and FMS is described by patients:

It's invisible, with no concrete thing to look at, like a big lump on your arm. Not only is it invisible to everybody else, but I begin to question whether it exists.

My body just crumbled. It was out of my control and scary. The early symptoms, then the inability to drive or learn, and then I just couldn't function. Am I going to be incapacitated? Am I crazy, or dying? What is going on?

I feel like I have permanent jet lag.

I gained weight for no reason that I know of; I can't control it, and I was used to controlling my life.

I do the things that I know are good for me, expecting they will help. Sometimes nothing helps.

Life is passing me by.

I ache from head to toe. Other times the pain moves around. It's invisible, but I live with it every day. People think they understand, but they don't—or can't.

I used to look forward to every day. Now I wake up totally exhausted and think, "Oh shit, I'm awake."

On a good day I feel like I've got this thing licked for good. I figure if it comes back I can handle it; I guess it's denial. On a bad day I think I'll never in my whole life feel good again. I feel useless, worthless, drained, fat, and stupid. I hate being sick. I hate myself and figure that anyone who loves me is even crazier than I am.

Michelle Akers, symptomatic with CFS since 1991, continued to play on the U.S. Women's National Soccer Team by attending to lifestyle and nutritional needs, taking in IV fluids, and sitting out a season trying to recover. The relapses continued, and she finally disclosed her illness in 1996. Interviewed on CNN in October 1999, Akers described CFS as "unimaginable to any of us until we experience it ... like just feeling totally empty on the inside. There's no reserve, no energy. It's like a black hole in the very depths of your soul."

"[CFS] is capable of destroying the *experience* of life," writes Hillary Johnson. "For me, [CFS] has been the most wrenching, discouraging episode of my life, changing my relationship with the world... [like] endless mononucleosis with a touch of Alzheimer's disease." In Part II of her *Rolling Stone* article, she described fruitless attempts to maintain a positive attitude; most often her mood was black and gloomy.

And everybody says, "I'm sick and tired of feeling sick and tired. I can't take another day of this."

Wondering each morning how we will feel that day, we pay close attention to the nuances of our physical and emotional functioning, alert for the development of new symptoms or for old symptoms subsiding. Others may accuse us of paying too much attention to our symptoms, but if we're not vigilant, we can invite a crash.

A good day (or week or hour) is a treasure. We attempt to spend our limited energy wisely and savor the pleasure of feeling good, or even halfway decent. We are on leave from being sick but can be called back at any moment. Ever alert for signs of relapse, we must be careful not to overdo, to cut our good time short.

On a bad day (or week or hour), time is interminable, life is bleak, and our goal is just to survive. Basic, routine activities, such as getting the mail and making minor decisions, become major tasks of enormous complexity. Kyle says, "I feel overloaded, overwhelmed. There are many days when I feel like I can't handle one more thing. I've made so many major decisions in my life. Now even the simplest thing is a major decision."

It is impossible to prepare for continual readjustment—to plan in advance or make major commitments. Every plan is tentative, carefully qualified with "maybe." We make "iffy" plans with others who are ill: "Would you like to come over on Saturday night about 8:00, if we're both feeling okay?" And the response: "Sure. Maybe. I'll let you know on Saturday at 7:55."

When we feel sickest, we don't even care about getting together with friends or doing other things we used to enjoy. Lacking motivation and goals, we feel lazy and awful. We're too drained and achy to *want to* want to do anything.

Uncertainty and unpredictability are hallmarks of the new lifestyle that we grudgingly adopt. These themes permeate every aspect of our lives: self-image, self-esteem, career, finances, education, relationships, and recreation. Our family, career, and social roles change; our feelings are unpredictable; and our bodies function strangely. Others don't understand. Friends, family, and doc-tors are puzzled by our altered behaviors and feelings. No longer able to contribute as we once did, we feel dependent and demand-ing. We lose a large degree of control over our lives. We feel sabo-taged.

Andy Rooney described having the flu as wanting only one thing: to recover. He noted how difficult it was to do such simple things as turn over and get up to use the bathroom. "I'd lie in bed wondering how I'd feel if this were a disease I'd never get over." That's where we're stuck—with an illness that might get better, or better and then worse, or just stay the same. Everything we've ever planned is up for grabs.

ECONOMIC EFFECTS

Loss of wages and benefits as medical expenses soar presents practi-cal and emotional hurdles. Chronic illness creates financial depend-ency on others: spouse, parents, friends and family, and perhaps on disability benefits. Dependency often brings feelings of embarrass-ment, frustration, and helplessness. Self-esteem plummets along with income and one's identity as a productive worker.

The effects of CFS/FMS on patients' ability to participate pro-ductively in the workforce have been drastic. Many who once worked full-time now work part-time or not at all. Men who are unable to work suffer the stigma of the inability to fulfill the tradi-tional male role as breadwinner, wage earner, achiever. Women who fought their way up the ladder to success and independence now find themselves disappointingly dependent on their spouses or fam-ilies for support. Young adults seeking independence are thrust backward into the role of dependent children. Giving up the roles and goals that helped to define us and gave our lives meaning is dif-ficult. And, on a more practical level, the financial crunch can be devastating.

Since so many of us had been strong, responsible people who still appear healthy, others' expectations of us remain constant. They are continually disappointed in our failure to function as we had previously.

Betty describes her boss's disappointed and disappointing reac-tion: "He kept saying, 'You've always produced for us.' I said, 'I can't right now. I can't concentrate. I can't absorb what I read.' He said,

'It's just a virus, so just work for a couple of hours and go home and rest and you'll do all right.'" Betty's reply: "I can't let him down. I can't let my family down. I can't let anybody down." But she was letting everyone down, including herself. Quitting her job and learning to relax was a difficult but eye-opening experience, since her department did continue to function in her absence. She learned to pace herself and rest as needed. Six months later, Betty felt somewhat better but not nearly ready to return to work. The good news: She no longer felt responsible or guilty for her inability to work.

Others comment:

I was at the height of my career when this thing struck.

I'm the kind of guy who never fell apart, a good problem solver and hard worker. Now I can't do the kind of job I can feel good about, so I don't work at all. It's a big hurdle for a Type A, workaholic, hard-driving, very successful, polyphasic thinker who loves what he does. These are abrupt and difficult changes.

My worst fear is being dependent.

My security got taken away.

I'm terrified that it will never go away and I will lie in bed the rest of my life with only the TV, magazines, and pets. There is no joy or fun in my life; I'm a burden. I can't participate in work or community activities. I can't get out of bed.

My life has become centered only in work because that's all I have energy to do.

I will have to retire earlier than I had planned, and I don't know how I will make it.

Such reactions are common in those who are unable to function at previous levels and whose careers, educational plans, and incomes have been drastically altered. The challenge of chronic illness is to continue meaningful activities but not to the point of jeopardizing chances of recovery—and to determine where to draw that line.

To continue what you are doing to whatever degree is comfortable for you at a given time requires difficult evaluations, flexibility, common sense, and guesswork. It means being honest about what is feasible, and shedding unrealistic, heroic self-expectations.

If unable to work, we enter the ranks of the disabled. Viewing ourselves in this light heightens the loss of our productivity, our contributions—our very identities. On good days we may feel ready to reenter the workforce, but when symptoms flare, we realize the impossibility of doing so. The accompanying stigma, coupled with the tedious and often adversarial process of attempting to obtain disability benefits, creates a heavy toll. Reliance upon insurance companies and the government for support is difficult to accept for those who are career-oriented.

The application process for disability benefits is long and frustrating, the paperwork is overwhelming, and the standards for determining disability are often unfair in the absence of "objective evidence," particularly a diagnostic test. Highly stressful, protracted battles with the Social Security Administration and private insurers shatter our naivete—the assumption that benefits were waiting for us should we require them. Relapses often occur during this process, which requires stamina and persistence. Once benefits are granted, we are subject to periodic reviews and must live with the uncertainty that benefits may be withdrawn.

EFFECTS ON SELF-IMAGE

Self-image is the way we view ourselves. Self-esteem is how we feel about ourselves, our sense of personal value and worth. Both are dramatically altered as we experience the new and unwelcome changes that accompany CFS/FMS. Having become strangers to ourselves, we must redefine who we are and determine what we can do.

Before becoming ill, Lorna was an outgoing, vivacious woman, self-described as "always up—the achiever, the giver, the caretaker. I was successful; I felt I could do anything I wanted to do. Now I have mood fluctuations, I become depressed, and even think of suicide. I feel guilty and vulnerable. I've lost my identity and my self-esteem."

Paula's self-esteem plummeted as her helplessness increased. "I've always been fiercely independent, radically so. I never needed any help, and after I became ill it was difficult for me to ask for any-thing. I kept struggling to try to do it all and got angry at the expec-tations of the people around me, but this is what I'd trained them to expect: that I could do it better than anyone. All of a sudden, I couldn't. My whole lifestyle, my mindset, the core of my identity. . . . I'm not who I was."

We feel a loss of control regarding our plans for the present and the future. Helplessness feels alien, uncomfortable, and dangerous; it is highly correlated with depression. Distorted self-statements compound the problems of chronic illness:

I want to be productive. I used to think I could be perfect if I tried hard enough. I was this superperson. Under stress, I just pushed harder. It worked for all those years.

I feel so stupid now. My brain isn't the same anymore. I can't even do simple things, like type. I don't think I've lost my sense of humor, but I have to fake it; life has become a lot more serious. I can't joke because my brain can't come up with anything smart. Things are fragmented. Sometimes I even have trouble talking, putting sentences together. I'll be in the middle of the most profound thing in the world, and I'll forget what I was saying.

I was successful, aggressive, fast moving, and I thrived on it. My pro-fession was lucrative. But I can't function like that any more. I can hardly function at all, period. I do the best I can, but I'm not the same guy I used to be.

I don't know what I'm capable of doing. I wish someone could tell me what to do and what not to do. Then I wouldn't feel guilty about all the things I'm not doing.

I was taught to be strong. Now I don't have the strength to get up off the floor. I feel I have failed my family, my coworkers, myself.

The uncertainty is awful. Will I be an invalid for the rest of my life? [Is it coincidence that invalid is spelled the same as invalid?]

The worst thing that could happen has happened: The functioning of my mind is impacted. I can handle physical discomfort, but cognitive impairment is frightening and horribly upsetting.

I can't lead a normal life. I live a one-dimensional life where I go to work and come home, spend the evening in my recliner, and go to bed at nine o'clock. I have no social life.

I can't handle the uncertainty of not knowing if I'm going to be me again. I feel like my brain will never be the same and I'll never be the same person I was before, even if I recover.

I was trained to be "fine." You're supposed to always be fine.

We define ourselves largely in terms of what we do. Indeed, this is usually the first question new acquaintances will ask each other: "What do you do?" How do we answer that embarrassing question when we can no longer function in previous roles? Options: *I sleep. I stay in bed a lot. I do what I can. I work part-time. I collect disability payments. I complain a lot.* Who am I without my former roles? Without something specific to *do*, we are unsure who to *be*.

Our self-messages are often negative and irrational, reflecting changes in self-image and self-esteem. We compare and catastrophize, damaging an already fragile sense of self with irrational beliefs:

I can't do anything now. I am not me any more.

I'll always be this way; I'll never get better.

I brought this on myself. It's my fault that I'm sick.

If I could think positively or do the right thing, I could banish this illness.

I should fake it, play the "I'm fine" game. I'm acceptable only when I'm well and productive.

I need to be taken care of; that's a sign of weakness.

I shouldn't complain.

I shouldn't be so down, so depressed.

I'm supposed to be strong, capable of anything, able to handle the responsibilities of the world.

I used to think I was smart, but now I'm stupid.

My life is over.

We might do well to remember that each of us has already coped with tremendous stress, misfortune, and pain. We've been to hell and back, and back and forth again, and have survived with strength and endurance.

FEELINGS

Feelings are pure emotion, irrational by definition. It's helpful to know how others in similar circumstances react so we don't feel so alone and crazy. We may feel...

▸ **Guilty.** Did I cause my illness? Did I choose to become ill? Is this "mind over matter"? Am I being punished for a wrongdoing? Am I somehow keeping myself from getting well? Is there something else I should be doing, or something I'm not doing right? I can't work any longer, or I don't work as productively as I should. I'm spending too much money on treatments that don't help. I shouldn't have so many needs. I'm letting everyone down, disappointing them. Maybe I'm just copping out. I don't have fewer responsibilities when I'm sick, just extra guilt for not carrying them out.

▸ **Misunderstood.** No one else really understands what I'm going through, except others who have it too. Those close to me may try to understand, and think they understand, but they really can't.

▸ **Overloaded.** Even simple tasks overwhelm me. I can't make decisions. I can't sort things out. I can't trust myself to judge the degree of a problem or to know how to react in proportion to its significance. I don't always know when I'm distorting.

▸ **Diminished.** I'm so much less than I once was. My physical and cognitive abilities have shrunk my identity and sense of self-worth. I don't feel as if I have a place in the world anymore.

▸ **Depressed.** I've lost so much—my career, hobbies, social activities, the ability to participate in life. Sometimes things are so bleak, disappointing, and pointless. I feel incapable and unlovable. Sometimes I cry over nothing; other times I need to cry but can't. There's nothing I value or enjoy. Life is just an interminable string of empty moments. Everything takes too much effort; nothing is worth doing. I'm not spontaneous or creative or fun loving any more. I'm a blob.

▸ **Desperate.** There's no hope. I've tried various remedies and interventions, even weird stuff, and nothing has worked well enough. Maybe nothing ever will. If only I knew what to do, I'd do it—whatever it was.

▸ **Suicidal.** Why don't I just die now? There's nothing left; my life is the pits. If I can't lead a useful life, I might as well not exist. I'd rather die than continue to exist like this. I need to get well or die. Virtually everyone with a debilitating chronic illness has considered suicide. Marc Iverson, founder of the CFIDS Association of America, commented in 1990: "I have known a number of individuals with this disease who have chosen death.... CFIDS steals so much of their lives that life is simply not worth living."

▸ **Isolated.** Sometimes I don't want to be alone, but I don't want to be with anyone either. Others can't possibly understand my feelings; I have no way of explaining them. Come closer; go away. I live in a private hell. An invisible wall separates me from the rest of the world.

▸ **Crazy.** Is this real? Have I lost my mind? This is a hall of mirrors from hell, distorted and freaky. Once levelheaded and able to cope, I've gone off the deep end. Awake and asleep, my thoughts are distorted. I'm not normal now, not myself anymore, and I don't understand this person I've become.

▸ **Sad.** I've lost so much. This is so difficult. I've been taught to look on the bright side, but right now there isn't one. Everything hurts—my body, my heart, my spirit.

▸ **Stunned.** I can't believe this is happening to me. I cannot accept this illness.

▸ **Deprived.** I live with so many limitations. What's left? I want a normal life back. My life has been pulled out from under me; so much has been torn away.

▸ **Uncertain.** Will this ever be over? Will I ever feel good again? When? How will I feel tomorrow? How will I feel in an hour? Why did this happen? Do I dare make any plans? Do I dare to have hopes and dreams?

- **Confused.** I don't understand what's happening to me. I can't make sense out of this predicament. I can't trust myself to think or react rationally and logically.

- **Helpless.** I feel out of control, like a victim. I'm physically and emotionally vulnerable. I'm being held hostage by something unpredictable, mysterious, and elusive. I'm trapped inside a body that doesn't work right and won't cooperate. I've lost faith in my abilities, my competence. I don't have the resources to fix this or even to adapt. The rules keep changing and all I can do is react.

- **Dependent.** I'm useless, worthless. I am forced to rely upon others to do the things I used to do. I was in the driver's seat; now I'm a passenger. I used to be a giver; now I'm a taker. It's not okay to be so needy.

- **Self-absorbed.** I become so wrapped up in how I'm feeling that I lose awareness of how others feel or what they need. I lack the energy to care. That's not like me. My entire focus is inward; I'm preoccupied with this illness and what it's doing to me.

- **Debilitated.** I have no energy. I feel used up. The vital part of me is gone.

- **Angry.** Why do bad things happen to good people? Why me? I hate this; it's unfair. I've tried so hard, and I've done so well; why am I being punished? This illness doesn't follow the rules. I *hate* this illness.

- **Weak.** I'm a wimp now. My body is weak; my mind is broken. I'm inadequate.

- **Afraid.** What will happen to me? Will I become sicker? Will I develop new, worse symptoms? Lose even more control? Will I get cancer? Die? My head is filled with frightening possibilities without answers. Nobody can assure me the worst won't happen. I fear that which I can't identify and don't understand.

- **Numb.** I feel dull, flat. This may be a temporary escape from emotional pain, but I can't feel pleasure either. I feel nothing.

- **Resigned.** It will always be like this. It's hopeless and endless. They'll never find a cure, or even a remedy. I might as well get used to it. My life as I knew it is over.

▶ **Hopeful.** Maybe there will be a breakthrough. Some people recover; maybe I'll be one of them. I just have to get better; I have to believe I will. Someday I'll look back on all of this....

▶ **Relieved.** It is possible to feel good, even if only for brief periods of time. I haven't forgotten how. There's hope.

The feelings vacillate unpredictably and uncomfortably, often triggered by symptom fluctuations. All these feelings are natural reactions to chronic illness; we must learn to recognize and express them. There are no shortcuts: Feelings don't go away when ignored; they go underground. Unexpressed emotions fester and ultimately spill out, often in inappropriate and damaging ways. Repressed feelings may further compromise the immune system.

EXACERBATIONS AND REMISSIONS

Acceptance is undone by nasty surprises.

— *Cheri Register,* Living with Chronic Illness

Although some exacerbations seemingly come out of nowhere, most are triggered by physical, emotional, or environmental catalysts such as these:

▶ Overexertion: periods of intense or increased physical activity.

▶ Changes in weather, temperature, barometric pressure, altitude, humidity, or general climate (especially abrupt or severe changes) in about 80 percent of cases.

▶ Emotionally stressful events, such as family problems and increased demands at work or elsewhere. (General stress is an exacerbating factor in about 94 percent of patients.)

▶ Exposure to environmental allergens or toxins.

▶ Changes in diet or water source.

▶ Hormonal or immunologic changes.

▶ Pregnancy (which also causes remission in some cases).

▶ Other illnesses or infections.

▶ Physical trauma, including surgery, accidents, and other injuries.

▶ Effects of medications.

▶ Air travel (in about 50 percent of cases).

Toni Jeffreys wrote in *The Mile-High Staircase*:

I sank down rather less gracefully than a dying duck. . . . Once again I was hauled up those stairs to bed. I was quite hysterical . . . with the horror of finding myself back in the nightmare. Every cell was crying out. My body was leaden. My head was in agony. I cried and screamed with what little strength there was left. And then I lay staring at the familiar hateful bedroom wall. . . .

Patients comment about their relapses:

I have to be careful to guard against exhaustion. I'm unable to determine an appropriate activity level. When should I crusade? When should I rest? What can I handle?

During a job interview, the room spun. I couldn't concentrate. It was a draining experience. When it was over, I wanted to go home and collapse, and they wanted me to do an extra test. By then I was totally out of it. I had been feeling better and then I realized that a focused, short period of stress could quickly catapult me into that deadened zone. I was wiped out for days.

I took my doctor's advice, got out of bed, and went back to the office. It was very poor advice; I got worse again. I was not ready to go back and would have been better off in bed.

Some days I feel calm and relaxed; things are going well and the world is rosy. But on "downer" days, the world is black. I can't put forth any energy. I just want to feel good again.

It's a crapshoot. One minute I'm having a life, not thinking about my illness. I'm not normal or well, but I'm making it! The next minute I'm flat on my back, in agony. Everything can change that fast. I can never count on the good moments lasting.

This is such an up-and-down thing; you feel like you're getting better and you feel like you can handle it, and then—Boom! Problems again, you start from scratch again, you lose hope again. How many times can you go on the roller coaster?

◆◆ Warning Signs ◆◆

Some crashes are preceded by warning signs: increased fatigue, pain, visual disturbance, or slowed motor activity. Although it's tempting to deny the indicators of a tailspin, noticing the signals and slowing down may decrease the severity and duration of the relapse. The sooner we pay attention to the body's request for a time-out, the less severe the relapse is likely to be, although sometimes it doesn't seem to matter what we do. The symptoms return full force.

It's tempting to assign blame when exacerbations occur. In the absence of a cause or a scapegoat, we may blame ourselves. "It is quite common to feel ashamed or guilty when the illness worsens," writes Cheri Register. "Most of us would rather believe that mind has authority over matter, if we can only learn how to enforce it." So we heap self-blame on top of the devastating disappointment of the crash, creating a bitter stew of fear, guilt, betrayal, and helplessness. Our feelings run the gamut from hope to desperation, from guilt to anger, as our lives bounce between harmony and chaos.

◆◆ Ah! Remissions ◆◆

The exacerbation is a black hole. I'm acutely aware of every second—difficult, dark, empty, painful. Then when the sun breaks through, the pain becomes a blur. I wonder where I've been all that time. I am so grateful to have the kind of day that I once considered only average.

The freshness and energy of remission are invigorating. Hope is rekindled; life matters again. We readily readapt to the pleasant sensations of living and are able to appreciate beauty and joy. Unwrapped from our cocoons, we are able to see beyond our own boundaries.

We are more aware of others and better able to tend to their needs. We reexperience the joy of giving spontaneously, willingly, and lovingly. Tempted by the fantasy that a reprieve grants permission to make up for lost time, we may overdo, expending excessive energy that puts us back into bed. A moderate activity level is difficult to achieve.

We learn to savor the moment, pushing back fears of relapse as we enter a period of tentative optimism. Ever cautious, we're alert for signs that the grace period is over. When the misery inevitably returns, we're back in the black hole, hoping for another reprieve.

EFFECTS ON RELATIONSHIPS

With the onset of CFS or FMS, others in our lives are puzzled but often sympathetic. Yolanda says, "When I first got sick, everyone was concerned, but now it's last year's news. Since it's not fatal, they think it should be gone by now." As time goes on, they may begin to doubt the existence of an invisible malady. As their doubts compound our own, we feel betrayed. The unfortunate labels "fibromyalgia" and "chronic fatigue syndrome" further detract from our credibility.

Two aspects of chronic illness are the obvious, physiological, tangible signs, and the hidden difficulties. The obvious signs are usually taken seriously, while the most distressing aspects are invisible. When there is a discrepancy between the two (feeling awful but appearing okay), others have difficulty grasping the true nature and severity of our illness. Seeing is believing. With no bandages, casts, or spots, we are presumed well, or at least suspect.

Since we may look fine while feeling horrible, others' expectations of us remain about the same, as they harbor erroneous assumptions:

You're sick? You look fine to me! (The severity of one's illness is directly proportional to its degree of visibility.)

No big deal; it's not terminal.

We should just get on with our lives as before and stop paying attention to symptoms, worrying, and pampering ourselves (i.e., resting so much).

It's an emotional disorder.

It must be curable. You get sick, you take medicine, you get better, right? Health will be restored with the proper resources—willpower, determination, the right diet, medicine, or exercise program.

If you complain, you're being negative. If you don't complain, you obviously feel okay.

A double bind: to tell or not to tell? How do we decide whether to fake wellness or to describe the feelings and symptoms honestly? We want our "invisible" illness to be acknowledged, but sometimes it's simpler to play the game and ignore it—the more socially acceptable option. Always aware of our symptoms and the reactions of others, our "I'm fine" act fools others into believing we are.

Our attempts to disguise or minimize symptoms may backfire. Well-intentioned others often make insensitive comments such as:

Maybe this illness is all in your imagination.

Do you still have that illness?

I read that chronic fatigue syndrome and fibromyalgia don't really exist.

You're lucky to stay home from work and have all that free time.

Cheer up. Things could be worse.

Everyone has the your symptoms. We all get tired, achy, and confused.

I think you just enjoy being sick—especially all the attention you get. You could get better if you really wanted to.

I know just how you feel.

And the silent, pervasive message: *You're not allowed to be sick.*

People react in a variety of ways to chronic illness, depending upon their own psychological makeup and issues, their perceptions of illness, and their belief systems. Our society encourages denial of all things unpleasant, especially those we fear or cannot readily understand. A lingering and debilitating yet invisible illness can be a trigger for the need to avoid contact and establish distance. Our pain and helplessness—and the fact that what's happened to us could happen to them—causes others to back away, while we feel unloved and abandoned. We have difficulty comprehending that their reactions have more to do with them than with us.

◆◆ Effects on Spouses and Partners ◆◆

Pledging "in sickness and in health," we are unable at the time to comprehend the full implications of the phrase. Initially, a shared tragedy will bring partners closer together, but as time goes on and the problem endures, the marriage may not. The divorce rate for couples in which one partner has a chronic illness is estimated at 75 percent (Pitzele 1986).

The ill partner requires attention, costly medical services, and financial and emotional support. These increased needs, coupled with the inability to contribute emotionally or financially as in the past, require significant relationship adjustments. Well partners bear the burden of increased workloads, while their needs may remain unexpressed because, after all, they are healthy.

Sacrifices become necessary. Life with a sick person becomes monotonous and dull. Plans must be canceled, dreams and ambitions put on hold. Many major decisions are dictated by the illness, but the caregiver is expected to remain understanding and patient. One partner said, "It's awful being around a person who's always depressed and lethargic. She doesn't accomplish anything; she feels lousy all the time. I want to be understanding but I'm too overwhelmed."

Spouses complain about the dual financial burdens of decreased income compounded by high medical bills. While desiring to help, they may distrust many health practitioners and costly treatment programs, often expensive "quack remedies" of questionable value. An understandable but unreasonable attitude may develop: "With me spending all this money, the least she/he could do is get well." Some partners become determined to pursue treatment regardless of cost. All are fed up with the illness that has destroyed their family's emotional and financial stability.

Pre-illness relationship problems are compounded. Changes in role expectations—the part each spouse is expected to play—are often not discussed. To push on grimly and silently seems heroic, as unexpressed but mounting pressure and resentment damage the relationship.

Despite changes in stereotypical male and female roles, men continue to be regarded as the primary wage earners and women as the family's emotional caretakers. When one spouse is ill, the other may need to take on both roles, creating a sense of guilt in the ill partner.

Hard-driving female achievers may be thrust back into an uncomfortably dependent relationship. Having achieved educational and career goals, accompanied by satisfaction, competence, self-esteem, and independence, a woman may be thrust into a role she has resisted: the dependent wife.

A partner who is a "fixer" may offer suggestions and advice, becoming angry if the ill spouse does not cooperate. If the ill spouse complies but the remedy is unsuccessful, the fixer may feel the need to place blame for this failure. Some problems are just not easily fixed, even when motivation is strong. Often the fixer is unaware that what the partner needs is support and understanding rather than well-intended but often ineffectual advice.

Chronic illness can become the primary focus of a relationship. Priorities must be balanced so that illness does not dominate the relationship.

Patients may experience a substantially diminished sex drive and insufficient energy to be sexually active. Some enjoy sex as a brief respite from illness, a time when they can forget and enjoy, but others find that sexual exertion triggers relapses, forcing them to weigh desires against consequences.

There's also the confusing "come close, go away" syndrome. The ill partner may crave the comfort of touch but be unable to tolerate the additional sensory input or may experience even gentle touch as extremely painful, causing the partner to feel rejected and alienated.

A once-active and contributing partner who is now depleted deprives the healthy spouse of a challenging companion. Communication becomes strained and difficult as cognitive dysfunction increases. The well partner may retreat, resulting in loss and loneliness for both.

At times the need to communicate is strong, but the words won't come. This is in part the result of an inability to express these new feelings, compounded by cognitive difficulties: impaired concentration, memory, and word-finding abilities. "I know what I want to say," reports Kyle, "but I get confused and my point gets lost, and it starts a fight." The words are jumbled, the message is distorted, and both parties become frustrated.

Many spouses learn to understand and handle illness-related stressors, while others find their tolerance and understanding wearing thin. In the face of preexisting relationship problems compounded by the effects of a chronic illness, some relationships are strengthened; others do not survive.

Even when significant others are caring, the illness remains a lurking enemy in the household, producing tension and disruption. Even with the knowledge that the problem is the illness rather than a lack of love, old problems escalate and new ones develop. It's tough to hang together with chronic illness in the way.

◆◆ Effects on Families ◆◆

Family priorities shift to accommodate the changes accompanying CFS/FMS, as feelings of confusion, anger, and resentment develop. The ill parent may feel guilty for creating problems and being a burden. Healthy family members may feel guilty because they were spared and resentful that the patient was not. The exacerbation-remission roller coaster renders family life unpredictable. Family members may be reluctant to express their own feelings and needs.

Restoration of homeostasis, or balance, presents a challenge. Adjustment requires flexibility, tolerance, clear communication, and problem solving. Family members must accommodate changing needs and new responsibilities. They must learn to be helpful to the ill family member without going to either extreme of denying the problem or becoming overprotective.

One patient's young son said, "When are we going to get Mommy back?" She used to take him to the park, where they would play and laugh together. Now she cries often, and her husband has assumed many of her former responsibilities. She says her whole family feels robbed.

Bill felt that he could no longer be an adequate father to his children:

> I can't discipline my kids appropriately or spend as much time with them. It's one of the saddest things I've ever experienced. They're energetic, always jumping around, wanting to do stuff. I can't do it. I do push myself because I want them to have a good experience, but my wife still carries an extra burden.

We worry that our children will be deprived of what they deserve and would have had if we weren't ill. Looking back on their childhoods, will they feel cheated? Probably—but all children do, and must learn that many of their expectations will not be met. We may become overly concerned with pleasing our children, but they, too, are subject to life's disappointments and must learn to cope.

Relationships with extended families change. As adults, we increasingly regard our parents as peers, but illness changes the traditional roles. Parents fall back into former parental roles with concomitant worry, advice giving, and sense of responsibility. They still want to make it all better and may try to deny the illness because of their own feelings of helplessness.

A curious role reversal takes place. Parents may lead active lives despite the inevitable difficulties that accompany advancing age, while their chronically ill children experience symptoms and deficits that, in the scheme of things, are supposed to happen to parents first. "I *feel* older than my parents *are*," we may think. "I have many of the same problems with my illness that they have with advancing age." We may feel ashamed to rely on our parents again: "Here I am again, needing more parenting—emotionally and financially." Illness interrupts the natural life cycle by making us dependent, middle-aged children.

Paula's role as her mother's primary source of support didn't end when Paula became ill:

> *It's been hard for me to say "I need." I'm still in a supportive role with my mother, who is just beginning to understand that I can no longer do many things. I always tried to live up to her expectations, but now she has to understand that there's something going on that I have no control over and has had to change her expectations. Now she says, "Are you up to it?"—a request rather than demand. Our relationship has improved.*

Illness presents a challenge in all family relationships. It shakes up the status quo and demands change. Those families who work together, drawing on collective resources to meet new challenges, become stronger as a result.

◆◆ Effects on Friendships ◆◆

Illness renders us different from our friends and alters our roles in friendships. Although we need support and understanding, we pull back at times during relapses and because of isolative tendencies. We are needier, often unable to participate in social events and preoccupied with our health status. Like other relationships, friendships may be strengthened in the process or may be shattered, unable to withstand the changes:

My friends have been tolerant and supportive. They take good care of me and yell at me to rest and take care of myself.

I have found out who my real friends are: those who understand, not those who want me to push too hard.

My personal life has gone down the tubes. I was dating and now feel unable to do that. People are afraid of catching something from me.

I lost most of my friends and feel devastated.

Most of us experience a combination of reactions from others. Special efforts at communication are required, which is difficult when energy is limited. Friendship becomes a balancing act between their needs and ours, and our needs often have grown to astounding proportions. The test of a friendship is its degree of flexibility—how well it can withstand change and allow for communication about what both parties are experiencing. Can our friends accept our limitations without judgment? Do they accept that we are ill despite the absence of obvious signs? Will they accept us when we are at our worst? Will our friends love us even when we are unable to love ourselves?

Each friendship is unique. Friends may disappear, stick with us unconditionally, or crumble after the early stages, distancing as the illness lingers. The survival of relationships requires continued readjustment and rebalancing.

12

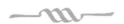

CFS and FMS in Children

This is NOT a "benign" disease. The loss to the minds and bodies of children who are too dysfunctional to attend school regularly is inestimable.
— *Michael Goldberg, M.D.*

Lisa, formerly a bubbly and energetic fourth grader, began to take naps after school, complaining of being tired and not feeling well. She became reclusive over time and stopped participating in family activities. She neglected her chores and became "overly sensitive to everything." Lisa complained of headaches, muscle pain, fatigue, and gastrointestinal problems. "I've always gotten sick a lot, but it was never like this. I can't get better. Nothing makes sense. I used to be smart, but my brain doesn't work right anymore. I cry too much. I feel like an old person." Ultimately, Lisa was diagnosed with both FMS and CFS by her pediatrician. She attends school, although her attendance record is spotty and she takes naps every afternoon.

John, an intelligent, perceptive fourteen-year-old, is the son of parents with FMS. He has been ill since childhood. Unable to attend school, John is bored with homebound instruction. His most troubling symptoms are pain, fatigue, depression, and cognitive impairment. He views his life as bleak and doubts he will have a productive future. John is trying to individuate from his parents and hates being dependent upon them. He is frequently irritable and even self-destructive, having hurt himself several times. Following a suicide attempt, he said, "I don't really want to die. I want to be normal, do normal things, and not feel sick all the time." Four years later, John is able to work and spend time with friends, although he remains symptomatic. "I don't know how I made it," he says.

Fran had to drop out of college during the first semester of her freshman year. She got sick after midterms and never recovered. An infectious disease specialist diagnosed CFS. "I might have it for the rest of my life," she says. "I have hobbies, but I'd really like to go back to school with my friends. They're all ahead of me; I feel left out and cheated. I don't know if I'll ever be able to have the life I wanted." Fran has decided to take one course at a time on the Internet, hoping eventually to earn a college degree.

The incidence and impact of CFS and FMS in children have been greatly underestimated, and no systematic studies have been conducted on this population. Some physicians distinguish between CFS and FMS in children; others believe the two are manifestations of a similar or identical illness. Children with CFS/FMS are often referred to as YPWCs (young people with CFIDS/CFS/FMS). The prevalence rate is not known, since many children remain undiagnosed by their pediatricians; prevalence studies rely on information supplied by parents, whose reporting may be inaccurate; many pediatricians miss or dismiss this diagnosis; and young children have difficulty describing their symptoms (Jordan et al. 2000).

Chronic illness is especially difficult for younger children, who have not yet fully developed their capabilities or identities. Those with a gradual onset may not recognize themselves as ill since they cannot remember ever feeling well. Having incorporated their symptoms into their concept of normalcy, they may assume that other children feel as they do. Assessing a child's full potential is difficult when symptoms have been present long-term.

INCIDENCE

Girls and boys are equally likely to develop CFS and FMS, and they have about the same number of symptoms. Girls are more likely to suffer from headaches, sore throat, and lymph node pain, whereas boys more often report memory and concentration impairment and postexertional malaise (Jordan et al. 1998). Fatigue is often less prominent in children than adults.

CFS/FMS are believed to be rare in very young children. Some parents believe their children were born with it, raising the question of possible transmissibility through pregnancy, childbirth, or nursing. Most physicians do not see or diagnose CFS or FMS below the age of five due to the infrequency of the illness and the difficulty in diagnosing the very young.

As in adults, the type of onset varies. Illness may develop after a flulike condition from which the child never fully recovers, or it may be gradual with no obvious precipitating event. Adolescents often have an abrupt onset following acute viral illness. Onset at puberty is common, perhaps related to hormonal changes.

The medical histories of children who develop CFS and FMS may include complaints of pain; frequent, recurrent minor illnesses (e.g., upper respiratory infections, sinusitis, ear infections, bronchitis); a family and personal history of allergies and sensitivities; and a low-energy state that may be perceived as "laziness."

SYMPTOMS AND DIAGNOSIS

The most prominent symptoms in children are fatigue (particularly after exertion), headache, abdominal discomfort or irritable bowel, depression, sleep disorder, body pain, dizziness, lymphatic pain, and neurocognitive problems. Unlike for adults, the symptoms may be almost equally severe, with symptom changes from day to day.

Children's vocabulary may be inadequate to describe such symptoms, especially fatigue, pain, malaise, decreased stamina, weakness, nonrestorative sleep, exhaustion following activity, cognitive problems (e.g., attention deficit, memory impairment, difficulty with words and numbers), mood changes, and neurological problems (e.g., feeling off-balance, altered perception). They have particular difficulty recognizing cognitive symptoms since their abilities are still developing. Although some children may complain about their symptoms, some do not, especially if they perceive them as normal or somehow their own fault. Their symptoms may be as severe as those in adults but less obvious because children are quite adaptable.

Since children often have difficulty describing what's wrong, parents should be alert to the following symptoms, especially if there is a family history of CFS or FMS:

‣ changed or atypical behavior, e.g., an active child who now shuns activity

- weakness and exhaustion, particularly following minimal or no exertion
- intellectual dysfunction: slowed thinking, diminished ability to concentrate, memory problems, sleepiness at school, acquired dyslexia, or a drop in grades
- sleep disturbance: insomnia, change in sleep pattern, restlessness during sleep (including frequent movements such as kicking), nightmares or strange dreams, or nonrestorative sleep
- complaints of pain affecting muscles or joints, particularly that which may be deep or burning, localized or bodywide.
- headaches
- gastrointestinal distress (e.g., abdominal pain and nausea)
- depression: tearfulness, appetite changes, or sense of hopelessness and helplessness
- moodiness, irritability, and frequent crying
- personality change, from energetic to inactive or from outgoing to introverted and isolated
- behavioral disorders at home or in school

CFS/FMS may underlie many scholastic, behavioral, and social problems. However, a child's complaints may be misinterpreted as any of the following:

- school phobia
- laziness
- attention deficit disorder (which may be present secondary to CFS/FMS)
- learning disabilities
- growing pains
- juvenile arthritis
- underachievement
- parental neglect
- attention-seeking behavior
- psychiatric illness: depression; anxiety with or without panic disorder; conversion of emotional distress to physiological symptoms

- separation anxiety; overdependency on parents
- manipulative behavior, such as malingering (faking)
- hypochondria
- Munchausen syndrome, or Munchausen syndrome by proxy (a feigned illness due to the child's—or a parent's—imagined symptoms and desire for treatment)

Children who are school phobic, faking symptoms, or seeking secondary gains would display symptoms on school days but not weekends. They would be unable to perform schoolwork and household chores but quite able to play. By contrast, children with CFS/FMS are symptomatic on weekdays and weekends (although those attending school may become more symptomatic as the school week progresses), with both play and work significantly affected. Like adults, children experience boost-and-crash cycles, engaging in activity and relapsing as a result.

Atypical behaviors and symptom complaints signal that something is wrong. When a previously active child becomes sedentary and loses interest in life, there is a reason. A full evaluation should be performed to determine the cause.

Children may be seen by many doctors before a CFS/FMS-knowledgeable doctor makes a correct diagnosis. Because adult criteria for CFS and FMS were not developed to apply to children, physicians must be alert for typical manifestations in the young.

ABNORMALITIES

Routine laboratory test results vary, much as they do in adults, but are typically within normal limits. Abnormalities in children have not been studied, but certain abnormalities may be found. Autonomic dysfunction may be present as evidenced by orthostatic intolerance (an abnormal drop in blood pressure when standing). Neurocognitive testing may reveal characteristic deficits, and results may be helpful in developing special learning plans when appropriate.

EFFECTS ON CHILD DEVELOPMENT

A child's chronic illness significantly impacts personal and social development, schooling, and the family. Social development and school attendance are disrupted, with resulting identity confusion, a sense of differentness, and uncertainty regarding future educational and vocational options.

Self-confidence is often undermined in a child whose school performance deteriorates without an understandable basis, who has difficulty remembering and concentrating, and whose grades plummet.

Children may be shunned by peers who regard them as outcasts or "losers" due to poor school performance and inability to participate in activities. Disrupted social development presents a tremendous challenge to the child who feels alienated by unsympathetic classmates, teachers, families, and physicians.

Feeling frustrated and misunderstood, some children present behavior problems. Adolescents may resort to drug use or suicide. Psychological counseling is often beneficial.

Most teachers and school administrators lack an adequate understanding of CFS/FMS and its effects. Parents frequently become advocates, educating the educators about the child's illness and seeking appropriate changes, including special school-related accommodations that are mandated by law for children with special needs. An individualized learning plan must be developed for children who are unable to learn in traditional ways, cannot attend school regularly, or require home tutoring.

EFFECTS ON FAMILY

Parents of chronically ill children may feel helpless and guilt ridden, and can be helped with education, improved communication, and the services of well-informed health professionals. Children need to be told that the illness is not their fault, that it is very real and treatable. They need reassurance, support, and encouragement to assuage their fears.

Family disruption may be significant. Children with CFS/FMS, who are often unable to participate in family activities or perform chores, may require greater flexibility due to their symptom fluctuations, and siblings may resent such "preferential treatment" and extra attention. Sick children need extra praise for their accomplishments but also need to be held to reasonable standards of behavior and responsibility.

TREATMENT

As with adults, treatment is mainly symptomatic, beginning with attention to sleep disorders. Children with altered circadian rhythms may function best at night, falling asleep late and sleeping until midday or afternoon.

Successful adaptation to illness may maximize these children's chances for maximum wellness. They may benefit from learning time-management skills, participating in exercise and activities (as tolerated), good nutrition, and taking rest breaks during the day. Detection and treatment of food allergies and sensitivities (often manifested as behavioral changes), strategic planning of activities and study time to correspond with higher-energy times of the day, special learning techniques tailored to cognitive deficits, and other coping techniques contribute to successful adaptation.

PROGNOSIS

The prognosis seems to be more favorable for children than adults. The majority of children experience partial or full recovery, although some remain quite ill and a few grow worse over time. Those who become asymptomatic remain at risk of relapse. No single factor predicts the course of the illness, but in the case of CFS, the prognosis seems more favorable in those with acute illness onset, epidemic (rather than sporadic) onset, and least amount of school missed. Despite social, academic, and emotional challenges, children are remarkably adaptable and many do well over time.

PART THREE

What You Can Do

13

Medical Care

Men of the cure have been more cruel than the disease.

— *Miguel de Cervantes,* Don Quixote

The needs of chronically ill patients present unique challenges for health care providers. Most of our symptoms are variable, unquantifiable, and difficult to treat. No standard tests or therapies exist for CFS or FMS. We react unpredictably to many medications, and what helps one patient may be useless to another. We have brief, positive responses to many therapies that then lose their effectiveness. Our ongoing needs and continued symptoms, unpredictable reactions to medications, and need for validation make us a frustrating lot to deal with.

In seeking treatment for problems that are invisible and difficult to explain, we often feel rejected by the medieval medical system on which we rely. In a frustrating quest to be treated as sane people with crazy-making illnesses, we may continue to seek treatment from a system that doesn't welcome us or become hopeless and give up. The fortunate ones among us have found exceptional physicians who understand and accept that we are ill, which in itself is therapeutic.

The physicians who are skeptical about our illnesses need to review medical history. Polio was once dismissed as "hysterical paralysis," ulcers were attributed to stress, and multiple sclerosis was "all in the patient's head," an hysterical disorder. Rheumatoid arthritis was a psychological disorder, and pernicious anemia was "tired blood." Tuberculosis was caused by depression, inadequate diet, and poor ventilation. And the *Titanic* was the "unsinkable ship."

Many doctors continue to say, "I don't believe in CFS or FMS," usually signifying that "If I can't test for it, it's not there." Doctors often cannot comprehend what they cannot see or measure, for they identify specific disorders by known markers or etiologies. An illness cannot achieve legitimacy in the absence of an identified cause or marker (a consistently measurable abnormality among patients). Routine laboratory work yields normal results, and so we are pronounced "fine" in a "well until proven sick" bind. Doctors should be prepared to acknowledge the limitations of our current state of knowledge. To reject the illness is to reject those who suffer.

When physicians lack a biomedical model that explains patient complaints, they revert to catchall psychiatric diagnoses: depression, somatization disorder, or malingering. As we experience significant losses in our lives, we are characterized as recipients of special fringe benefits available only to those claiming to be chronically ill: cushy disability benefits and pleasant leisure time. We may be accused of enjoying medical attention that is often unpleasant or unavailable. We are accused of adopting fashionable illnesses, participating in "fad epidemics," and avoiding productivity and responsibility.

Patients suffer not only with illness but at the hands of a rejecting and dismissive medical community that should know better. As researchers continue to document abnormalities, physicians will no longer be able to malign or ignore syndromes that do not fit neatly into their belief systems.

THE STATE OF THE HEALTH CARE SYSTEM

Medical consumers are no longer satisfied with perfunctory care and no longer regard the physician as a demigod who makes all the decisions and fixes everything. Tired of being treated like numbers (often numbers representing laboratory test results), patients are becoming their own advocates, expecting to be listened to and taken seriously, and asking questions rather than simply complying with recommendations. Medical consumers are now more likely to examine options, recognizing that standard medical practice is only one of many alternative sources of available health care.

◆◆ Physicians ◆◆

A surprising thing often occurs when doctors cannot hold an abnormal test result in their hands: they tend to think that there is nothing wrong with the patient.

— *Benjamin H. Natelson, M.D.*

CFS/FMS patients are often skeptical and defensive, having been damaged by cruel and dismissive attitudes. Whether your illness is chronic or acute, you want to know that your physician is concerned about you as a patient, but foremost as a human being. Just as consumers are becoming aware of more effective ways of dealing with the medical system, the medical system is becoming more impersonal, with policies dictated by insurance companies that have a disincentive to authorize the care we need. The physician can become either part of the problem or part of the solution.

A doc-in-the-box, mechanistic approach to patient diagnosis and care is unacceptable. Overreliance on advanced technology and data has replaced, rather than complimented, careful listening skills. Although we cannot expect doctors to be aware of all the nuances of every current health problem, we should expect them to be attentive, thorough, and willing to explore.

Careful diagnosis requires a complete medical history, a thorough medical examination, and a willingness to listen to the patient with an open mind. Diagnosis of illnesses in the absence of standard laboratory tests relies upon the knowledge, attitude, and skill of the medical professional. We should no longer accept an opinion that we are not ill, or not as ill as we think we are. We will not continue to be ignored, dismissed, or shuffled off to psychiatrists for problems that are "all in our heads."

◆◆ The Insurance Industry ◆◆

The insurance industry has largely taken over the practice of medicine, and the bottom line is the dollar, not the patient or the health care practitioner, for whom this system is counterproductive. At a time when patients are becoming more consumer oriented and insistent that their needs be met, doctors are finding it increasingly difficult to spend adequate time with their patients, now seeing more patients for less compensation. They are given disincentives to make referrals to specialists.

At the mercy of insurance companies, medical professionals, and laboratories, patients feel insecure. Unqualified personnel regularly make life-and-death decisions about patients, approving or disallowing claims with impunity. Our lives are in their hands, but this situation presents a conflict of interests. Their bottom line has a dollar sign in front of it, with patient needs regarded as an incon-

venience. Health-care reform is overdue, but the insurance companies are a powerful force with a strong lobby rivaling that of the
tobacco industry. Only marginally responsible for how they do business, insurance companies deny coverage for treatments and disability, and if the patient is too sick to fight back, so much the better.

Any physician who has weathered the changes in medical practice, with insurance company clerks dictating how to practice and
what doctors are allowed to do, has to be highly dedicated, independently wealthy, or certifiably insane.

CONCEPTS OF ILLNESS AND WELLNESS

We tend to view illness as the result of a germ, a sign that the body
has gone biologically awry, needing to be fixed by a pill or a procedure. But illness is not simply an interaction between a "bad" germ
and a "good" body. When exposed to a germ, some people become
ill and others do not. The larger picture must be considered: genetic
makeup; environmental conditions; nutrition; our thoughts, beliefs,
and feelings; social interactions; addictions; emotional stress and
pain; care or abuse of our bodies; and how we live our lives.

The very concepts of illness and wellness are poorly understood. "We know health well in its absence," writes Andrew Weil.
Apart from suggesting merely the absence of illness, however, the
term "wellness" connotes a harmony of mind, body, and spirit, and
an appropriate style of living and self-care—proper nutrition, rest,
and exercise. Attention to these aspects of health has generated
many unfortunate health fads; we seek magical remedies in our
instant-fix society. But the wellness we seek eludes us; it cannot be
purchased or easily achieved. We are impatient for relief but forced
to accept that there is no quick fix, and no *one* fix. The only reliable
"treatment" is self-care—seeking balance, slowing down. Though
medical professionals can help us augment the healing process, we
must dismiss notions of magical panaceas.

THE SPECIAL PROBLEMS OF CHRONIC ILLNESS

Wildly expensive medical care has made little advance against
chronic and catastrophic illness while becoming steadily more
impersonal, more intrusive.

— *Marilyn Ferguson,* The Aquarian Conspiracy

Doctors prefer to work with easier-to-diagnose and easier-to-treat illnesses. They are trained to cure people, and that's what they like to do. When they can't fix what's wrong, they become frustrated, their professional identities threatened. Once a series of expensive diagnostic tests has yielded negative results, the physician faces difficult choices. The temptation to dump us on some other specialty, usually psychiatry, is strong.

We are a huge inconvenience to professionals, particularly those with the attitude that unexplained symptoms and normal test results should not be taken too seriously. We don't get better, we don't go away; we just keep coming back with the same old complaints and additional new ones.

Patients who feel rejected and neglected either continue with their doctors, while harboring resentment, or seek medical attention elsewhere. Switching from one doctor to another or fragmenting care among several is common among the chronically ill.

Doctors would like us to cooperate by getting well, and we'd love to comply. However, physicians must learn to treat chronic illnesses without blaming themselves or their patients for remaining ill.

PATIENTS TALK ABOUT MEDICAL TREATMENT

Most initial doctor visits involve recitations of symptoms and the inevitable question, "What's wrong with me?" These inquiries may be met with a variety of discouraging responses, including accusations of hypochondriasis, depression, anxiety, inappropriate lifestyle, neurosis, inability to handle stress, laziness, or a "bug." Physicians are becoming more comfortable stating, "I don't know what's wrong with you. Let's see how we can identify the problem." Or, "It sounds to me like you have CFS/FMS. I'd like to refer you to someone who specializes in your illness." Or, "There is no cure, but treatment can help your symptoms."

Some patients report upsetting experiences:

I've been sent to a separate specialist for each of my symptoms. None of them understands that all these things seem to be connected. They won't listen when I tell them this is all one illness.

The neuropsychologist who tested me was mad at me; he said a third grader could do better than I could on the tests. He thought I just didn't want to work any more. I had a cushy job that I loved, and I was making a lot of money. Why would I want to stop? And my doctor believed everything this guy reported to him; he didn't believe me.

The nurse in my doctor's office said, "You must know you're causing these problems yourself." I told my doctor about it . . . but he didn't seem to care.

The advice I got was, "Just adapt to it. Rest a lot. Learn to manage stress. Persevere and be patient."

DIFFERENT SYSTEMS OF MEDICINE

Of the plethora of available treatment approaches, we typically begin with allopathic medicine, the dominant model in our society. Many health consumers have become increasingly disgruntled with this approach, turning to other types of medical practice and sometimes to dangerous "fringe" therapies. The greatest benefit is often obtained with a synergistic combination of intelligently chosen treatment modalities.

◆◆ Physical Approaches to Healing ◆◆

◆ **Allopathy** Most mainstream doctors in the United States practice allopathic medicine, which relies upon the use of pharmaceuticals and technology. Allopathic medicine excels at treatment of acute illness or trauma. Sophisticated technology allows access to the internal workings of our bodies, in many cases with noninvasive procedures. Many allopathic doctors are sensitive, caring, and open-minded; others are rigid, cynical, and resistant to new ideas.

Some doctors are more preoccupied with their machinery than with the health of their patients; they are said to treat test results rather than individuals. Studies have demonstrated the power of touch in mobilizing healing, but technology pushes doctors further away from their patients. The awe in which we hold hard science leads to reliance on objective measures, which, although extraordinarily helpful, are rendered useless in the absence of the human aspects of healing and the integration of test results with other sources of information.

The allopathic model clings to the antiquated notion of mind-body duality, drawing artificial distinctions between illnesses of the mind and those of the body. Dismissing the role of consciousness in wellness and illness may increase the distance between doctor and patient.

Allopathic medicine is often accused of falling short in dealing with chronic illness. Drugs can offer symptomatic relief, but deeper causes of chronic problems are less easily detected or treated. Allopathy has also been criticized for a lack of attention to preventive medicine and health maintenance, although patients often do not follow advice regarding preventative measures.

Allopathic medicine has both strengths and shortcomings. "Although disenchanted with establishment medicine," wrote Locke and Colligan in 1986, "we must be aware of the danger of turning wholeheartedly to other forms of treatment. The risks of alternative practices are in some cases ignored or minimized."

♦ **Osteopathy** Training for allopaths (M.D.s) and osteopaths (D.O.s) is similar, and their medical degrees are legally equivalent in all states. Osteopathy emphasizes structural aspects of the body (bones, muscles, and joints) and the body's innate capacity for self-healing. Osteopathic physicians are licensed to prescribe drugs and perform surgery, with added training in manipulative therapy for treatment of pain and structural disorders. Osteopathy has come to resemble mainstream allopathic medicine, and fewer D.O.s now practice therapeutic manipulation. Whereas many mainstream M.D.s viewed D.O.s as "pseudodoctors," or practitioners of alternative medicine, osteopaths have gained greater acceptance over the years. Although allopathic and osteopathic medical facilities are usually separate, cooperation between the two branches of medicine is most beneficial for patients as it becomes increasingly evident that medical skills and attention to the whole patient rather than the type of diploma are the truly relevant aspects of quality medical care.

♦ **Homeopathy** Homeopathic doctors seek to treat the whole body, to balance and strengthen it, and to identify symptom patterns in each patient. Homeopaths emphasize individual manifestations of illness, seeking to stimulate healing by tapping the body's innate healing powers rather than by simply medicating symptoms. Laboratory tests and diagnostic labels are not of paramount importance. Seen simplistically, homeopathy is based upon the principles that "like cures like" and "less is more." Rather than treating with pharmaceuticals, the homeopath seeks to isolate substances that produce symptoms like those the patient is experiencing. These substances are then highly diluted and administered so that the body will react against them, thus fighting the symptoms. The mechanisms responsible for the efficacy of homeopathic treatment remain speculative.

Some disenchanted mainstream physicians have "converted" to homeopathy in part because allopathic medicine has been ineffective in combating prevalent chronic and degenerative diseases. However, most mainstream medical practitioners regard the practice of homeopathy with suspicion, and the American Medical Association (AMA) has taken an exclusionary view of homeopathy, which lacks governmental licensing or regulation. Training involves a three- to four-year program, but some practitioners are poorly trained, having attended only a series of weekend seminars. Homeopathic treatment is quite expensive and is not generally covered by medical insurance. As with most treatments, homeopathy is helpful for some patients and not others.

◆ **Naturopathy** Naturopathy is based on ancient medical practices and includes Oriental medical approaches, botanical interventions, homeopathy, nutrition, and other modalities. Naturopaths rely on the body's innate healing ability and on curative properties of certain natural substances in the environment, such as plants and molds, the origins of many pharmaceutical products. Although the healing power of nature is certainly real, naturopaths lack a consistent, shared, methodical approach to treatment, and many of their practices are scientifically unproven. Some patients have reported excellent results with naturopathic healers, while others have not been helped. Some states license naturopathic physicians.

◆ **Traditional Chinese Medicine** An ancient practice steeped in tradition, Chinese medicine is often portrayed as a fad or a "New Age" approach to healing. Its integrated approach, more subtle than that of Western medicine, blends physical and spiritual healing. The body is viewed as an energy system, and illness as a result of blockages in the flow of energy (*qi* or *chi*) along circuits called meridians. Treatment is not diagnosis-based but instead aimed at correcting energy imbalances so that energy can flow freely, improving body functioning. Practitioners are licensed in some states.

Chinese medicine takes a long-term, preventive approach that is also helpful for chronic illness. Western medicine is acknowledged by practitioners of Chinese medicine to be more appropriate for trauma and acute illness. A combination of Eastern and Western medicine may be the accepted treatment modality of the twenty-first century.

◆ **Acupuncture** Acupuncture is a Chinese medical treatment in which fine needles—sometimes along with heat, electricity, oils, or lasers—are inserted at various energy points along the body's meridians. Acupuncture is used to treat specific symptoms, restore energy, and enhance feelings of well-being. While its mechanism of action is not fully understood, acupuncture is believed to stimulate the body's production of neurochemicals. Acupuncture has been practiced for centuries and is becoming a standard component of integrated medical treatment. Acupressure is a similar therapy in which a trained practitioner applies manual pressure, rather than needles, to certain points on the body.

◆ **Ayurveda** An integration of philosophy and medicine, ayurveda has origins in ancient India. It encourages a wholesome lifestyle, incorporating diet, herbal preparations, massage, meditation, and behavior. The whole person rather than the diagnosis is the focus of treatment, which seeks to enhance and integrate the three life forces: movement, digestion, and structure. The practice of ayurveda is not licensed or regulated by federal or state agencies.

◆ **Other Physical Therapies** Many other treatment approaches, including massage, physical therapy, craniosacral therapy, chiropractic care, occupational therapy, and nutritional therapy, are beneficial when used adjunctively with medical care. Each method of treatment has advantages and limitations, and the patient's belief system plays a large part in determining success. The availability and growing popularity of alternative approaches indicate that there is no one correct approach.

◆◆ Mental and Spiritual Approaches to Healing ◆◆

When investigating nonphysical approaches to healing, a certain level of suspicion is healthy—we must not accept new therapies blindly—but we should also guard against rigidity and immediate rejection of anything new or unusual. Any tool that mobilizes hope is helpful in reducing feelings of helplessness and victimization.

Alternative treatment approaches vary widely in success rates, and some claims are exaggerated and unfounded. Many systems of practice lack credentialing organizations, and individual practitioners may differ radically in approach, theory, competence level, and cost. Medical insurance does not usually cover treatments considered experimental, and since there are no standard approaches to treating CFS or FMS, all interventions are deemed experimental.

Types of treatment range from beneficial to harmless to dangerous—and many are quite expensive. An outbreak of a new illness or increased attention to an existing one invites the development and aggressive marketing of a flurry of treatments, often touted as cures. Safety claims may be fabricated, especially when products are labeled as "natural" (poison ivy and arsenic are natural, too). Despite claims of "miracle cures" and wildly successful therapies, no treatment miracles have emerged.

◆ **Positive Thinking, Faith Healing, and the Like** In the growing movement of patient empowerment and the belief in the healing properties of the human body, the potency of positive forces is respected. In such diverse healing systems as shamanism, Christian Science, and folk healing, intervention is believed to be a supernatural, or at least superhuman, phenomenon. Such approaches are oriented toward the intervention of forces beyond the usual range of human understanding and the limitations of technological and cultural beliefs.

Faith in any method is a strong factor in its success. For example, healing rituals produce positive results in communities with strong spiritual beliefs and support.

Skeptics abound, especially in cultures that place a high value on science and logic. Our society faces a dilemma: We reject overreliance on technology that reduces the patient to a label or number but have difficulty embracing practices that lack scientific validation. We are skeptical of such procedures as hypnosis and guided imagery, but less so when technology such as biofeedback equipment is introduced to demonstrate scientifically measurable results.

The need for surgical intervention in the case of appendicitis is obvious. However, interactions between an intangible illness and an unobservable intervention encourage disbelief even when results are successful. The practices of prayer, imagery, belief in the supernatural or invisible, innate healing sources, or any type of spiritual medicine is alien to our culture. Although we tend to believe in the "power of positive thinking," we have difficulty believing that it can truly affect healing. Can faith and belief transcend and heal physical symptoms? If not, how can we explain the apparent success of some of these methods?

◆ **Psychology and Psychiatry** Although the fields of psychology and psychiatry are attaining more realistic and legitimate status in our society, the need for therapy is often as suspect as its practice. Mental health or behavioral health practitioners vary in approach, education, training, and personal style. Therapeutic goals often include personal growth, insight, behavior change, enhanced self-esteem and efficacy, problem solving, and emotional support. Some issues may require only short-term therapy, while more complex, deep-seated issues may require long-term treatment.

In my experience as a psychologist who treats chronically ill patients, I find that a number of interventions are helpful, but the type and duration of therapy depends on individual needs rather than a one-size-fits-all approach. Cognitive behavioral therapy (CBT), a recent focus of attention in chronic illness, is indeed a potent therapeutic tool for many patients. CBT helps an individual to identify faulty, irrational beliefs; to challenge them; and to develop more rational, productive beliefs and behavioral changes. This process is quite helpful with depression, coping skills, and adoption of more healthful behaviors, but it is not a panacea for the chronically ill.

DEVELOPING A POSITIVE DOCTOR-PATIENT RELATIONSHIP

If you expect your physician to pull you out of this, forget it. You're the best treatment you've got. Use your doctors to help you.

— *Arthur Schimelfenig, Ph.D.*

Teamwork is essential to effective treatment. Physicians are experts in the field of medicine but are human beings first, and all of us are experts regarding our own bodies.

Unfortunately, physicians often receive little or no training in communication skills. Doctors are confronted daily with patients' fears and insecurities, which may be increased or alleviated during visits. When communication is abrupt and cursory, the patient is left with unanswered questions, misunderstandings, and additional fears that may negatively affect the treatment outcome. To doctors who give orders rather than offer explanations, "difficult" patients are those who ask many questions and expect to participate in their health care. Doctors who demand patient compliance, ignore patient input, and act too busy to care are "difficult" doctors.

We want doctors to be something more than mechanics. We expect them to pay attention to our concerns and treat us with compassion as well as competence—a lot to ask, but the only path to successful treatment. We appreciate new technology but abhor its overuse. Treatment of the whole patient is essential—not just test results, isolated symptoms, or body parts, but the whole human being. We benefit most from doctors who communicate well, behave respectfully, and consider alternative approaches to healing and medicine, exercise, and nutrition. All healing is scientific, according to Bernie Siegel, M.D., even when we cannot explain how the healing occurs.

Patients and doctors each have responsibilities in their relationship. A true partnership between doctor and patient combines the perceptions and strengths of both based on a foundation of communication, trust, and mutual participation.

◆◆ Patient Responsibilities ◆◆

▶ Be a well-informed consumer of medical care. Make sure in advance that you see physicians who are experienced in diagnosing and treating CFS/FMS. You're the customer; shop carefully for your experts.

▶ Although your decision to see a particular doctor should not hinge solely on cost, you have the right to know up front what the charges will be.

▶ Request extra time with the doctor when scheduling your appointment, if necessary. Expect to be charged for the additional time.

▶ Keep careful track of your appointments and give a twenty-four-hour notice (barring emergencies) if you cannot keep an appointment. Arrive on time. If the doctor is habitually late, discuss this problem not with the staff but with the doctor, who is ultimately responsible for scheduling.

▶ Arrive prepared. At your first visit, you may want to offer a list of past and current diagnoses; date and type of illness onset; a concise relevant medical history; past treatments and results, including beneficial and adverse effects; and the reason for your visit. Make copies of previous medical records and test results available to your new physician. If this is your first visit, you may prefer initially to remain fully clothed and meet the doctor in the office rather than an exam room.

▶ Bring to each visit a list of current symptoms and concerns, your questions (limited to a few per visit), and all medications and supplements you are taking.

▶ Maintain a medical file containing a copy of records from each doctor you have seen. Organize them systematically; you will probably need them for reference.

▶ Be well informed about CFS/FMS. Offer new or interesting information to your doctor, making it clear that you are sharing information rather than telling your doctor how to practice medicine. Physicians cannot keep up with every new medical development but should be open to reasonable amounts of new information.

▶ Ask questions when you need information about your illness, prognosis, medications, or other treatment options. Specific questions will generate clearer answers.

▶ Listen attentively during your discussions and take notes. Ask questions until you are sure you understand the answers. Since information that makes sense at the time can be difficult to remember later, consider bringing someone to appointments with you to corroborate or expand on your history, offer observations, clarify information, and take notes.

▶ State your needs and concerns assertively. If you have a complaint about medical care, bring it to the attention of your doctor in a straightforward, businesslike manner. Complaining is not productive, but direct, reasonable requests often are.

▶ Become aware of the role you are playing as a patient. Are you the dependent child, expecting your doctor to be the magical healing parent? Develop an adult-to-adult relationship based on mutual respect and your need for a competent, caring medical professional—not a parent. Differentiate between obedience (doing what you are told without questioning) and cooperation (working as a team with your physician).

▸ Refrain from punishing your doctor for sins of past professionals. You may have been dismissed, denied, and maligned by others, but do not make assumptions or become unnecessarily defensive with a new doctor because of past experience.

▸ Recognize that medicine is not a hard science and that diagnoses and treatment plans are judgment calls based on objective and subjective information. Let go of unrealistic expectations that a single therapy will cure a long-term, complex illness.

▸ Be honest. Don't fake feeling better than you do just to please the doctor. Although doctors like their patients to get well, you do yourself a disservice by pretending.

▸ Communicate your satisfaction to the doctor when you are pleased with your medical care. Specific praise is most meaningful and helpful.

◆◆ Health Care Practitioner Responsibilities ◆◆

▸ Jump off the pedestal. Let your patients know that you don't view yourself as omniscient.

▸ Talk to your patients. Tell them what you think; tell them when you don't know or aren't sure—that you don't have all the answers. Initially you may disappoint them, but in the long run you will be doing them (and yourself) a service. Offer explanations and information and explore alternatives with the patient.

▸ Listen to your patients without preconceived notions. Their statements will be at least as informative as their lab test results, and your willingness to listen demonstrates your caring.

▸ Take your patients seriously. Patients often overhear doctors talking about them or other patients in a flippant manner. This behavior is insulting, hurtful, and trivializing. Please recognize that you are dealing with human beings, not cases. No one wants to be "the appendectomy in Room 402."

‣ Avoid the labels "somatizer," "hypochondriac," "neurotic," and "crock." All symptoms have origins and should be taken seriously. If you don't understand what's going on, say so, but don't battle with the patient regarding the existence of a "real" illness.

‣ Avoid assuming a parental role that fosters childlike dependence and, ultimately, resentment in your patients.

‣ Let patients know you cannot effect a quick cure or alleviate all of their suffering but will do your best to help them to feel better. If you are unable to diagnose or treat them, tell them and discuss options.

‣ Recognize that some patients will return visit after visit without improvement. This is not your failure or theirs; it is characteristic of the illness. It is natural to feel disappointed if there is no change (or negative change), but avoid making statements that cause the patient to feel guilty for the lack of progress, and avoid blaming yourself for your inability to solve a puzzle that has stumped the experts.

‣ Keep an open mind about newly emerging concepts and treatments. Patients have a strong network and will hear of various treatments that sound unusual; consider such options only if they are not likely to cause harm.

‣ Your patients have emotional needs that are inseparable from their medical needs. They need your understanding and support and need to have their suffering acknowledged although it can't be "fixed." A simple statement such as "I realize this is really rough for you" can be quite comforting. While you are conceptualizing the disease, the patient is often experiencing confusion and fear.

‣ If patients are using their time with you to discuss emotional issues, offer a referral to someone who can help them in that area. Explain the purpose of any referral for psychological or psychiatric treatment so your patient doesn't feel "psychologized," dumped, or dismissed.

- Offer your patients guidance and encouragement to take responsibility for their own care in the realm of lifestyle modification (activity level, diet, physical modalities, adjunctive treatment, support groups, and so on). Patients often feel "disciplined" (shamed or scolded) by doctors, reinforcing dysfunctional parent-child roles. A preface such as "I know it's really hard to give up some of the things you really like, but..." encourages the patient to perceive the suggestion as positive motivation rather than an order. Patients are often fearful that their doctors will "yell at them" to promote compliance; empathetic guidance works better.

- Show respect for your patients by keeping to your appointment schedule as closely as possible. Barring emergencies, excessive lateness is not acceptable. Discuss scheduling problems with your office staff.

- Allow patients to share information with you. Some of your CFS/FMS patients are more knowledgeable about their illness than you are. Many have read extensively, networked, and contacted support groups to obtain information.

CHOOSING A DOCTOR WISELY

The worst way to find a doctor is to consult the yellow pages for a name that sounds good or a location that is convenient. Here are a few more successful methods:

- Consult your local support group for a list of recommended doctors and other professionals. You may need to see several types of specialists, but have one physician consolidate and oversee treatment.

- Consult *The American Medical Directory: Physicians in the United States* in the reference section of your public library or use respected online resources to obtain information about individual physicians, including type of practice, training, credentials, and board certification.

- Once you have chosen a candidate, ask if and how the doctor treats CFS and FMS and how long she or he spends with each new patient. If the answers are satisfactory, make an appointment to interview the doctor. You are in a "hiring" situation. Prepare pertinent questions in advance.

‣ Use referrals and information about a doctor as a starting point, and then trust your instincts to determine whether you can work well with and trust this professional. Ask yourself these questions:

– Is this professional knowledgeable about CFS/FMS, including treatment options?

– Do I feel comfortable with this doctor? Is this someone in whom I can confide?

– Do I feel listened to and understood? Am I being given the doctor's full attention, free from distractions?

– Are there likely to be power struggles? Is this person abrupt or arrogant?

– Does this doctor have an open, accepting, positive attitude?

– Do we share the same treatment philosophy?

– Is a sense of hope being conveyed to me?

– Is this doctor willing to admit uncertainty, to say "I don't know" when appropriate?

‣ Be realistic. No physician will meet all criteria, so decide which qualities are the most important. Don't expect inappropriate favors from a doctor, such as falsifications on insurance forms or frequent telephone calls in place of office visits.

◆◆ If You Are Dissatisfied with Your Doctor ◆◆

Many patients complain about poor doctor-patient communication. The highly motivated patient who addresses specific problems directly will probably obtain better results from the health care system.

Examine your complaints for validity, and discuss the problems openly with the doctor, not a staff member. Ask questions and request changes in a considerate, positive way, focusing on each specific problem and the desired outcome or solution options, and evaluate the doctor's response. Because most patients feel more comfortable grumbling to others than discussing problems directly with their doctors, your doctor may be surprised to hear of your dissatisfaction. Your doctor may have requests of you as well; listen objectively before launching a defensive reaction.

If you can agree on changes to be made, allow a reasonable time for them to take place. If the problem is not corrected, consider switching to another doctor.

If you have switched several times and are still dissatisfied, your expectations may be unrealistic. Perhaps no doctor can provide what you're seeking. However, do not compromise on reasonable standards.

UNPOPULAR TRUTHS

CFS/FMS patients fall through the cracks of medicine. When we are ill, we are expected to do one of two things: get well or die. We do neither. We continue to be sick despite the many therapies available, presenting an impossible challenge to those who would like to cure us.

There is no magic bullet, no universally successful form of treatment. We would like to believe there is a single causative that we can fight and eradicate, but the true picture is complex.

In the absence of a cure or even a standard therapeutic regimen, we continue to challenge our physicians to make us well, or just better. We are not popular patients; our symptoms are numerous and diverse, we don't tolerate medications particularly well, and each of us responds differently. There is no true "normal"; what is typical of one person may be atypical for another. Each of us is unique and complex, functioning differently and responding individually to treatment. We plague relatively helpless physicians with scores of symptoms that they can only palliate, if that. Most of us have become savvy, well-educated health consumers with many questions. We are a difficult lot to treat.

Any treatment carries the risk of harm, no one has all the answers, and the doctor does not necessarily know best. Few medical professionals offer the combination of knowledge, experience, warmth, and understanding that we crave. When a treatment fails to help, there is no one is to blame, no appropriate target for our anger and frustration. The bottom line is this: We are responsible for our own medical decisions and care.

Medicine is not a perfect or an exact science, and treatment is a trial-and-error process. Healing remains an art, a combination of scientific knowledge, skills, and intuition.

GOOD DOCS: PROFESSIONAL PARIAHS

I know that these people were well, and now they're sick, and they're staying sick. So I have to hang in there and be diligent about it, regardless of what the rest of the world thinks.

— Daniel Peterson, M.D, speaking about the Incline Village
CFS outbreak in the early 1980s

Although many patients have expressed disgust, bitterness, distrust, and anger at their physicians, many have found excellent physicians who are knowledgeable, understanding, and helpful. The qualities deemed most important by patients are competence, honesty, warmth, concern, willingness to listen, being down-to-earth, and willingness to spend adequate time and explore treatment alternatives. Physicians who acknowledge and treat such illnesses as CFS and FMS risk judgment by their colleagues and are often viewed by their colleagues as pariahs or "fringe" doctors. Patients greatly appreciate doctors who are brave enough to stand up for their beliefs and for us. Many conduct time-consuming studies and share their knowledge with patients and professionals at medical conferences.

Medicine is riddled with challenges, and exceptional physicians are up to the task. We are not an easy bunch to treat; each of us represents an experiment. Physicians who study and treat CFS and FMS are of a special breed; they are willing to endure the censure and even ridicule of their rigid, conservative colleagues to provide needed care. Outstanding health practitioners are to be commended for accepting and believing their patients rather than following the skeptical professional flock.

Patients who have a close rapport with their health professionals fare best. In a vulnerable and compromised state, we need to trust our physicians and regard them as allies in the struggle. Those of us with CFS and FMS are grateful to the exceptional doctors who have respected us, listened to and believed us, and treated us with compassion. A growing number of concerned health care providers have devoted long hours to research and treatment. Those who are dedicated to practicing the art as well as the science of medicine are truly special. We respect and appreciate them beyond measure.

14

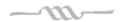

Treatment of CFS and FMS

There are many different approaches, many claims, and many theories. The bottom line is that no approach consistently produces long-term results for the majority of patients. We need a breakthrough.

— *Scott Rigden, M.D.*

When diagnosed, many CFS/FMS patients assume every illness has a cure, or at least a standard treatment regimen. Expectations turn to disappointment as we learn that there is no universally successful treatment. The subsequent search for treatment options begins with the search for an open-minded physician who is willing to coordinate a multifaceted treatment plan that integrates synergistic therapies.

Since no established treatment protocol exists, we learn to be good medical consumers, not too closed-minded to experiment, but sensible enough not to be gullible to every patient testimonial for the latest fad treatment. We must not be easy prey for the unscrupulous, or for the well-intentioned folks who would have us try every remedy that comes along. We must become experimental scientists, choosing wisely among alternatives, giving each a fair trial, and not assuming that our treatment at the time of remission was the sole cause of improvement. We must learn to be self-protective to the point of being wary or cynical.

All treatment is potentially dangerous if misused. The current trend toward the use of "natural" products is based on the false assumption that "natural" equates with "safe." Any substance that enters the body can alter its functioning.

Most doctors rely on pharmaceutical drugs as a primary treatment modality. Many medications ease suffering and save or prolong lives, but they can create new problems as well. Any substance powerful enough to affect body chemistry is capable of causing serious side effects or severe complications. Many of today's "miracle" drugs (if only we knew which!) will be deemed worthless or even harmful in the future. Some pharmaceutical products, once considered safe, later produce tragic results with indiscriminate use. Little is really known about the synergistic interactions of drugs taken simultaneously. Our best bet is to take a careful yet open-minded approach to treatment.

Our concern about the risks of experimental treatment decreases in inverse proportion to symptom severity. We try out various medications, weighing risk, fear, and uncertainty against our degree of desperation. In the dark about the long-term effects of a drug, and yet weighing relief against an unknown future, we are likely to use what might bring welcome relief. We often choose to try promising therapies rather than wait for the results of scientifically valid, double-blind studies to ascertain their safety and effectiveness as we continue to suffer. In the absence of standard therapies, we justifiably feel like guinea pigs, since every treatment attempt is an experiment.

Much available information about treatment results is anecdotal, that is, based upon individual experiences or informal trials with small numbers of patients. Anecdotal reports provide interesting leads as to what might be helpful, but we get only small bits of information. We need more systematic, scientific trials, which are expensive and (sometimes unnecessarily) time-consuming, and in the meantime we need symptom relief. Physicians, in a similar bind, want to use medications wisely but cannot wait years for results of experimentation when their patients are ill *now*.

Lack of a standard treatment regimen creates difficulties for patients and health care practitioners. Deciding which treatments to try is confusing and frustrating. Evaluating their effects is almost impossible, given the unpredictable course of the illness and changing responses to medications. Well-intentioned friends and family members offer advice and admonitions. ("There is a stigma now about taking drugs," said one patient. "My mother and husband think I shouldn't need or take them. The next minute they read about the latest 'breakthrough' and want me to try it.") Given the number of failed therapies and disappointments, we are tempted to give up and go cold turkey, but as much as we would like to "just say no" to drugs, our need for relief is intense.

When a particular treatment seems to be effective, we are often told this is just a "placebo effect," as if the placebo response were synonymous with voodoo. It is actually the power of belief, our confidence in a treatment or a physician that triggers mobilization of our internal resources. Belief in the curative power of a treatment can be as potent as the treatment itself; the interaction of the mind (our set of beliefs) and the body's physiological response together determine a therapy's success. Although a scientific rationale for a treatment's apparent effectiveness is not always available, positive belief and hope help create physiological change. Paul Cheney, M.D., views the placebo response as an expectation of wellness that causes the emission of polypeptides from the central nervous system, improving immune function. "The most important thing is to pick a therapy you believe in and proceed with a positive attitude," writes Bernie Siegel, M.D. Norman Cousins described the placebo as "the doctor who resides within." Instilling hope is one of the practitioner's most valuable functions. Knowing that there are more options to try, that relief is possible, and that I have good doctors on my side has often kept me going.

An entry from my journal states: "Another new medicine, and renewed hope. I'd sell my soul for a magic pill. And then some weird-ass reaction to the medicine or none at all, and there goes the hope...until I hear about the next minor miracle, which, against my better judgment, I will probably try. Do I feel better because I'm hopeful, or do I get hopeful when I'm feeling better? Both, I suspect." One's belief system constantly evolves; we cannot simply self-impose an effective healing philosophy. Developing an understanding of the complex mélange of hope, behaviors, new therapies, and an emerging belief system is a challenging process.

When something seems to help, the properties of the treatment, combined with the relief and sense of hope, interact in a psychological-physiological process. If it is helpful without causing undue harm, the treatment is of value. If a treatment is initially effective but later loses its beneficial effects, we may discontinue it for a period of time and then try it again. If beneficial effects are not felt the second time around, it may have been another one-shot wonder.

When a treatment makes symptoms worse, we may be told that we are having a "healing crisis" and that our discomfort results from the detoxification process. Although some medications cause initial temporary side effects, it is unclear whether a so-called healing crisis, especially when protracted, is a positive sign.

The spectrum of treatments is amazingly diverse. Symptom severity and our degree of desperation often determine how aggressive treatment will be. Physicians favor particular treatment approaches, tailored to the needs of the individual and evolving as new therapies develop. Even promising drugs yield variable results: significant alleviation of symptoms in some patients, modest improvement in others, and no response or adverse effects in the remainder. One person's miracle is another's poison.

FACTORS THAT MAKE CFS AND FMS DIFFICULT TO TREAT

An old adage states, "An illness for which there are many treatments has no cure." The corollary is, "When there is no cure, there will be a multitude of treatments."

— *Jackson Parkhurst, letter in* The CFIDS Chronicle

CFS and FMS are difficult disorders to treat, for many reasons:

‣ There are no FDA-approved or universally successful therapies—no magic bullets.

‣ Patient responses are variable and idiosyncratic.

‣ Exquisite medication sensitivities are common.

‣ Pathophysiology remains undetermined, so we can treat effects (symptoms) but not cause.

‣ Little research has been conducted. The government does not consider us a priority, and research into supplemental or alternative therapies is scarce due to lack of profit incentive.

‣ Responses to treatment may vary over time; a treatment may be helpful now but not next week.

‣ Treatment success may vary with the length of time one has been ill and other undetermined factors, helping some subgroups but not others. These subgroups remain largely undefined.

‣ Medications regarded as effective in treating "typical" pain may not help FMS pain.

‣ Symptoms wax and wane regardless of medications used, rendering assessment of treatment effectiveness impossible.

‣ Side effects of treatment may resemble illness symptoms, such as sedation, lethargy, confusion, mental fuzziness, emotional instability, and feeling "wired" or overenergized. Are we to attribute these symptoms to the intervention or the illness?

‣ Medications and other therapies work best when used additively and synergistically, making it difficult to ascertain what is helping.

‣ Competitive inhibition (medications and foods competing for the same enzyme system) potentiates or inhibits metabolism of therapies, modifying their effects.

◆◆ Limitations of Treatment Studies ◆◆

Before pharmaceuticals are made available, they must be studied for safety and effectiveness, although errors do occur. Controlled scientific studies have both great value and serious limitations, such as flaws in methodology and criteria for inclusion, small numbers of patients studied, and erroneous conclusions. Medication trials offer useful information—and sometimes misleading information; results may be nonreplicated or contradictory. In addition, studies of CFS/FMS treatments have these limitations:

‣ Data may be skewed in the direction of "normalcy" by large numbers of patients who cancel testing appointments due to illness, inability to drive, and conflicts with medical appointments, and those who break the study protocol, turning elsewhere for treatment.

‣ CFS/FMS patients have idiosyncratic responses.

‣ CFS/FMS patients may take longer than expected to respond to medications, and most trials are short-term.

‣ Response to medications may change over time.

‣ Symptom changes are not necessarily related to the substance being studied.

‣ Trials usually study one intervention at a time to limit the number of variables, but synergistic use of therapies is more effective. Treatments are usually studied in isolation, which limits our knowledge of synergistic benefits and dangers.

‣ Overreliance on technology often outweighs participants' subjective responses.

‣ Symptoms of CFS/FMS cannot always be distinguished from side effects of a treatment.

SUGGESTIONS FOR PATIENTS AS CONSUMERS OF HEALTH SERVICES

Unable to afford the luxury of passivity, we must become informed consumers who actively participate in our own treatment. Check consumer resources at the library, reputable online resources, and support group publications. Discuss potential therapies with your medical care practitioners, combining treatment interventions in a complementary fashion. In addition:

‣ Seek input from open-minded but cautious health professionals.

‣ Avoid unnecessary and potentially costly or harmful treatments, particularly fad treatments.

‣ Do not substitute any new product for medical care.

‣ Use common sense: Be open-minded but extremely cautious.

‣ Apply the same precautions to over-the-counter medications, herbs, vitamins, and supplements ("natural pharmaceuticals") as you would to prescription medications.

‣ Ask questions:
  – What does the treatment consist of?
  – What benefits can be expected?
  – How soon should I expect results?
  – What is its cost? Is a generic equivalent available? Acceptable?
  – Is it compatible with my other medications and supplements?

- Have scientific studies been conducted? (Obtain copies of them.)
- What are possible side effects and risks? What can I do to minimize side effects?
- For how long is treatment recommended? Will symptoms return upon discontinuation?
- If I am not obtaining benefit, how long do you recommend I wait before discontinuing?
- Does this drug need to be taken consistently to produce results, or is it used as necessary (PRN)?

COMPLEMENTARY AND ALTERNATIVE TREATMENTS

Patients with poorly understood illnesses lacking standard treatment protocols often seek complementary and alternative medicine (CAM) when they feel that conventional medicine has failed them. When considering a complementary treatment, ask questions about scientific studies, including its success rate, side effects, cost of treatment, and likelihood of medical insurance reimbursement; alternatives to be considered; the practitioner's credentials, training, and prior experience treating CFS/FMS patients with that product; and expected length of treatment.

Many so-called alternative therapies are quite useful even though their mechanisms of action are not well understood. (We do not know how many pharmaceuticals work, either.) Complementary therapies—which span many disciplines and cultures, including numerous therapeutic practices and interventions that have not been scientifically studied—include home remedies (herbal therapy, vitamins, or homeopathy), relaxation therapies (massage therapy and guided imagery), chiropractic, yoga, biofeedback, ayurveda, aromatherapy, nutritional therapy, reflexology, traditional Chinese medicine, macrobiotics, hypnotherapy, herbal medicine, naturopathy, and shamanic practices.

Integrative medicine combines therapies synergistically to achieve maximum benefit for the patient. CAM often involves the judicious use of pharmaceuticals, homeopathic preparations, herbs, vitamins and other supplements, physical modalities, psychotherapy, diet and nutrition, manual healing, and spiritual approaches.

All therapies have side effects and risks, and none is helpful to everyone who tries it. Clinical trials may be nonexistent, practitioners may not be credentialed, product labels may be misleading, and results may vary. Although the Office of Alternative Medicine (OAM), a branch of the National Institutes of Health, funds research on the safety and effectiveness of complementary therapies, funding is limited and most therapies have not been studied.

Lack of standard therapies for chronic illness breeds desperation, leaving us vulnerable to false claims for touted cures. In trying new therapies, we often cannot tell whether changes (improvements or exacerbations) result from the treatments or illness-associated symptom fluctuations. Inflated claims may render therapies tempting, and the research finding of the moment may allow us to believe once again that the breakthrough has been found; we are, however, typically met with disappointment.

♦♦ Intelligent Use of Supplements and Herbs ♦♦

Supplements, including herbs, do not require FDA approval. No specific standards or regulations have been established regarding their quality, effectiveness, or safety. Amounts of active ingredients vary greatly from one product to another, depending on where they are grown, proper identification of contents, different plant species, and which parts of the plant are used. Standardized or guaranteed products are more expensive, since assays are performed on such products to verify that they contain what the labels purport. A Good Manufacturing Practices Certification Program has been established by the National Nutritional Foods Association (NNFA), requiring third-party inspections to verify that the manufacturing facilities are up to NNFA standards, but membership is optional.

When using supplements and herbs, these guidelines may be helpful:

▶ Exercise caution. Obtain reliable, objective information about any therapy, whether traditional or complementary.

▶ Discuss alternative therapies with your doctor. Unsupervised therapy can be dangerous.

▶ Find out whether your alternative practitioner will work with your physician.

- Do not abandon your conventional therapy. Use CAM therapies adjunctively.

- Supply your health care providers with a list of all the medications you are taking, including over-the-counter remedies, vitamins and other supplements, herbs, and birth control pills.

- Buy supplements and herbs from a well-known source. Contaminated preparations may cause serious complications.

- Seek reputable, accurate sources of information; do not rely on health food store clerks for information.

- Optimal dosages of most herbs and supplements are unknown. Active ingredients may be present in inadequate amounts due to inferior preparations. Beware of using too much of an herb, for example, when it is contained in multiple products.

- CAMs can be used synergistically for maximum benefit. However, certain combinations are toxic, so seek reliable information before combining supplements.

- Choose a product to fill a specific need, buying supplements and herbs individually rather than in combination formulas.

- Start medications one at a time to assess your response, and then add others for a synergistic effect.

- Talk to people who have used the treatment; firsthand knowledge is invaluable. Ask about its advantages, disadvantages, risks, side effects, costs, and the results they obtained, including long-term outcomes.

- Investigate any treatment provider's background, philosophy, training and credentials, and experience in treating CFS/FMS patients.

- Ask about the cost of a full course of treatment. Some alternative therapies cost thousands of dollars, and most are not covered by health insurance.

- Document your experience. Keep a detailed log: whom you consulted, what you took or did, and all changes you observed.

- Remember that "natural" doesn't mean "safe." Some natural preparations have serious side effects and may even be life-endangering. For example, echinacea is counterproductive for a largely upregulated immune system.

‣ Avoid herbs during pregnancy. Do not give them to children except under the guidance of a qualified health professional.

‣ Remain open-minded but skeptical. Consider every treatment potentially helpful—but suspect until proven safe and effective.

‣ If you are sensitive to medications, consider starting at one-fourth the normal dose.

Physicians and other health professionals may sell products at their offices. This practice has been criticized by the Ethics and Human Rights Committee of the American College of Physicians' American Society of Internal Medicine as "ethically suspect" when done for the doctor's own financial interest. This board recommends doing so only if the product is sold at or near the physician's own cost and has "immediate relevance to the patient's need for care."

INTEGRATED TREATMENT OF CFS AND FMS

Scott Rigden, M.D., strongly advocates functional medicine, which focuses on biochemical individuality, metabolic balance, ecological context, and unique personal experience. Functional medicine integrates knowledge across a wide range of academic disciplines, including biochemistry, botanical medicine, clinical ecology, endocrinology, environmental toxicology, gastroenterology, genetics, hepatology, immunology, immunotoxicology, natural medicine, neurology, neurotoxicology, nutritional physiology, psychoneuroendocrinology, and psychoneuroimmunology.

Effective treatment is eclectic, spanning all the following treatment modalities:

‣ Lifestyle modification: self-care, therapeutic changes, relaxation, activity, coping skills, nutrition, and quality-of-life issues

‣ Medications and supplements: vitamins, supplements, herbs, and OTC and prescription medications

‣ Psychological interventions: emotional support, coping strategies, stress management, problem solving, and cognitive behavioral therapy

‣ Spirituality: belief system, life philosophy, and sense of meaning and purpose

◆◆ Lifestyle Modification ◆◆

◆ **Education** Learn about CFS and FMS and treatment options from books, newsletters, audiotapes and videotapes, seminars, Internet resources, medical and patient-oriented publications, and professional speakers at support group meetings.

◆ **Activity Level Monitoring** Too little activity leads to deconditioning, while overdoing leads to increased pain and relapse. Learn to manage energy as you do money. The tendency to overdo usually outweighs the tendency to underdo, requiring that we prioritize. How do I choose to spend my energy? What needs to be done, and what can wait? How can I attend to my responsibilities to others while taking care of my own health needs, rather than focusing on one at the expense of the other?

Identify counterproductive behavioral patterns and learn to schedule rest and relaxation intervals, whether or not you feel fatigued. Complete tasks in small steps interspersed with rest periods rather than one big chunk. Be aware of early signs of fatigue or increased pain, and stop. Focus on the progress achieved in reaching short-term goals, rather than viewing less accessible long-term goals as the only acceptable level of accomplishment.

Fatigue is exacerbated when levels of expended energy exceed the amount of energy available. When these are roughly matched, fatigue symptoms lessen and energy increases over time—not an easy balance to find or maintain.

Activity pacing is the most onerous challenge facing CFS/FMS patients. The overdo/crash cycle, although counterproductive, is difficult to break. Efforts to learn one's tolerance threshold for activity are hindered by unpredictably fluctuating energy levels and the temptation to overdo to "make up for lost time." Given the pathetic state of treatment research and the high number of failed therapies, lifestyle modification remains the number one successful therapeutic approach to CFS/FMS. It's also free—and extremely unpopular.

◆ **Stretching** Stretching techniques are taught in classes, physical therapy, on videotape, and in books.

  ▶ Prior to stretching, muscles should be warmed, either actively by gentle exercise or passively with a heating pad, warm bath, or hot tub.

❯ Stretch to the point of resistance and then hold the stretch, making sure to breathe. Do not stretch to the point of pain.

❯ Sustain the stretch for 60 seconds. Work toward this point gradually, starting with 10 to 15 seconds of stretching followed by 10 to 15 seconds of rest.

❯ Stretching throughout the day is preferable to one longer session.

◆ **Exercise** Exercise prevents deconditioning and muscle atrophy, builds strength and endurance, increases blood circulation, enhances cardiac fitness (if you can tolerate more vigorous exercise), and increases pain threshold over time.

❯ Warm up first by stretching.

❯ Gentle, moderate exercises such as tai chi, yoga, and Pilates are usually well tolerated.

❯ Follow a slow, incremental program. If you are not in the habit of exercising, start on a "decent day" with a 3-minute gentle exercise routine. If you don't relapse within 48 hours, try exercising for 3 minutes daily, eventually adding another 3-minute session later in the day. Increase to 4 minutes twice a day. If you tolerate it well, move to 5 minutes. Build gradually from there. Some people can work up to 10 to 20 minutes twice a day, while others can tolerate only a few minutes. Don't push; find your own level. This is not a competition.

❯ Start with range-of-motion, weight-bearing, nonaerobic exercise, progressing to aquatic exercise and aerobic exercise if tolerated.

❯ Suitable exercises are walking (outdoors, around the house, or on a treadmill), bicycling or exercycling, swimming, and water aerobics. (If you take a class, don't push to "keep up" with the group.)

❯ Work toward musculoskeletal fitness before cardiovascular fitness, which requires more exertion.

❯ If at any point you experience symptom exacerbation or relapse, cut way back and build up slowly.

◆ **Ergonomics** Ergonomics involves learning to sit, stand, and move in ways that do not place undue stress on the body and that minimize the risk of injury. The mainstays of good body mechanics are proper posture, frequent shifts in position, and avoidance of eccentric movements. For comfort at home and at the office:

- Stand with shoulders back and relaxed, head erect, and arms resting comfortably.

- Pay attention to posture, sitting and standing with your back straight and your head held upright rather than tilted. Do not slouch, and avoid swaying your back.

- Become aware of muscle tension in your back, and practice standing, sitting, and reaching without increasing the muscle tension.

- Try to use your whole body when performing tasks.

- When lifting, bend at the knees and allow your legs—not your back muscles—to do the lifting.

- Request help if an object is too large or heavy for you to lift comfortably.

- Swivel your chair or turn your entire body when reaching for something.

- Avoid repetitive motion.

- Switch among tasks to avoid remaining in one position for too long.

- Use furniture with good support, and assume a comfortable, relaxed position.

- Use pillows and other devices for proper support of the back, neck, shoulders, and arms.

- Use an adjustable task chair with good lumbar support.

- When using a computer, try these suggestions:

  - When typing, tap the keys lightly. Try to move only your fingers when typing, rather than your wrists. Use an ergonomic keyboard if it is comfortable for you.

  - Support your wrists with wrist pads. Support your feet by using a footrest.

  - Keep your elbows angled at 90 degrees and your arms close to your sides.

  - Pay careful attention to posture; avoid slouching over the keyboard.

- Position the top of the monitor at eye level.
- Make sure good light is available, eliminating glare.
- Learn stretches you can do while seated, and do them often.
- Don't remain in one position for too long. Take frequent breaks, moving around to improve blood circulation, and stretch hands, fingers, wrists, neck, shoulders, and back.
- Practice deep breathing.

‣ When traveling by car or train, shift position often. Stretch and walk or move around. Use neck and back pillows for support, repositioning them frequently to increase comfort.

◆ **Sleep Hygiene** Sleep hygiene is the development of habits and methods of promoting quality sleep by rebuilding a normal sleep schedule and bedtime routine to reset one's biological clock.

These techniques work synergistically with sleep medications:

‣ Try to go to bed and awaken at the same time each day. Going to bed at a reasonable hour allows the advantage of the deep sleep that occurs during the first half of the night, such as higher levels of growth hormone and other hormones needed for optimum rest and repair.

‣ Avoid substances that can produce sleep disturbance: alcohol, caffeine, nicotine, some blood pressure medications (beta blockers), some asthma medications, antidepressants (especially SSRIs, or selective serotonin reuptake inhibitors), steroids, and diuretics (which can interrupt sleep due to increased need to urinate).

‣ Exercise early in the day.

‣ Exposure to sunlight during the day and dim lighting at night help to regulate circadian rhythms. Lower the light level in the later evening, and sleep in a darkened room or use a sleep mask.

‣ Relax in the evening: Take a warm bath, listen to mellow music, or use relaxation techniques.

‣ Avoid naps if they disrupt sleep-wake rhythms and make nighttime sleep more difficult.

‣ Don't overeat or undereat in the evening. A bland snack or warm beverage before bed may help sleep.

▶ Create a cool and comfortable sleep environment, where noise and other interruptions are minimized.

▶ Put worries aside. Do not allow "should haves" or planning for the next day to disrupt sleep. Keep a pad and pen nearby to write down things to do that you might otherwise forget, and then dismiss such thoughts.

▶ If you use television or radio before going to sleep, set a timer to turn them off to avoid their stimulating the brain and interfering with deep, restful sleep.

▶ If you are unable to sleep after twenty to thirty minutes, get up and do something low-key, nonstimulating, and boring. Return to bed when you become drowsy.

◆ **Diet and Nutrition** Ours is a nutrition-conscious age in which "natural" products are widely touted and self-proclaimed nutrition experts abound. We are bombarded with a wealth of information and misinformation about nutritional products, often with contradictory and inflated claims. Medical schools paid little attention to nutrition in the past, yet we often turn to our physicians for nutritional advice. Fortunately, research in this area is flourishing.

▶ Obtain information from a credentialed dietician or physician, not health food stores, fad diet books, or media ads.

▶ Eliminate foods to which you are sensitive or allergic. Use test results along with personal experience to determine which foods make symptoms worse. Foods that are not well tolerated due to allergies or sensitivities often include dairy products, wheat, gluten, eggs, corn, nuts, soy, and such food additives as MSG, sulfites, nitrites, nitrates, preservatives, and coloring and flavoring additives.

▶ Individual experimentation is the most accurate method for determining food intolerances. An elimination diet combined with careful record keeping may help you uncover food allergies and sensitivities. Symptoms of food intolerance include malaise, mood alteration, digestive disturbances, food cravings, and repetitious eating patterns.

▶ Those with food intolerances may benefit from a rotation diet, in which a food is consumed only once every few days.

▶ Most patients do best with a low-fat diet high in protein, vegetables, and fruits with small amounts of complex carbohydrates that are high in fiber (fruits, whole grains, and certain vegetables). Complex carbohydrates are metabolized and released into the bloodstream more slowly. Benefits often include general well-being, improved energy, mood enhancement, and weight loss.

▶ Small, frequent meals may be preferable to three large meals per day.

▶ Avoid or limit the "big five": caffeine, nicotine, alcohol, sugar, and aspartame (NutraSweet). (Small amounts may be tolerated.)

▶ Sugar and other simple or refined carbohydrates (honey, molasses, white flour, white potatoes, corn, and alcohol) may increase pain, drain energy, adversely affect cognition, and contribute to yeast overgrowth in susceptible individuals.

▶ Carbohydrate cravings are especially common during exacerbations when energy is low. Although a psychological basis for these cravings has been proposed, evidence suggests that the source is largely biochemical, possibly related to abnormalities in neurotransmitter levels and metabolism. Consumption of simple carbohydrates may increase pain, cognitive dysfunction, and fatigue, causing a "boost and crash" cycle (in which the blood sugar level rises and then plummets quickly and dramatically).

▶ Carbohydrates may be best tolerated in the evening.

▶ Decrease consumption of fats, particularly saturated fats, and processed foods.

▶ Wash fresh produce in water containing a teaspoon of bleach (such as Clorox) and rinse thoroughly; remove outer leaves or peel skins to remove pesticide residues and parasites.

▶ Use vitamins, minerals, and supplements appropriately.

◆ **Stress Management: Relaxation** Relaxation techniques are discussed later in this chapter on pages 261–262.

◆ **Emotional Support** Sources of emotional support include your team of health care providers, family members, support groups, and friends. Ask family members and close friends to gain a basic under-standing of your illness by reading an article or a pamphlet. Illness is often isolating; involve others in your life.

◆ **Avoidance of Environmental Toxins** The immune system and the body's detoxification pathways must work overtime to deal with environmental pollutants and chemicals. Avoiding all toxic sub-stances is impossible, but we need to exercise caution to minimize adding to total body load. Sensitivities to chemicals are common, including perfumes and colognes, petrochemicals (e.g., gasoline, exhaust fumes), hairsprays, pesticides, formaldehyde, and cleaning products.

"Sick home" improvement is necessary for those with environ-mental sensitivities. Although most people are not in a financial position to build a new, low-toxicity house, many modifications can be made in existing homes to create a more healthful environment. Helpful changes include having adequate ventilation using air-handling systems with activated carbon filters, using HEPA (high-efficiency particulate air) room air filters or purifiers, frequent dust-ing and vacuuming, avoiding cleaning products to which you are sensitive, keeping knickknacks and "dust catchers" to a minimum (including old books and stuffed animals), replacing carpeting (which is a breeding ground for dust mites) with ceramic tile or wood flooring, using low-toxicity paint, sealing the door between the garage and house, eliminating pesticide use, using chemically inert building materials (stainless steel, glass, stone, and solid wood) in place of particleboard, eliminating room-freshening sprays and other scented household products, and sealing off any materials that contain formaldehyde. Nontoxic building materials, cleaning products, and pesticides are readily available, and tolerance can be ensured by experimentation. Many manufacturers of such products supply free samples to those who are chemically sensitive.

◆ **Belief System, Outlook, and Faith** Spirituality can boost immu-nity, promote healthful behaviors, add to one's support system, and help develop a sense of meaning and faith. Those with a positive belief system may have a better prognosis. A more positive outlook may be achieved through meaningful work or projects, modification of previously enjoyed activities, hope, humor, and awareness of abil-ities—not just dis-abilities.

◆ **Psychological Support** Many patients do not "need" psychotherapy but find it helps with illness acceptance and adjustment, coping
skills, support, self-esteem, depression, anxiety, and individual and
family issues secondary to FMS/CFS illness.

Cognitive behavioral therapy (CBT) is a valuable adjustment
tool but by no means a cure-all, as some studies have suggested.
Useful in treating depression, anxiety, phobias, panic disorders, and
eating disorders, CBT is not a cure for any illness, nor is it suitable
for all CFS/FMS patients, but it can be valuable as part of a multidisciplinary program that tailors therapy treatment to the individual. Nancy Klimas, M.D., describes CBT as learning to "do what
you can, accept what you can't, and get on with your life."

The purpose of CBT is to improve quality of life by challenging
irrational and destructive self-messages, unrealistic goals, and mal-
adaptive behaviors. CBT can help with coping and stress-reduction
skills, productivity, lifestyle management, and appropriate activity
levels. Effective in relieving depression and anxiety, CBT helps
patients to challenge irrational beliefs that give rise to feelings of
inadequacy, hopelessness, and helplessness. It empowers them to be
in charge of handling the effects of their illness, increasing their
sense of control and efficacy.

TREATMENT OPTIONS

The primary goals of CFS/FMS treatment are improving sleep,
relieving pain, increasing energy, and relieving the most troublesome symptoms. Patient responses are variable, idiosyncratic, and
often paradoxical (achieving the opposite of the expected effect).
What helps one patient does not necessarily help another, and our
responses vary over time. Medications that help most people may
not help those of us with CFS or FMS. The following discussion of
treatments—which, although lengthy, is hardly exhaustive—is presented as information rather than advice. Some of the information
is technical and may be of greater relevance to the practitioner than
to the patient. Therapies should be initiated *only under medical
supervision.*

Explanation of abbreviations: OTC indicates over-the-counter treatments that are available without a prescription, IM indicates

administration by intramuscular injection, and IV indicates intravenous administration. The trade name of the medication is given first, with the generic name in parentheses.

◆◆ Getting Organized ◆◆

Organize your medications and keep them where you will see them frequently—not in damp areas such as the bathroom or kitchen. Trays of seven individual daily containers with four compartments for each day (morning, noon, evening, and bedtime) can be filled in advance for an entire week.

Keep a symptom calendar. Using a calendar with large squares, note how you are feeling each day (a scale of 1 to 10 works well), along with symptoms, medication changes, and unusual activities (travel, major weather changes, toxic exposure, and other stressors). Setting it up may take time, but jotting daily notes is quick and easy. Keep the calendar simple and legible; it may help you or your doctor identify symptom-treatment-activity correlations and patterns as well as disability documentation.

Prepare for medical visits. Make notes in advance regarding symptoms, all current treatments (pharmaceuticals, hormones, vitamins, supplements, and physical modalities), and questions, which are best confined to two or three per visit. Keep your own copy so you can jot down notes during your visit.

VITAMINS AND MINERALS

Vitamin-mineral supplements (most available OTC) should be of good quality, preferably sugar free. They should contain adequate amounts of vitamins B, C, E, and beta-carotene, and include zinc, potassium, and magnesium. Because vitamins and minerals may be poorly absorbed, taking supplements in addition to following a healthful diet is often advisable.

Antioxidant therapy involves products that reduce the harmful effects of free radicals, molecules that can cause cell injury or death and contribute to the development of many illnesses. Common antioxidants are vitamins E and C, beta-carotene, bioflavonoids, ginseng, ginkgo biloba, silymarin, and grape seed extract (proanthocyanidin).

Vitamin A maintains the mucous linings in the body. Beta-carotene is its precursor, converted by the body into vitamin A.

B vitamins are associated with brain metabolism, memory, and mood. Vitamin B_{12} (cyanocobalamin or hydroxycobalamin), injectable by prescription or OTC for oral and sublingual forms, increases energy and stamina, enhances absorption and metabolism of foods, and may correct several types of CFS/FMS dysfunction. B_{12} should be accompanied by a full complement of B vitamins (IM, or oral OTC).

Vitamin C (IV by prescription, oral OTC) is beneficial in treating a number of chronic disorders. It serves numerous functions in the body, including immune enhancement and maintenance of tissues and capillaries. Ultra-high-dose vitamin C, often administered intravenously, is controversial. If vitamin C produces gastrointestinal problems, the dose should be decreased and then increased gradually.

Vitamin E, a fat-soluble antioxidant, decreases LDL ("bad" cholesterol), maintains membranes and tissues, and may increase glutathione utilization.

Calcium citrate and calcium glycinate are the best-absorbed forms of calcium. Calcium helps to maintain bone density and strength and is an important preventative measure against bone loss (osteoporosis), particularly for those who are inactive and therefore at risk. Calcium may help prevent muscle spasms and cramps. **Vitamin D,** a potent, fat-soluble antioxidant, helps calcium absorption.

Magnesium (IM, oral or elixir OTC) helps cellular energy production. **Magnesium malate, magnesium lactate,** and **magnesium glycinate** are the best-absorbed forms. IM magnesium injections yield mixed results and are quite painful. Magnesium malate helps with pain relief. Blood levels of magnesium are often deceptively normal, not reflecting whether it is depleted in the tissues. Magnesium purportedly works at the NMDA receptors and helps pain and can be used synergistically with calcium and zinc. If nausea or diarrhea occurs, reduce the dose and increase gradually.

Potassium decreases blood pressure, especially important when taken with other supplements that decrease potassium or if one is dehydrated.

Chromium decreases blood sugar, insulin, and cholesterol levels.

Selenium may decrease risk of cancer and is best used adjunctively with vitamins C and E.

Vitamin infusions, often a combination of C, magnesium, and B vitamins, or "Meyer's cocktail," may provide a temporary energy boost.

Chelation therapy: Chelation means "to combine with and dissolve." A crystalline acid (EDTA), injected intravenously over several hours, chelates (binds) heavy metals in the bloodstream, which are then excreted through the kidneys. It is used to treat a range of illnesses including cancer, arthritis, heart attacks, strokes, multiple sclerosis, and Parkinson's disease. The FDA and other professional associations deem chelation therapy worthless for purposes other than heavy metal accumulation. It has never been tested in other diseases in a well-designed, properly controlled clinical trial. This expensive therapy carries significant risk of kidney damage and is considered potentially lethal without adequate supervision.

Essential fatty acids, or EFAs (fatty acids not naturally produced by the body), supply linoleic acid and alpha-linolenic acid and have anti-inflammatory properties. They help maintain normal membrane structure and regulation of cell function, mediate cytokine effects, modulate the HPA axis, and may have antiviral properties. Anecdotally, EFAs improve pain, fatigue, and depression. They may decrease muscle fatigue, morning stiffness, and joint tenderness; help the digestive, cardiovascular, and immune systems; and assist reproductive functioning, metabolism, and brain functioning. Omega-6 fatty acids are found in sunflower, safflower, and corn oil; evening primrose oil; and black currant seed oil. Omega-3 fatty acids are found in fish oil and flaxseed powder or oil.

Herbs, or natural pharmaceuticals, have been used for centuries to treat various illnesses. The scientific basis for their action is often unknown, but many of our pharmaceuticals are based on the active ingredients in botanicals. Used judiciously, some herbs offer tremendous benefit, while others do little or nothing or may cause harm. Dosages must be appropriate to the individual. Herbs may be prepared as tinctures, teas, or powders. Few scientific studies have been conducted, and the effects of herbs are not well established. Herbs are usually used synergistically. Herbal treatment can be expensive and is not covered by medical insurance, but many have found it quite effective. Examples of herbs and supplements used to treat CFS/FMS are integrated with other treatment approaches in this chapter.

Most herbs are contraindicated during pregnancy and nursing and in children under the age of twelve. Many are contraindicated for those with hypertension or clotting abnormalities. Since herbs are contraindicated in certain conditions and may cause harmful effects if used inappropriately, they should be used only with the guidance of an expert who has proper training and experience.

SYMPTOMATIC TREATMENT

In America you just fix what shows.

— *Gallagher*

◆◆ Anxiety ◆◆

Regular relaxation, meditation, and minor tranquilizers, such as the benzodiazepines Klonopin (clonazepam) and Xanax (alprazolam), are helpful for treatment of anxiety. BuSpar (buspirone), an anti-anxiety agent unrelated to benzodiazepines, is nonaddictive but usually less effective. Because low-dose clonazepam (a long-acting benzodiazepine) improves neurological functioning and sleep, it is generally the drug of choice for treating both anxiety and sleep disorder. Small amounts taken during the day may increase alertness and enhance cognitive functioning. Benzodiazepines are addictive; sudden discontinuation is accompanied by withdrawal symptoms. For the treatment of occasional anxiety, these medications can be taken as needed. Maintenance doses of certain antidepressants prevent panic attacks.

Kava kava (available OTC) reduces anxiety, stress, tension, and insomnia, encouraging a sense of tranquility. It has sedative and sleep-enhancement effects but should not be used for more than three months without medical advice. Side effects include dry, flaking, discolored (yellow) skin; scaly rash; red eyes; puffy face; and muscle weakness. Kava should not be used with central nervous system (CNS) depressants such as alcohol, barbiturates, sedatives, and certain antidepressants. It adversely affects motor reflexes and judgment necessary for driving.

✦✦ Cognitive Functioning, Stimulants, and Neuroprotective Agents ✦✦

Acetyl-L-carnitine, essential for mitochondrial function, is postulated to reduce fatigue and improve cognition. It is available both OTC and by prescription as Carnitor (levocarnitine). Results are mixed; adverse effects are rare.

Alpha-lipoic acid, another powerful antioxidant, is believed to have the ability to regenerate other important brain antioxidants including vitamins E and C and glutathione. It acts as a coenzyme in Krebs cycle reactions, affecting carbohydrate metabolism.

Caffeine (trimethylxanthine), called "America's favorite drug," is relatively safe in those able to tolerate it. A mild diuretic, it occurs naturally in many plants and is often added to foods and drinks. Moderate use early in the day may stimulate energy, alertness, and cognition. It increases feelings of well-being and relieves vascular headaches. However, it may be poorly tolerated by CFS/FMS patients, is addictive, and may create a yo-yo effect (a need for more caffeine as its level drops). Caffeine may cause irritability, prevent falling asleep, and interfere with deep sleep. Withdrawal from caffeine should be gradual to avoid headache and irritability.

Calcium channel blockers (for example, nifedipine, nicardipine, nimodipine, and verapamil) are used to treat angina, hypertension, arrhythmias, and migraine headaches. They act as stimulants by increasing blood flow to the brain and may have a mild positive effect on energy and stamina as well as cognition. Side effects include dizziness, headaches, gastrointestinal upset, and weakness.

Coenzyme Q10 (OTC) is a mitochondrial coenzyme used in cellular adenosine triphosphate (ATP) production. Found in every cell of every living being, CoQ10 increases the efficiency of cellular energy production. It is believed to have antioxidant and immune-enhancing qualities and to act as a free radical scavenger. Often used synergistically with other medications, CoQ10 may be swallowed or used sublingually. Some patients report general improvement, cognitive improvement, increased energy level, and increased muscle strength. Vitamin B_{12} may help as well.

Cognex (tacrine HCl), developed for treatment of dementia associated with Alzheimer's disease by boosting CNS acetylcholine concentrations, may benefit cognitive abilities in CFS/FMS patients. However, Cognex has not been well tested in these disorders. Its primary side effects are gastrointestinal symptoms, dizziness, and liver toxicity.

DDAVP (desmopressin acetate), a synthetic version of the hormone vasopressin, may enhance cognition and alertness and is used to treat certain blood disorders. Available as an oral preparation and a nasal spray, DDAVP may increase stamina and endurance while decreasing malaise. This medication may cause headache, runny nose, sore throat, drowsiness, dizziness, nausea, stomach ache, or flushing of the face.

Diamox (acetazolamide) is used to treat seizure disorders, glaucoma, and altitude sickness. It may increase alertness and energy. Diamox has diuretic properties and may cause such side effects as potassium depletion, tingling in the extremities, weakness, decreased appetite, fatigue, and malaise.

DMAE (dimethylaminoethanol) is a supplement said to enhance acetylcholine synthesis, increasing alertness, memory, energy, sleep, and mood. This supplement has not been tested or widely used in CFS/FMS patients. DMAE is a natural food component, found especially in fish, and is also a natural metabolite of the human body. It helps memory and learning ability and raises blood choline levels.

Ephedra, or ephedrine (ma huang), is a stimulant that may cause chest pain, anxiety, heart attack, and stroke, with caffeine heightening such effects. It should be avoided.

Ginkgo biloba is a strong antioxidant that improves blood circulation to the brain, enhancing memory and decreasing tinnitus (ringing in the ears) related to decreased blood flow. Ginkgo improves brain metabolism, reduces platelet aggregation, and improves cognition. Benefit is usually felt within three to eight weeks. It can be used indefinitely, and its efficacy may increase over time. Since ginkgo may prolong bleeding time, it should not be taken with anticoagulants or antiplatelet agents. It may potentiate blood thinners and other medications.

Ginseng, a central nervous system stimulant, is an "adaptogen," helping the body adapt to stress. Many types are available, including Siberian, American, and Panax ginseng. Siberian ginseng has been noted as a regulator of numerous body functions, including cholesterol, blood pressure, blood sugar, and thyroid and adrenal function. American ginseng contains trace minerals and is believed to enhance cognition and mood. Panax or Chinese ginseng is an antioxidant that increases energy and helps the body cope with stress. Good-quality ginseng is diffifcult to obtain. Ginseng may increase immune abnormalities, cause overstimulation, and increase blood pressure, heart rate, and blood sugar; therefore, it should be used with caution, if at all.

Guarana root (available OTC) has been used for headache, cognition, and appetite suppression, typically on an as-needed (PRN) basis. It is purported to provide an energy boost lasting four to six hours, similar to that provided by coffee. Side effects include gastrointestinal distress, nervousness, and restlessness, particularly in those who are sensitive to caffeine.

Huperzine A (Huperzia serrata) (available OTC) is an extract from a club moss that inhibits the neurotransmitter acetylcholine esterase, enhancing cognition. Side effects are not widely reported but may include dizziness.

Hydergine (ergoloid mesylates), an antioxidant used to treat dementia, improves short-term memory and alertness. Side effects are rare but include headache and nausea.

Ionamin (phentermine HCl), a central nervous system stimulant used in the treatment of obesity, enhances energy and cognition. Side effects include insomnia, nervousness, and increased blood pressure.

Klonopin (clonazepam) is an antiseizure medication. Although it is used to promote sleep, small doses during the day raise the threshold to stimuli and improve alertness and cognitive functioning in some cases. Higher doses produce drowsiness, light-headedness, and dizziness. Because clonazepam is habit forming, it should not be discontinued abruptly.

N-Acetyl-L-Cysteine (NAC) is an antioxidant purported to protect against toxins such as heavy metals and environmental pollutants.

It increases brain glutathione, especially in combination with vitamins C and E. Side effects such as gastrointestinal symptoms, rashes, and fever are associated with intake of large quantities.

NADH (nicotinamide adenine dinucleotide) (available OTC), a coenzyme that triggers energy production through ATP (adenosine triphosphate) generation, may improve energy levels, endurance, and strength and alleviate depression. In addition to antioxidant properties, NADH stimulates production of the neurotransmitters dopamine, noradrenaline, and serotonin and may alleviate depression.

Naphazoline HCl, in eyedrop form, is available in several strengths OTC or by prescription. It increases alertness and cognition in some CFS/FMS patients. Side effects, although rare, include headache, hypertension, cardiac irregularities, nervousness, nausea, dizziness, weakness, and sweating.

Nicotine transdermal patch (available OTC), used for smoking cessation, is a vasodilator that increases blood flow, enhances mental clarity and cognition, increases energy and strength, and exerts analgesic effects by releasing nicotine steadily. Side effects include burning at the application site, increased appetite, and tachycardia. Initially, headache, dizziness, and light-headedness may be experienced. Using one half of the lowest-strength patch is often recommended. Cigarette smoking is not recommended while using "the patch."

Nootropyl (piracetam), available from compounding pharmacies, helps memory, alertness, and attention, possibly by improving brain metabolism and stimulating ATP. Side effects include mild anxiety, agitation, and headache.

Oxygen administration produces mixed results, with some patients reporting improved cognition.

Phosphatidylserine (PS) (available OTC), a naturally occurring phospholipid in the brain, can be taken in supplement form to improve cognition, particularly memory loss, and decrease "brain fog." PS is expensive, and results are mixed.

Pitocin (oxytocin), used to induce labor contractions and to treat lactation deficiency, may improve cognition and stamina while decreasing pain and creating mood improvement, although its use in CFS and FMS has not been studied well. Side effects are reportedly rare.

Provigil (modafinil), used to treat narcolepsy, is a "wakefulness-promoting agent" that increases energy and concentration and decreases postexertional fatigue. Usually well tolerated, it may improve sleep (a rebound effect at the end of the day) and help sleep apnea. Adverse effects include anxiety, headache, nausea, nervousness, and insomnia.

Pycnogenol (pine bark or grapeseed extract) (available OTC) stimulates energy and has anti-inflammatory and potent antioxidant properties. It stabilizes red blood cell membranes and is believed safe.

Selective serotonin reuptake inhibitors (SSRIs) are antidepressants that enhance cognition in some patients. The SSRIs include Prozac, Paxil, and Zoloft (further discussed in section on treatment of depression). They may cause increased alertness, but over time may increase fatigue and decrease alertness. Side effects include visual disturbance, sexual dysfunction, gastrointestinal symptoms, and initial insomnia and nervousness.

Selegilene, or deprenyl, an antioxidant purported to have immune modulating and antineurodegenerative effects, may increase alertness and enhance libido.

Vinpocetine (available OTC) (a purified extract of the periwinkle plant) is a well-tolerated cerebral vasodilator and antioxidant. It increases cerebral perfusion, reduces the tendency of red blood cells and platelets to aggregate (stick together), enhances glucose use in brain cells, has anticonvulsant activity, and increases brain levels of ATP. Vinpocetine should not be combined with blood-thinning drugs except on the advice of a physician. No serious side effects are reported.

Yohimbe (available OTC), an African plant with reported aphrodisiac qualities, is is an herbal stimulant. Because it can cause such side effects as nervousness, anxiety, and sleeplessness, Yohimbe should be used with caution.

Prescription stimulants include Cylert (pemoline), Dexedrine (dextroamphetamine), Ritalin (methylphenidate), and Concerta (methylphenidate). Other medications with stimulating and/or cognitive-enhancing effects include Symmetrel (amantadine HCl), Tegretol (carbamazepine), Depakene (valproic acid), Depakote (divalproex sodium), and low-dose Trexan (naltrexone HCl). Some of these medications are quick-acting, and others must be taken for several weeks before effects are felt. Because these drugs may cause overstimulation, patients are advised to be cautious about the temptation to overdo, thereby precipitating a relapse.

Quantitative EEG (brain mapping) and neurotherapy. Although electrocardiograms (EEGs) often appear normal, those with cognitive problems may have an abnormal increase in slow-wave activity. Using digital technology, quantitative EEG is a noninvasive measurement of electrical patterns at the surface of the scalp that reflect cortical electrical activity, or brain waves, which occur at various frequencies (EEG bands). Many patients display unique functional brain abnormalities during cognitive challenges. Brain mapping documents cognitive decline and improvement, tracking treatment efficacy. Sensors placed on the patient's head are linked to a system that offers visual or auditory feedback as the patient learns to increase brain wave activity. Various neurofeedback protocols are used, and many sessions may be required for optimal results. Some programs may be used at home. Results are purported to include improved concentration and short-term memory, reduction or resolution of headaches, improved sleep patterns, improved balance and physical stamina, decreased sensitivity to sound and light, increased attention span, and fewer letter or word reversals. Neurofeedback is in its early stages and has not been formally tested but holds promise in normalizing brain waves and creating cognitive improvement.

◆◆ Depression ◆◆

Finding the right antidepressant or combination of antidepressants and the most effective dose is a trial-and-error process. Sometimes numerous medications must be tried, but most cases of depression are responsive to treatment.

Antidepressants fall into several categories according to the neurotransmitters (brain chemicals) they affect. They are nonaddictive and must be taken regularly to be effective. Full antidepressant effect is not experienced for several weeks. Antidepressants may be enhanced by the use of other medications and psychotherapy.

Tricyclic antidepressants (TCAs), notably Sinequan (doxepin), have antihistaminic and anti-inflammatory properties. Low-dose TCA administration often improves sleep and decreases pain. Because of drug sensitivities, TCAs are initially administered in tiny doses and increased to the patient's optimal dose. If one does not tolerate a drug in this class, others can be tried. Common side effects include dry mouth, constipation, and weight gain.

Selective serotonin reuptake inhibitors (SSRIs) include Prozac (fluoxetine), Zoloft (sertraline), Paxil (paroxetine), and Celexa (citalopram). Less sedating than TCAs, they may initially provide an energy boost and are usually taken in the morning. SSRIs may decrease irritability and mood swings and offer pain relief and improved cognition. They usually cause fewer side effects than TCAs, with any initial anxiety or "wired" feelings subsiding over time. However, SSRIs may later cause fatigue and weight gain.

Other antidepressants: Several antidepressants that are structurally unrelated, not fitting into any of the established classes, include Desyrel (trazodone), Effexor (venlafaxine), Remeron (mirtazapine), and Wellbutrin (bupropion). Wellbutrin is helpful for fatigue, emotional swings, and depression, with fewer side effects than most other antidepressants. Remeron is helpful for sleep and anxiety. It has fewer side effects than many of the others, and it blocks receptors associated with decreased sex drive, nausea, nervousness, headache, insomnia, and diarrhea. Luvox (fluvoxamine) may be better tolerated than SSRIs. Serzone (nefazodone) may improve sleep and cognition, without causing the sedation, insomnia, or sexual dysfunction associated with SSRIs. Effexor, Serzone, and Wellbutrin are weight-neutral, causing neither gain nor loss.

5-HTP (5-hydroxytryptophan) is an amino acid extracted from seeds of the *Griffonia simplicifolia* plant that crosses the blood-brain barrier and may help with pain and sleep disorders. It is converted to serotonin in the brain, possibly affecting dopamine and norepinephrine levels. It may take a month or longer to work and should not be combined with SSRIs.

Monoamine oxidase inhibitors (MAOIs) are somewhat effective in CFS/FMS but are rarely used due to significant side effects and strict dietary restrictions.

St. John's wort (Hypericum perforatum) extract has been used for many years to treat depression and mild to moderate anxiety, but treatment studies yield conflicting results. St. John's wort may have antiviral properties and is thought to ease myalgia. It should not be taken with SSRIs or other antidepressants. It may cause reductions in levels and therapeutic efficacy of other medications and interferes with absorption of iron and other minerals.

Substance P antagonists have potential application in the treatment of depression, anxiety disorders, posttraumatic stress syndrome, obsessive-compulsive disorder, and panic disorder. In preliminary trials with CFS/FMS patients, effects were felt quickly but no change in pain levels was noted.

◆◆ Edema (Swelling) ◆◆

Edema, or swelling due to pooling of fluid in body tissues, is particularly noticeable in the hands, ankles, feet, and face. It may be reduced with diuretics, although their extended use is not advised. Many physicians do not prescribe diuretics even for short-term use. Decreasing sodium intake while increasing fluid intake is an effective nondrug treatment for swelling.

◆◆ Gastrointestinal Problems ◆◆

General measures for relieving gastrointestinal problems include the following:

‣ Reduce stress and anxiety.

‣ Do not rush meals or gulp air.

‣ Chew food thoroughly.

‣ Avoid alcohol, caffeine, and nicotine.

‣ Eat plenty of fiber.

‣ Avoid excessive use of laxatives and enemas.

‣ If you are lactose-intolerant, use enzyme products or switch to reduced-lactose dairy products.

‣ Identify food intolerance by eliminating a food for ten to fourteen days and then reintroducing it heavily, noting any reactions. Offending foods should then be completely eliminated from the diet.

▶ For candidiasis or systemic yeast infection, an anti-*Candida* diet relieves digestive problems, especially bloating and gas.

▶ Testing for gut pathogens, including parasites, is recommended for severe, intractable gastrointestinal problems.

Diarrhea can be treated with OTC preparations including Metamucil, Kaopectate, Donnagel, or Imodium (loperamide HCl), and adequate fluid intake is important. Activated charcoal capsules are effective but should not be taken within 1 hour of other medications, as they may render them less potent. Geranium (American cranesbill) or teas made of agrimony leaves, bilberry fruit, or slippery elm bark help stop diarrhea. Prescription medication, such as Lomotil (atropine and diphenoxylate), may be necessary for more severe cases.

Heartburn, or reflux of stomach acid, can be helped by H_2 blockers, antacids, not eating close to bedtime, and avoiding spicy foods if not well tolerated.

Intestinal gas and bloating can be relieved by activated charcoal capsules; the enzymes papain, bromelain, pepsin, and trypsin; and OTC products containing simethicone. Avoid offensive foods, such as dairy products, certain raw vegetables, beans, and sugars, including fructose and sorbitol. Beano drops (digestive enzymes) and Angostura bitters decrease the gassiness associated with gas-producing foods.

Nausea may be treated with Tigan (trimethobenzamide HCl) or Phenergan (promethazine), which causes drowsiness. Antivert (meclizine HCl) is prescribed for nausea accompanied by dizziness or balance problems.

Muscle spasms in the intestinal tract are decreased by such antispasmodics as Librax (chlordiazepoxide HCl and clidinium bromide), Bentyl (dicyclomine HCl), Donnatal (phenobarbital, hyoscyamine sulfate, atropine sulfate, and scopolamine hydrobromide), and Isordil (isosorbide dinitrate). Ginger capsules, activated charcoal capsules, stale popcorn, and pressure-point wristbands may be helpful.

Constipation is relieved by psyllium seed, cascara sagrada, senna, aloe (the anhydrous aloin type), and other OTC products, often used in combination.

Inflammatory bowel syndrome (IBS) is treated with benzodiazepines, Zantac (ranitidine HCl) or other acid blockers, calcium channel blockers, TCAs, and, in severe cases, Lupron (leuprolide acetate). Chamomile has sedative and antispasmodic effects. Upset stomach is helped by oral cayenne.

Enzymes are special proteins in all plant and animal cells that sustain every organ and system, acting as catalysts for chemical reactions in the body. Only a fraction of existing enzymes have been identified. **Enzyme deficiencies** result from certain illnesses, aging, improper diet, and sun damage. Digestive enzymes such as bromelain, an anti-inflammatory, help IBS symptoms. Ginger capsules settle the stomach, promote peristalsis, and help nausea and vomiting. Modestly antibacterial, ginger stimulates circulation and should not be taken with blood thinners or anticlotting drugs.

Goldenseal, an immune stimulant, reduces inflammation of mucous membranes, including the gastrointestinal tract. It is used to treat digestive problems, including infections and *Candida* overgrowth, and has fairly good effect against intestinal parasites. Goldenseal is also used for menstrual problems and PMS and treatment of eczema, mouth ulcers, and respiratory infections. It should not be used in pregnancy or by hypertensives.

Peppermint, an antispasmodic for abdominal cramping and irritable bowel, is often taken in the form of enteric-coated tablets. Peppermint tea eases upset stomach and nausea.

Chronic liver toxicity, resulting from overloaded liver-detoxification pathways, is frequently associated with multiple sensitivities, with even minor toxic exposure generating symptoms in some individuals. Those with extreme gastrointestinal sensitivities and symptoms may suffer from leaky gut syndrome, an allergic reaction to protein molecules that leak across the intestinal wall. Antibodies produced in reaction to these substances activate the immune system inappropriately. Enterohepatic resuscitation is achieved with a nutritional detoxification plan of diet and supplementation. Avoidance of offending foods, bland diet, and diet rotation are helpful in treatment. Liver function is helped by milk thistle (silymarin).

◆◆ Hormone Therapy (Endocrine Problems) ◆◆

Hormones are chemical messages produced by special cells in glands and other organs of the body. Levels of many types of hormones are low in CFS/FMS patients.

Estrogen and testosterone should be supplemented if low.

Hydrocortisone supplementation is controversial. Low doses may produce modest benefits that are not worth the attendant risks. Glucocorticoids are not recommended for CFS/FMS patients.

Thyroid hormone controls metabolism by converting calories to energy. Hypothyroidism is common in CFS/FMS patients. Many physicians treat hypothyroidism when symptoms are present and test results are low or low-normal. Hypothyroidism slows the heart rate and is characterized by symptoms of sluggishness, fatigue, modest weight gain, dry skin, hair loss, brittle nails and hair, cold intolerance, irritability, confusion, and depression. Natural replacements such as Armour Thyroid supply both thyroxine and triiodothyronine, whereas synthetic thyroids (Synthroid and Levothroid) replace thyroxine alone.

DHEA (dehydroepiandrosterone) and pregnenolone, endogenous hormones, are excreted primarily by the adrenal glands. A potent steroid precursor, DHEA has not been studied well in humans, although a neuroendocrine role is suggested. Clinically substantiated (yet controversial) for replacement therapy in patients with low serum levels, DHEA is reported to slow or reverse the aging process, improve cognitive function, promote weight loss, and increase lean muscle mass. Side effects include heart palpitations and mild hirsutism and complexion problems in women. Long-term effects remain unknown. Pregnenolone may help with energy, immune function, and mental clarity.

Growth hormone (GH) is produced by the pituitary gland and is vital to most body tissues, particularly for proper brain and immune function. GH enhances energy level and cognition, augments stroke volume, and improves exercise capacity and muscle strength. Low GH levels are common in CFS and FMS. Treatment consists of daily injections of Genotropin (somatropin); levels normalize quickly, but response to therapy is delayed with improvement apparent at the six-month mark. When treatment is discontinued, symptoms return. GH treatment is expensive and remains experimental.

Oxytocin, a hormone and neurotransmitter, is produced during the nursing of babies, by orgasms, and by nonsexual social bonding. No lab test exists; deficiency is suspected in the presence of pallor and cold extremities. Jacob Teitelbaum, M.D., suggests treating DHEA deficiencies before using oxytocin. Available in sublingual and nasal spray forms, oxytocin treatment has a dramatic effect in some patients, helping with fatigue, pain, libido, and cognition. Blood pressure should be monitored.

Relaxin, a polypeptide similar to insulin, is secreted by the ovaries in females and in the seminal tubules of males. Samuel Yue, M.D., finds that relaxin treatment decreases fatigue and muscle tension and spasm, restores sleep quality, improves cognition, increases growth hormone secretion, improves cardiac function, stabilizes the autonomic nervous system, and regulates sex hormones. However, relaxin research is in its infancy.

♦♦ Endometriosis ♦♦

Endometriosis seems to affect a higher percentage of those with CFS and FMS than the general population, for unknown reasons. Treatment includes medication (e.g., progestational agents) and surgery in severe cases.

♦♦ Fever ♦♦

Aspirin, ibuprofen, and acetaminophen are often used to bring down fever. Some doctors caution against this practice except with extremely high fever, since an elevated temperature is one of the body's natural ways of fighting infection. In fact, a slightly elevated body temperature may be detrimental to viral reproduction, when this is a factor, and thus benefit the patient.

♦♦ Headache ♦♦

"Brain swelling" headaches are often helped by Diamox (acetazolamide).

Muscle tension headaches may respond to NSAIDS, Botox (botulinum toxin type A), Fiorinal (butalbital, aspirin, and caffeine), Midrin (acetaminophen, isometheptene, and dichloralphenazone), or Norgesic or Norgesic Forte (orphenadrine, aspirin, and caffeine). White willow, an analgesic anti-inflammatory, helps headaches and rheumatic conditions due to its aspirinlike compounds.

❖❖ Migraine ❖❖

❖ **Prophylactic Therapy for Migraine** Along with avoidance of migraine-triggering foods, a variety of medications (including NSAIDs, antidepressants, beta blockers, and calcium channel blockers) are used for prophylactic therapy. In addition to the therapies that follow, angiotensin-converting enzyme (ACE) inhibitors, vitamin B_{12}, certain antibiotics, and other medications are being investigated as potential migraine preventatives.

Beta blockers used to reduce the frequency and severity of migraine attacks include Blocadren (timolol), Corgard (nadolol), Inderal (propranolol), Lopressor (metoprolol), and Tenormin (atenolol). Anticonvulsants include Depakene (valproic acid) and Depakote (divalproex sodium). Certain antidepressants effectively prevent migraines and other types of headaches. The most effective include the tricyclic antidepressants Elavil and Endep (amitriptyline) and Vivactil (protriptyline); the SSRIs Prozac (fluoxetine), Zoloft (sertraline), Paxil (paroxetine), and Luvox (fluvoxamine); Serzone (nefazodone); and the MAOI Nardil (phenelzine). Tiagabine, a GABA reuptake inhibitor, is being studied for possible prophylaxis of migraine.

Ergots (ergotamine preparations) have significant side effects, including rebound headaches.

Ergotamine tartrate (ET) and dihydroergotamine (DHE) have been a mainstay for migraine treatment for many years. Dihydroergotamine (DHE), an alpha-adrenergic blocker with fewer adverse effects, is available for IV, IM, and intranasal use. Sansert (methysergide) is a synthetic ergot alkaloid with preventive and treatment applications.

Calcium channel blockers may prevent migraine and cluster headaches, although results are mixed, drugs must be taken for months before any benefit is realized, and side effects are numerous. They include Calan (verapamil), Cardene (nicardipine), Cardizem (diltiazem), DynaCirc (isradipine), Nimotop (nimodipine), Norvasc (amlodipine besylate), and Procardia SR (nifedipine).

◆ **Treatment of Migraine** When migraines occur, helpful behavioral interventions include taking a hot shower or bath; lying down in a dark, quiet room; applying an ice pack to the head or alternating heat and cold; using relaxation techniques; massaging the painful area vigorously; and drinking a caffeine-containing beverage. Acupuncture, acupressure, biofeedback, osteopathic or chiropractic manipulation, and herbal preparations may also help.

OTC medications should be tried first for mild migraines, especially when taken at the first sign of an impending attack. Most often used are the NSAIDs (oral or injectable) and preparations such as Excedrin Migraine Formula, which contain ibuprofen, acetaminophen, and caffeine (which some patients prefer to take individually). Stronger analgesics, such as barbiturates and opioids, may be required for pain relief. These should not be used on a frequent basis, as they may cause rebound migraines. Prescription drugs often used synergistically with analgesics include vasoconstrictors, benzodiazepines, and muscle relaxants.

Ergots (ergotamine preparations) are used for treatment as well as prevention of migraines. DHE (dihydroergotamine) may be administered orally or as a nasal spray, Migranal. Cafergot and Wigraine are available in suppository form. Parlodel (bromocriptine, an ergot derivative) may be helpful for menstrual migraines. Side effects include light-headedness and nausea. Dependency may develop if ergots are used often, and they have numerous side effects and are toxic at high levels.

Triptans (5-HT 1B/1D agonists, or serotonin agonists) cause blood vessels to constrict. They are nonsedating, and some are available in quick-acting forms: Imitrex (sumatriptan; oral, injectable, or nasal spray), Zomig (zolmitriptan; dissolves on the tongue), Amerge (naratriptan), Maxalt (rizatriptan), eletriptan, avitriptan, frovatriptan, and almotriptan. Side effects of the triptans vary, and many are transient.

Among the **newer drugs** showing promise in migraine treatment are IV or IM magnesium sulfate in those whose magnesium levels are subnormal; nose drops containing lidocaine, a local anesthetic; the epalons (e.g., ganaxolone), anti-inflammatory, steroidlike drugs that affect nerve cells; Haldol (haloperidol, by injection), an antipsychotic; nitric oxide-blocking drugs ; the blood thinner Coumadin (warfarin); Stadol (butorphanol tartrate), a narcotic nasal spray possibly associated with reports of addiction and deaths; and herbs including ginger and feverfew.

Nonoral routes of administration (injection, nasal spray, and suppository) are preferable when migraines begin with nausea or vomiting, which may be helped by Compazine (prochlorperazine), Phenergan (promethazine), Reglan (metoclopramide), or Tigan (trimethobenzamide HCl).

✦✦ Immunomodulation ✦✦

Allergy injections may be helpful when proper precautions are taken. Starting doses for CFS/FMS patients should be quite low compared to typical starting doses. Some allergists prefer to use preservative-free serum for those who are most sensitive.

Alpha interferon liquid in small, sublingual doses may benefit some CFS/FMS patients. It is taken for three to six months and then discontinued, with a subset of patients experiencing benefit, often following an initial relapse.

Ampligen (poly I-poly C12U) is a biological response modulator with antiviral and immunomodulating properties that normalizes the 2-5A synthetase/RNaseL antiviral pathway. It is manufactured for IV use only and is quite expensive. It is an investigational treatment therapy, and results of studies are promising despite some side effects (idiosyncratic reactions; intractable pain, liver toxicity, headache, and nausea; and initial exacerbation of symptoms). Significant improvement was found on Karnofsky performance scores, bicycle testing, cognition, increased activity level and exercise tolerance, sleep improvement, and general health perception as well as a drop in the low-molecular-weight enzyme (RNaseL enzyme dysfunction disorder occurs with overproduction of the abnormal LMW [low molecular weight] RNaseL, which damages the body by consuming ATP, the energy source within cells). The best responders seem to be those who test positive for 37kDa RNaseL, have been ill less than five years, are less than fifty years old, and have a postmononucleosis status. Ampligen has antiviral properties that may be effective against HHV-6, cancer, and hepatitis B and C.

Anticytokine drugs, which block the action of harmful cytokines, are being researched. Enbrel (etanercept), which blocks the action of the proinflammatory cytokine tumor necrosis factor (TNF), has shown promise in a preliminary study, reducing fatigue and pain while improving exercise tolerance. Other such drugs may play a role in future treatment.

Astragalus (available OTC) increases white blood cell production and strengthens the immune response.

Bitter melon (Momordica charlantia) (available OTC) in enteric-coated capsules increases natural killer (NK) cell function and numbers and regulates sugar metabolism.

Bloodroot (sanguinaria canadensis), found in some toothpastes and mouthwashes, is an immune booster that decreases plaque and gum disease and may have antitumor activity.

Colostrum (available OTC), produced by all mammals, confers immunity to infants through breastfeeding. Animune TF is made from bovine colostrum, which may assist immune functioning in humans.

Evening primrose oil (available OTC) is rich in essential fatty acids, which are critical precursors in the manufacture of anti-inflammatory prostaglandins.

Flaxseed oil (available OTC) contains essential fatty acids and can help eczema, menstrual disorders, rheumatoid arthritis, and atherosclerosis while decreasing inflammation of the mucous membranes.

Gamma globulin, a blood product containing antibodies, is used when total IgG is low, or in the presence of IgG subclass deficiencies. (IgG is one of several types of immunoglobins that are produced in the lymph cells to combat foreign substances.) Although expensive, inconvenient, and not always covered by medical insurance, IV gamma globulin is usually more effective than IM administration. Low doses do not produce significant effects, while high doses cause major side effects, including headache, nausea, malaise, phlebitis, and transiently abnormal liver-function tests. Benefits may be temporary. Results of experimental trials have been inconsistent due to the wide variability in dosages.

Garlic (available OTC), an antifungal, antibacterial, antiviral, and antiparasitic, may increase natural killer (NK) cell activity. Garlic is believed to have cardiovascular benefits, lowering cholesterol and blood pressure. Its active ingredient is allicin. Garlic is contraindicated in those taking anticoagulants.

Glutathione, a naturally occurring brain antioxidant, is important in the body's detoxification pathways and is believed to act as a strong antiviral and antimicrobial agent, fighting such opportunistic infections as chlamydia and mycoplasma. Intravenous glutathione therapy helps fatigue, IBS, pain, cognition, and energy. Undenatured whey, sold under various product labels, has been found to restore intracellular glutathione levels in a subset of CFS patients but is considered experimental.

Imunovir (isoprinosine) is an immune modulator with antiviral properties. Available for over thirty years, it has no serious side effects. Studies yield variable responses. Modest improvements in general health and energy include improved cognition, decreased ataxia and clumsiness, better motor function, and increased activity level.

Kutapressin, a porcine liver extract of polypeptides with a long history of safety, is an immunomodulator with lymphokine-inhibiting, antiviral, and anti-inflammatory properties. Kutapressin's effectiveness often begins after a series of injections. Relapse may occur upon discontinuation of treatment. Side effects are minimal, limited to local injection-site reactions. A primary drawback of Kutapressin is its high cost.

Licorice root (glycyrrhiza glabra) (available OTC) inhibits viruses, improves blood circulation, and aids digestion and adrenal insufficiency. It increases fluid retention and blood pressure but should be used with caution when treating neurally mediated hypotension as it may deplete sodium and potassium. Blood pressure should be monitored.

Lomatium tincture (available OTC) may be used for symptom exacerbation. It is an antiviral immune stimulant that helps chronic fatigue and respiratory problems.

Raspberry leaves (available OTC) brewed as a tea helps flus, colds, diarrhea, and other viral illnesses.

Shiitake, reishi, and maitake mushrooms contain oligosaccharides, potent immune stimulants.

Selective serotonin reuptake inhibitors (SSRIs) may play a role in the treatment of CFS and FMS that goes beyond its antidepressant effects. It may serve as an immune modulator, possibly increasing the number of natural killer cells.

Th1/Th2 cytokine balance: A Th2-type response is characterized by the production of cytokines such as interleukin IL-4, IL-5, and IL-10, and favors the function of B lymphocytes, the cellular factories of immunoglobulins. A predominance of a Th2-type response is therefore consistent with such pathologies as autoimmunity and atopy. A Th1 response favors the macrophages and natural killer cells, whose function is to destroy invading microbes and cancer cells. Typical Th1-type cytokines include IL-2 and interferon gamma. The goal of many immune therapies is to decrease Th2-type predominance to allow a stronger Th1-type response.

In a recent study, lymph nodes of patients were surgically removed and cultured with certain immune substances. Cells were then reinfused into donors to alter the balance of certain cytokines from a Th2 to a Th1 immune response. In altering the cytokine balance, sustained general clinical improvement was obtained with no adverse effects. Further studies are planned (Patarca-Montero, Klimas, and Fletcher 2001).

Transfer factor (TF) is a naturally-occurring substance that "teaches" immune cells to identify specific pathogens as threats, attack them, and remember them in case the same agent should attack in the future. One type of TF is disease-specific, conferring immunity to a particular pathogen, whereas the nonspecific type is used to improve overall immune functioning. TF is quite expensive, and its safety and efficacy in treating CFS/FMS are undetermined.

Trental (pentoxifylline), used to treat circulatory disorders, is an inhibitor of tumor necrosis factor (TNF), a troublesome cytokine in CFS and possibly FMS.

❖❖ Infections ❖❖

Antivirals are used only when evidence of active viral infection is present. These agents include Cytovene (ganciclovir), Famvir (famciclovir), Foscarnet (foscavir), Valcyte (valganciclovir), Valtrex (valacyclovir), Vistide (cidofovir), and Zovirax (acyclovir). A. Martin Lerner, M.D., hypothesizes that CFS results from cardiomyopathy caused by the Epstein-Barr virus and cytomegalovirus that can be successfully treated with Valtrex or Cytovene, respectively. Ampligen, discussed earlier, has been found to inhibit HHV-6 replication and may be effective against other viruses.

Antibiotics are used to treat only bacterial infections; overuse and inappropriate use of antibiotics encourages the development of resistant bacterial strains. Most strains of mycoplasma respond to such general antibiotics as hydrophobic tetracyclines (doxycycline, minocycline), Zithromax (azithromycin), floxacins (ciprofloxacin, sparfloxacin, levofloxacin, and so on), Biaxin (clarithromycin), clindamycin, and erythromycin, but not penicillins. Short-term treatment is rarely effective and may be harmful. Since an individual patient may be infected with several mycoplasma species that respond to different antibiotics, they are often administered in six-week cycles, interspersed with drug holidays. Recovery from long-established infections is typically slow. John Martin, M.D., believes that antibiotics may have immune-modulating effects.

Beta interferon has been used with moderate success in treating HHV-6 in patients with multiple sclerosis. Antivirals may be used synergistically with alpha or beta interferon.

Nitric oxide (NO) is a vasodilator, neurotransmitter, antimicrobial effector molecule, and immunomodulator that can inhibit the growth of certain viruses, parasites, and bacteria.

Herbs used to treat viral infections include garlic, a broad-spectrum anti-infective; raspberry leaf tea; yarrow to break up congestion and decrease fevers; marshmallow to soothe bronchial membranes in bronchitis and act as an expectorant; and eucalyptus leaves, whose vapors open congested airways. Olive leaf extract has antiviral (herpes, viral infections, flus, colds), antifungal, antiparasitic, and antibacterial properties, with the ability to inhibit the replication of viruses. Osha root is helpful for congestion and has antiviral and immune-stimulating properties.

◆◆ Multiple Chemical Sensitivity ◆◆

Although avoidance of offending chemicals is the best remedy for multiple chemical sensitivity, Neurontin (gabapentin), along with Zoloft (sertraline) or the antiseizure drug Lamictal (lamotrigine), helps patients tolerate previously difficult substances.

◆◆ Nasal Congestion and Sinus Pain ◆◆

Decongestants, available OTC or by prescription, reduce nasal and sinus congestion. They may cause a "wired" feeling and interfere with sleep.

Antihistamines are available OTC and by prescription. Most cause drowsiness, but certain newer prescription antihistamines such as Claritin (loratadine), Seldane (terfenadine), and Hismanal (astemizole) do not. Nasalcrom (cromolyn sodium), nasal steroids, and seasonal injections of long-acting steroids such as Depo-Medrol (methylprednisolone acetate) may be helpful. Many patients report increased allergic symptoms that are not relieved by allergy injections.

Nasal douching is an excellent, inexpensive treatment for sinus problems and allergic rhinitis. With the head tilted to the side and slightly back, a mixture of 8 ounces of warm water, ½ teaspoon of salt, and a pinch of baking soda is squirted gently several times into each nostril using a rubber bulb syringe. The solution exits via the other nostril or passes down the throat and out through the mouth. Afterward, the nose is blown gently. This procedure is initially messy, uncomfortable, and awkward but can be easily mastered with practice. It relieves nasal irritation, eliminates allergens from the nasal passages, and drains the sinuses.

◆◆ Neurological Interventions ◆◆

Paul Cheney, M.D., believes that Klonopin (clonazepam), a useful drug for brain injury, is neuroprotective and should be taken in small doses at night for sleep and very small doses during the day for increased alertness. He also suggests the use of calcium channel blockers and magnesium, which acts as a calcium channel blocker in neurological disease.

◆◆ Orthostatic Hypotension: Neurally Mediated Hypotension ◆◆

Orthostatic hypotension (OH) affects those with autonomic insufficiency common in diabetes, Parkinson's disease, FMS, and CFS. Therapies have not been as successful as hoped. Pharmaceuticals and other interventions for neurally mediated hypotension (NMH) include Florinef (fludrocortisone) to increase blood volume; Pro-Amatine (midodrine), a vasoconstrictor; increased salt and fluid intake; DHEA; and oxytocin. Epogen (erythropoetin) increases blood volume and causes increased production of red blood cells, according to preliminary studies. Biofeedback may have application in treating OH and NMH. *Ruscus aculeatus* (butcher's broom) may help OH due to its vasoconstrictive and venotonic properties that help reverse the poor venous tone, pooling of blood in the limbs, and lack of vasoconstriction of OH. Behavioral interventions include standing in a legs-crossed position, squatting, sitting in a knee-chest position, bending forward, or putting a foot on a chair while standing, rather than remaining in a fixed position, and increasing intake of salt (sodium chloride) and fluids.

◆◆ Pain ◆◆

"Just learn to live with it" is not an acceptable approach to pain management. Although total pain relief is rarely, if ever, achieved, patients must be offered a number of options by knowledgeable healthcare professionals.

— Steve Fanto, M.D.

The goal in pain treatment is to block pain signals while minimizing physiological side effects and disruption of one's quality of life. Treatment of pain must be individualized and comprehensive, combining pharmaceuticals and such adjunctive therapies as stretching, exercise, physical therapy, massage, relaxation techniques, meditation, acupuncture, acupressure, and attention to psychological issues. The health care practitioner must be sufficiently flexible to try various approaches to determine what works best, starting conservatively and building as necessary. A regimen should be developed that is appropriate for the individual as an adjunct to the use of medications.

Pain should be treated aggressively but carefully. Many physicians mismanage pain patients, underestimating their experience of pain and undertreating it, often staying at the lowest end of dosage range for safety. Fearful of addiction issues and censure by medical boards and colleagues, they may be reluctant to prescribe opioids, particularly in poorly understood or "questionable" chronic pain states. Pain is often treated more aggressively by rheumatologists, physiatrists, anesthesiologists, and psychiatrists than by general practitioners or other specialists.

Lifestyle modification is always helpful, including moderation of activity, ergonomics, proper posture, frequent shifts in body position, sleep hygiene, avoiding eccentric movements, relaxation techniques, and dietary changes if sensitivities are present.

◆ **Pharmacology of Pain Treatment** Pain treatment often begins with NSAIDs (nonsteroidal anti-inflammatory drugs) and other analgesics, progressing to weak opioids, and finally to strong opioids if necessary.

NSAIDs have analgesic, antipyretic (fever reducing), and anti-inflammatory properties (although FMS is not associated with inflammation). Often used adjunctively with tricyclics and anxiolytics, commonly used NSAIDs include aspirin; Advil and Motrin (ibuprofen); Indocin (indomethacin); Relafen (nabumetone); Aleve, Anaprox, and Naprosyn (naproxen); Voltaren (diclofenac); Daypro (oxaprozin); and Feldene (piroxicam). Some NSAIDs are available by prescription, others are OTC, and most are available as generics. If one NSAID is ineffective, another should be tried. NSAIDs are effective against pain but often do not significantly affect severe, continuing pain. Long-term use may cause gastrointestinal (GI) problems such as bleeding and ulcers. Newer NSAIDs, called COX-2 inhibitors, such as Celebrex (celecoxib) and Vioxx (rofecoxib), were developed to avoid GI side effects, but like other NSAIDs may harm the kidneys with prolonged use. It may take a week or two to determine whether the medication is helping.

Acetaminophen (Tylenol) is an analgesic but not an anti-inflammatory drug.

Ultram (tramadol), a weak opioid, is a newer non-NSAID pain reliever. Easily prescribed by physicians, it is a helpful and usually well controlled substance. Side effects include drowsiness, dizziness, headache, nausea, constipation, or a stimulatory effect, usually decreasing after several days. If side effects are particularly troublesome, they can be treated with appropriate medications, or the dose of Ultram can be decreased and then increased gradually.

Steroids should be avoided because they are not typically helpful for CFS/FMS pain and have serious side effects.

Opioids are the strongest and most effective pain medications and are quite safe, causing no end-organ damage or toxicity. In a natural approach to pain management, opioids mimic the chemicals made by the central nervous system to control pain.

Opioids fall into several categories:

- Morphine based: MS Contin, Darvocet-N, and Darvon-N. Tylenol Nos. 3 and 4 contain codeine
- Oxycodone based: OxyContin, Percodan, Percocet; Roxicet, Roxicodone, and Tylox
- Hydrocodone based: Vicodin, Anexsia, Lortab, Norcet, and Zydone
- Methadone (Dolophine): equivalent to morphine but short-acting (two to four hours)

Many of these preparations combine acetaminophen and other pain relievers synergistically, enhancing their pain-relieving properties. However, acetaminophen and other OTC pain relievers can have serious side effects when used on a long-term basis.

A pain protocol typically starts with NSAIDs, progressing to Ultram, and then to short-acting opioids, and, if necessary, to sustained-release (long-acting) opioids: OxyContin SR (time-release oxycodone); morphine-based MS Contin, OxyContin, Oramorth, and Kadian; or methadone. (Methadone, also used in addiction recovery, is more potent than morphine.) Long-acting pain medications help sleep continuity. Synergistic use of pain medications often provides maximum benefit. Initial side effects of opiates include constipation, "brain fog," and sedation, although some patients become energized. Of the drugs in this category, hydrocodone and oxycodone are usually most effective.

Many physicians are concerned about patient addiction; however, only about 5 percent of the general population is at risk of addiction, and it rarely occurs in the treatment of chronic pain. Pain patients are not typically fond of pain medication; virtually all would gladly give up their medications if only the pain would cease. Pain patients typically experience pain relief without a state of euphoria.

The attitudinal barriers of many physicians result from misconceptions of the nature of chronic pain and its treatment, fear of disciplinary action by regulatory agencies, negative views of those with chronic pain, and learned biases that are perpetuated in medical schools. Addiction, a neurobehavioral syndrome resulting in psychological dependence on the use of substances for their psychic effects, is characterized by tolerance (requiring higher doses to achieve the same effect); nontherapeutic or recreational use; compulsive use despite harm and interference with the patient's life; and behaviors such as seeking prescriptions from multiple doctors and making excuses for early medication refills. Pseudoaddiction, drug-seeking due to inadequate pain relief, is often mistaken for addiction.

The physical dependence and tolerance that are normal physiological consequences of extended opioid therapy for pain should not be considered addiction. An expected result of opioid use, physical dependence is a physiologic state of neuroadaptation with withdrawal symptoms if the drug is stopped or decreased abruptly. Tolerance may develop during opioid treatment. If opiates must be discontinued, they should be tapered gradually.

Patients may be reluctant to seek treatment for pain and may underreport it to their physicians, fearful of being regarded as drug-seekers. Physicians who treat pain disorders are expected to do so aggressively and without judgment. Suicide should be considered a greater danger than addiction potential, since inadequately treated chronic pain patients are at significant risk of taking their own lives.

Anticonvulsants/antiepileptics (AEDs) may be prescribed for the relief of acute and chronic pain. The traditional AEDs—Dilantin (phenytoin), Tegretol (carbamazepine), and Depakote (divalproex sodium) or Depakene (valproic acid)—are somewhat toxic. Newer AEDs have better safety profiles: Neurontin (gabapentin), Lamictal (lamotrigine), and Topamax (topiramate). The most common side effects are mild, transient sedation and dizziness, with possible renal dysfunction and weight gain at high doses. Dosage should be reduced if drowsiness and sedation are problematic. Klonopin (clonazepam) is effective for trigeminal neuralgia, myofascial pain, and migraine prophylaxis.

Tricyclic antidepressants (TCAs) may help to relieve pain and restore sleep at doses lower than those required to treat depression and with faster onset of action. Adverse side effects of TCAs include dry mouth, constipation, urinary retention, and daytime drowsiness, increasing with higher doses. The "morning hangover effect" usually disappears over time; medication may be taken earlier in the evening if this is troublesome. TCAs must be taken on a regular basis for effective pain relief. If one TCA is ineffective, another may help. Low-dose Sinequan or Adapin (doxepin), Elavil or Endep (amitriptyline), Pamelor or Aventil (nortriptyline), Desyrel (trazadone), and Flexeril (cyclobenzaprine) are most commonly used. Other antidepressants may be sedating, including Remeron (mirtazapine). SSRIs have not been studied systematically for treatment of chronic pain, although they may decrease pain perception and are well tolerated.

Benzodiazepines, such as low-dose Xanax (alprazolam) or Klonopin (clonazepam), affect mood, spasticity, seizures, and sleep. They help chronic pain syndromes characterized by muscle spasm, anxiety, or neuropathic pain (such as chronic, intractable temporomandibular joint dysfunction, myofascial pain, and migraine). The potential for tolerance and abuse with long-term use is mitigated by the low doses typically used in CFS/FMS treatment.

Muscle relaxants, used adjunctively with other therapies, relieve painful musculoskeletal conditions by relaxing the muscles and reducing muscle spasms. They include Flexeril (cyclobenzaprine), Norflex (orphenadrine), Parafon Forte (chlorzoxazone), Robaxin (methocarbamol), Soma (carisoprodol), and Baclofen (lioresal). Dantrium (dantrolene), Skelaxin (metaxalone), and Zanaflex (tizanidine) are nonsedating muscle relaxants.

◆◆ Novel Agents and Promising Pain Therapies ◆◆

Bromocriptine (parlodel), an ergot alkaloid that increases dopamine and decreases prolactin, may help pain levels in fibromyalgia.

Cayenne, believed to inhibit substance P, is taken orally or applied topically. It helps peripheral neuropathy, muscle cramps, and restless leg syndrome.

Dong quai has analgesic properties, according to anecdotal accounts.

Glucosamine/chondroitin products are used for treatment of joint pain. They get mixed reviews, with some patients reporting pain relief after about three weeks. Standardization is poor, making efficacy difficult to ascertain.

Anecdotal reports indicate that **growth hormone,** discussed previously, may reduce joint pain.

Guaifenesin, an expectorant found in cough medicines, increases removal of phosphates from the body. Paul St. Anand, M.D., hypothesizes that an inherited defect in phosphate excretion exists in FMS patients, inhibiting ATP production and leading to constant muscle contraction and lack of energy. According to St. Anand, patients feel initially worse; the time until benefit is felt is directly proportional to the length of time ill. He recommends avoidance of salicylates and other substances that block the effectiveness of guaifenesin, which is available in capsule form by prescription or OTC. This treatment is experimental and controversial.

Low-dose sublingual nitroglycerin, a vasodilator, may reduce pain. Higher doses do not add benefit.

Mestinon (pyridostigmine) may augment mental clarity and energy as well as analgesia.

Nitric oxide (NO), a vasodilator, neurotransmitter, and immunomodulator, may help pain and can be augmented by nitroglycerin.

N-methyl-D-aspartate (NMDA) agonists: NMDA is a glutamate (amino acid) receptor that amplifies pain perception. Treatment with IV ketamine, an NMDA agonist, provides increased muscle endurance and almost immediate pain relief that lasts for several days, sometimes up to a week. Unfortunately, side effects preclude administration on a regular basis. Dextromethorphan, contained in many OTC cough medicines, is a nonnarcotic, morphinelike substance that affects abnormal central nervous system processing. It is available in an OTC liquid form, Delsym, and can be compounded in pill form.

Toxins may be injected into the spine to kill specific nerve cells to block transmission of substance P. Poison extracted from frogs (the South American frog *Epibpedobates tricolor*) is chemically similar to nicotine, producing an analgesic effect when it attaches to nerve cells. This phenomenon requires further research to identify nontoxic substances that have the same effect.

Marijuana may exert a direct effect on the pain signals in the central nervous system and tissues. Cannabinoids have been used for centuries to provide pain relief with fewer side effects (and probably less pain relief) than opiates, but societal attitudes discourage their use. Marijuana is considered effective and nonaddictive. Tolerance does not develop, meaning that pain relief is obtained without the need to increase the dose.

Transdermal medicines are topical applications of preparations that are absorbed through the skin. **Topical medications** have the advantages of increased efficiency, fewer side effects, easier dosing, and not having to be digested. Almost any drug can be made into a transdermal patch. Examples include NMDA/calcium channel blockers (ketamine, orphenadrine, and dextromethorphan), NMDA/sodium channel blockers (carbamazapine; lidocaine; and Mexitil or mexiletine HCl), alpha agonists (Catapres, or clonidine HCl), and GABA or antiseizure medications (Neurontin, or gabapentin; Baclofen, or lioresal; and Klonopin, or clonazepam). Transdermal nicotine patches, often one-half of the lowest-dose patch, may help pain while enhancing cognition. Capsaicin and other analgesic creams and ointments are topically applied to areas of localized pain. Capsaicin cream must be applied routinely for several days or weeks before relief is felt. DMSO (dimethyl sulfoxide) can serve as an efficient means of transporting substances through the skin, and some patients blend it with pain medications to make topical salves.

Substance P antagonists may prove helpful in treating pain, anxiety, and depression, although trials have not produced encouraging results.

Axonal transport, an alternative to swallowing and digesting medications, relies on communication among nerves, allowing a drug to be delivered directly to pain-sensitive nerves. Side effects are diminished when medications are transported by mucous membranes, such as with nasal sprays, which are able to cross the blood-brain barrier.

Gene therapy: Pain-relieving genes can be injected into the spinal fluid or the tissue surrounding the spinal cord for maximum benefit. Effects are not permanent, peaking within a week and wearing off after about two weeks. Gene therapy is reported to be nontoxic. Further research is needed for this promising therapy.

◆◆ Complementary Pain Therapies ◆◆

Heat and ice: Ice is used for muscle spasm, while heat is more beneficial for chronic pain. Draping gel packs over juice cans in the freezer allows them to freeze in an arc shape, and bags of frozen peas or beans are easily formed to the body's contours. Heat increases blood circulation and relaxes muscles and may be applied with a hot-water bottle, heating pad, heat lamp, whirlpool, or hot bath. Since hot baths may increase fatigue and malaise, it is best to cool down afterward by adding cool water to the bath.

Hypnosis provides a state of altered consciousness, or trance. In this state, one is suggestible but still maintains control. Contrary to entertainment-type hypnosis, one will reject any thoughts or behavior suggestions that are undesirable. Hypnosis has a variety of applications, including relaxation, pain reduction, and achieving desired behavior changes. To avoid unscrupulous or poorly trained practitioners, check the credentials of any hypnotherapist, preferably a licensed psychologist or counselor. Professionals may teach self-hypnosis skills for continuation of beneficial effects beyond the office setting.

Relaxation therapy brings on deep relaxation to decrease stress and muscle tension, improve sleep, and help to create or restore a sense of well-being. Techniques include breathing exercises, progressive muscle relaxation, visualization or guided imagery, autogenic training, and hypnosis or self-hypnosis. Techniques may be learned from therapists, books, audiotapes, or classes, and supplemented by daily practice. Biofeedback may be used to assist learning. Calming techniques may be practiced at first with a relaxation tape and, once the relaxation response is mastered, without it, allowing application in "real life" stressful situations.

Acupuncture, based on Chinese philosophy and tradition, is an electrochemical process used to balance and regulate the activity of chi, the basic body energy that flows through complex pathways called meridians. Symptoms and disease are believed to result from blocks in the flow of chi. Acupuncture stimulates various points along these channels (which often correlate with common tender or trigger points) with the insertion of fine needles to restore energy flow, decrease pain, and release endorphins, creating a sense of well-being. Additional techniques may accompany needle insertion, such as burning of a substance called moxa near the skin, shiatsu, laser acupuncture, and electro-acupuncture. Electrochemical stimulation of the peripheral nervous system has a positive effect on the central nervous system (CNS), probably affecting neurotransmitters. The FDA has removed acupuncture needles from its list of experimental medical devices, reclassifying them as accepted medical equipment, a sign that acupuncture is entering the medical mainstream.

Trigger and tender point injections (TPIs) are believed to interrupt nerve junctions to relieve pain, restore meridian energy flow, and release endorphins. Trigger points must be located accurately prior to injection, since they are often distant from the sites where pain is felt. When the TP site is properly identified, tissue resistance is felt as the needle is inserted, with a sudden increase in pain, often radiating to other body sites. Pain relief may be immediate, with an increased range of motion following the injection. One area at a time is treated, often with a combination of a local anesthetic (lidocaine or procaine) for quick relief and a longer-acting corticosteroid for inflammation, with effects felt after two to five days. Good results are also obtained with use of a local anesthetic alone, phenoxybenzamine, saline solution, Botox (botulinum toxin type A), or dry needling (acupuncture needles alone to mechanically disrupt the TP). Infrared laser therapy may prove helpful for trigger point therapy. Acupressure can also be used to break up trigger points in less painful areas.

After the injection, the patient is usually encouraged to stretch the muscle to its fullest range of motion. A spray may then be used on the whole muscle to inactivate less severe tender points. In some cases, injections may be needed two or three times over six to eight weeks. There is some soreness afterward, which can be severe, and the benefits of the treatment may not be immediately apparent. When TPI is successful, pain relief may last several months.

Stretching and exercise help to relieve muscle pain and spasms while strengthening muscles, increasing range of motion while preventing deconditioning. Patients are encouraged to follow a slow, incremental program. Walking, swimming, modified water aerobics, and bicycle riding may be best tolerated. (See "Lifestyle Modification" on page 276.)

◆ **Physical Modalities for Pain Treatment** A wide variety of hands-on bodywork therapies are available to treat pain.

Biofeedback applications are relevant to a number of CFS/FMS symptoms, including muscle tension, pain, and headache. The basic principle is simple: to provide auditory or visual feedback when a desired physiological change is produced. Brain waves, blood flow, and muscle tension can be measured with electrodes taped to various body points, with sounds or lights offering feedback in regard to muscle tension or other relevant functions. By associating the desired state with positive feedback, the behavior change is learned and reinforced, becoming easier to achieve over time. Ultimately, the patient is able to produce the response without the aid of equipment and apply the techniques in daily life.

Blockades such as facet blocks, epidurals, and peripheral nerve blocks are more aggressive forms of treatment for complicated pain problems and should be performed by experienced, skilled anesthesiologists with expertise in pain treatment.

Physical therapy, tailored to the individual, can help with pain reduction, range of motion, flexibility, and vascularization (improved blood flow), optimizing functional ability and preventing deconditioning. Ultrasound and electrical stimulation, stretching, and various devices may be used. Patients are usually taught self-management skills for home therapy between—and ultimately in place of—sessions with the therapist. The physical therapist should be knowledgeable about FMS/CFS pain states and experienced in working with FMS/CFS patients.

Spray and stretch: Tender points are sprayed with an anesthetic coolant, usually fluorimethane, and then muscles are stretched to the fullest range possible, followed by muscle warming and additional stretching. This technique provides pain relief, decreased muscle spasms, and increased range of motion. Such sprays are environmentally damaging to the ozone layer, and chemically sensitive patients may not be able to tolerate them. Sprays should not be used near the face.

Occupational therapy (OT) teaches proper body mechanics related to work and home environments, addressing physical comfort, avoidance of harmful or repetitive movements, and maximal productivity. Special movements, implements, and environmental adaptations increase functional ability.

Postural training can help one reeducate misaligned joints and muscles to decrease pain. Harmful postures and movements are often the product of lifelong habits that can be unlearned and replaced with more comfortable body mechanics.

Magnet therapy has received media attention, but few studies have been conducted. Anecdotal reports do not indicate substantial benefit.

Massotherapy, or massage, offers a multitude of benefits: pain relief, increased circulation, removal of toxins from the body, "unlocking" tight muscles, and encouraging relaxation. Believed to stimulate the sympathetic nervous system, massage may be combined with ultrasound or the use of hot and cold packs and other modalities. Types of massage include Swedish massage for relaxation; myofascial massage, deep-tissue work to relieve pain and tightness; reflexology, the stimulation of points on the hands and feet that correspond to body organs; and shiatsu, the application of strong pressure to points along meridians corresponding to lymph channels, often painful but ultimately relaxing. Since vigorous massage can cause symptoms to flare, it is best to start with one of the gentler types. A massage therapist should be knowledgeable about CFS/FMS and experienced in this area, and be willing to accept patient input regarding preferences and pain and comfort levels.

Craniosacral therapy is a gentle, noninvasive technique to restore normal rhythmic movement of the cerebrospinal fluid and the cranial bones, which is disrupted in CFS/FMS. Restoring normal rhythm is believed to have a positive effect on the central nervous system. Although no formal studies have been conducted, many anecdotal reports are positive.

Osteopathic or chiropractic manipulation may help to decrease pain. Techniques typically include spinal adjustment, massage, electrical stimulation, and ultrasound. X-rays are rarely needed. Results may be temporary, and repeated visits may be necessary to correct misalignments.

✦✦ Parasitic Infections ✦✦

Parasitic infections are treated with antiparasitics such as Flagyl (metronidazole) and Yodoxin (iodoquinol), antibiotics including Zithromax (azithromycin) and Bactrim (trimethoprim and sulfamethoxazole), and the herbs tricyclin and *Artemisia annua.*

✦✦ Sleep Disorder ✦✦

Often the primary focus of treatment, sleep disorders are helped with medications, relaxation techniques, and improved sleep hygiene (discussed on pages 225–226), as well as treatment of related disorders that may disturb sleep.

Sleep-related disorders that should be treated include myoclonus, restless leg syndrome, sleep apnea, bruxism, rhinitis (stuffy nose), acid reflux, frequent urination, anxiety, and depression.

✦ Sleep Medications Sleep medications are called "hypnotics." This group of medicines includes Ativan (lorazepam), Centrax (prazepam), Dalmane (flurazepam), Doral (quazepam), Halcion (triazolam), ProSom (estazolam), Restoril (temazepam), Rohypnol (flunitrazepam), Serax (oxazepam), and Xanax (alprazolam).

Before prescribing hypnotics, the health care professional must be aware of all prescription and OTC medications and supplements currently taken by the patient. Jacob Teitelbaum, M.D., recommends using small amounts of several agents as safer and more effective than using large amounts of only one. Some sleep medications—for example, Halcion, Restoril, and Serax—lose their effectiveness if taken continuously; these are best saved for difficult nights, for short-term use.

Side effects of many sleep medications include morning "hang-over," blurred vision, dizziness, confusion, nightmares, upset stomach, anxiety, and restlessness. Use the lowest effective dose, and consult your doctor if that amount is no longer effective. Since sleep medications vary in the length of time until sleep onset, ask a doctor or pharmacist when each should be taken.

Benzodiazepines are commonly prescribed for sleep, although some physicians discourage their use, feeling that they disrupt sleep more than they help it. Like narcotics, they may block stage 4 sleep, often deficient or lacking in CFS/FMS patients. "Benzos," often combined with low-dose tricyclic antidepressants for sleep, may decrease pain perception; however, they are habituating and addictive. Side effects include decreased REM sleep, daytime sleepiness, memory loss, anxiety, confusion, dizziness, nightmares, agitation, headache, and upset stomach, although most patients tolerate them quite well. Paradoxically, very small doses of benzos may increase cognition and alertness during the day. Of the benzos, low-dose Klonopin (clonazepam) is the most often used.

Nonbenzodiazepine short-acting hypnotics include Ambien (zolpidem), Sonata (zaleplon), and Imovane (zopiclone). These drugs may not pose as high a risk for drug tolerance or dependence as the longer-acting benzodiazepines. Sonata works even faster than Ambien and, unlike other hypnotics, can be taken for sleep after a patient has been in bed awhile without producing a morning "hang-over." Adverse side effects of these drugs are mild but can include nausea, dizziness, nightmares, agitation, headache, and daytime drowsiness. They may cause rebound and be subject to abuse, although the risk for dependence and tolerance is far lower than for benzodiazepines. Ambien is quite effective and well tolerated but considered habituating by some doctors, who are reluctant to prescribe it except for occasional use. Other physicians are comfortable prescribing it on a regular basis. Although Ambien does not interfere with sleep stages, it does not help to restore normal sleep patterns, either.

Antiepileptic agents may be used to improve sleep. Neurontin (gabapentin), for example, is calming; Depakene (valproic acid) is sedating and helpful for headaches that can disrupt sleep.

Tricyclic antidepressants (TCAs) are also prescribed for sleep. Sinequan (doxepin) is the most commonly used TCA. Because it is quite sedating, very small amounts are used, often in elixir form. Low-dose Flexeril (cyclobenzaprine) may be less likely to produce a morning hangover and has muscle-relaxing properties that also enhance sleep. If one TCA is ineffective, others may be tried.

Provigil (modafinil), a well-tolerated, wake-promoting agent that significantly improves fatigue and daytime sleepiness has the night-time "rebound effect" of drowsiness, promoting sleep.

OTC sleep aids are nonaddictive and often available as generics and in long-acting form. Sedating antihistamines are mild sleep inducers. Prominent among them are Benadryl and UniSom gel caps (diphenhydramine), UniSom tablets (doxylamine succinate), and time-release Chlortrimeton (chlorpheniramine). An additional benefit is treatment of nasal allergies; side effects include dryness of mouth and eyes.

5-HT, a serotonin agent, should not be used with high-dose SSRIs.

◆ **Herbal Sleep Remedies** Herbal or "natural" remedies help many individuals but have not been well studied.

Hops, brewed as a tea from fresh or freshly dried buds, helps with sleep and anxiety.

Kava kava contains pyrones and lactones. It has sedative and sleep-enhancement effects and reduces anxiety but may adversely affect motor reflexes and judgment for driving. Do not use kava for more than three months without medical advice. It may cause dry, flaking, discolored (yellow) skin, scaly rash, red eyes, puffy face, and muscle weakness, and is contraindicated in endogenous depression. Do not use kava with alcohol, barbiturates, or psychoactive agents.

Melatonin, a natural hormone, regulates circadian rhythms (the body clock) and is believed to be an immune system regulator and a potent antioxidant. It shortens sleep latency but does not lengthen total sleep time or alter sleep patterns. Decreasing light at the end of the day triggers increased production of melatonin, which tapers as morning nears. Melatonin is available in a sublingual form that takes effect more rapidly. It should be used nightly, rather than on an as-needed (PRN) basis. Recommended dosage levels vary widely.

It is believed nontoxic, with few side effects (in some cases, night-mares). Only small studies have been done with CFS/FMS patients; safety and efficacy have not been proven in trials, and long-term effects are unknown.

Valerian root is usually taken several times daily and at bedtime for alleviation of insomnia and anxiety. Results may not occur for two to four weeks. Valerian has muscle-relaxing properties, decreasing restlessness and improving perception of sleep quality. Morning hangover effects are rare, and valerian has no known addiction potential, nor does it interact with alcohol. Side effects are also rare: mild stomach upset, or a stimulating rather than sedating effect. Lemon balm is often combined with valerian root for sleep.

The **minerals calcium, magnesium, and zinc** may aid sleep. Magnesium helps pain, an additional benefit.

◆◆ Urinary Tract Symptoms ◆◆

Urinary problems include interstitial cystitis (IC), a common inflammation (not an infection) of the lining of the bladder that causes frequent and painful urination. Antibiotics are not helpful for this condition. Some physicians who treat IC with a solution of DMSO (dimethyl sulfoxide) held in the bladder for about ninety minutes report beneficial results. Minipress (prazosin HCl) is often helpful in the treatment of urinary tract disorders, especially prostate problems in men.

◆◆ Vestibular (Balance) Disorders ◆◆

Medications helpful in treating balance disorders include motion sickness medications—for example, Dramamine (dimenhydrinate), Antivert (meclizine HCl), and Transderm-Scop (scopolamine)—Nardil (phenelzine), B vitamin preparations (orally or by injection), antihistamines, stimulants such as Cylert (pemoline) and Ritalin (methylphenidate), tranquilizers, and antidepressants as "second-ary" medications to treat accompanying anxiety. Behavioral inter-ventions include minimizing stress; drinking adequate fluids while limiting sodium, caffeine, and sugar; exercising; taking safety pre-cautions to avoid injury; and, for acute vertigo, immobilizing the head, fixing the eyes on something stable, and remaining still until the nausea subsides. Become aware of triggers of balance problems (e.g., competing sensory input, fluorescent lights, bright lights, certain foods, activities, or body movements) and avoid or minimize them. Treatment for vestibular disorders may be provided by an otorhinolaryngologist, neurologist, or neuro-otologist.

◆◆ Yeast/Fungal Overgrowth: Candidiasis ◆◆

The phenomenon of generalized yeast infections or overgrowth of *Candida albicans* is a controversial issue. Some doctors believe that most CFS patients have this problem, and others believe that the condition is rare or nonexistent. Existing laboratory tests for candidiasis are expensive and unreliable, and there are no clear diagnostic criteria. Some popular literature lists myriad symptoms of yeast infection, including most CFS/FMS symptoms. However, the relationship between CFS/FMS and candidiasis remains unclear. Much of the literature about candidiasis and treatment approaches is anecdotal and unscientific, and thus regarded with skepticism by the medical community. Treatment consists of dietary modification and medication. Antifungals include Mycostatin (nystatin), Nizoral (ketoconazole), Diflucan (fluconazole), and Sporanox (itraconazole), which treat systemic yeast and fungal infections and may have immune-modulating properties as well. Although some practitioners regard fungal infection, particularly candidiasis, as significant factors in CFS/FMS, others have found antifungal medications and special diets ineffective. Nonprescription therapies include high-quality acidophilus containing FOS (a plant carbohydrate), olive leaf extract, slippery elm bark, L-glutamine, and grapefruit seed extract.

AIR TRAVEL

Traveling by airplane causes general relapses in many CFS/FMS patients and specific symptoms in others (e.g., migraine). The reasons for symptom exacerbation is unclear but may involve poor air circulation, resulting in air contaminated with microbes and the infections of other passengers; dry air and its dehydrating effects (compounding the possible contagion problem); prolonged sitting or immobilization; the reduced atmospheric pressure maintained in commercial airplane cabins; possible hypoxia (too little oxygen in the cells); the altitude of several thousand feet; the ultraviolet and ionizing radiation at high altitudes.

◆ Air travel tips:

▶ Hydrate throughout the flight with 8 to 16 ounces of water per hour. After your arrival, hydrate by soaking in the bathtub.

▶ Stretch and do sedentary exercise, shifting position frequently throughout the flight. (Try to be seated in an exit or bulkhead row with extra legroom.)

▶ Take frequent walks in the aisle.

▶ Medications: Klonopin (clonazepam) may help with effects of the vibration of the plane, Diamox (acetazolamide) with the altitude change, and oxygen, which must be supplied by the airline with advance notice. (Not all airlines supply oxygen.)

▶ Use sleep medications if you need to sleep during the flight, using proper neck support.

▶ Dress comfortably, preferably in layers.

▶ Elevate your feet when possible.

▶ Be careful about how you carry and lift luggage. Use a luggage cart.

▶ If you have difficulty walking long distances, request wheelchair service.

▶ If you have food sensitivities, request a special meal or bring your own.

▶ Don't eat a lot on a flight.

▶ Relax. Take it easy for the first few days following your arrival and after you return home.

SURGERY AND ANESTHESIA

Before consenting to surgery, patients are advised to investigate treatment options and to get a second opinion when surgery has been recommended. Recovery may be prolonged and may cause symptom amplification due to the stress and trauma of surgery as well as anesthetics and other medications.

Meet with your physician and surgeon beforehand. Advise them that you have CFS/FMS (which affects the central nervous system) and any other conditions such as neurally mediated hypotension, orthostatic intolerance, low red blood cell mass, low plasma volume, hypercoagulation, temporomandibular joint dysfunction, and mitral valve prolapse. List all medications, supplements, and herbs you take regularly, highlighting anticoagulants (blood thinners). Continue your medications unless advised otherwise. Make a list of all allergies and hypersensitivities to medications, foods, and other substances (e.g., latex or adhesives), and request that copies of your list be placed in your medical chart. Carry a list of your medical conditions, medications, and contraindicated drugs in case emergency surgery becomes necessary.

◆ Suggestions for surgeons and anesthesiologists:

▸ If the patient is highly allergic, consider performing skin tests in advance for agents you are planning to use.

▸ Hydrate the patient prior to surgery to avoid syncope and drop in blood pressure.

▸ If appropriate, supplement with magnesium and potassium before surgery to avoid cardiac arrhythmias during surgery.

▸ Do not use halothane (rarely used). Consider Diprivan (propofol) as an induction agent and nitrous oxide and Forane (isoflurane) as a maintenance agent.

▸ Versed (midazolam) is generally well tolerated, as is Inapsine (droperidol) as an antinausea medication.

▸ Avoid hepatotoxic induction agents to avoid liver damage, highlighting anticoagulants (blood thinners).

▸ Be cautious in using catecholamines (epinephrine), sympathomimetics (isoproterenol), and vasodilators (nitric oxide, nitroglycerin, beta-blockers, and hypotensive agents), which can cause syncope.

▸ Avoid histamine-releasing anesthetics such as thiobarbiturates (e.g., sodium pentothal) and muscle relaxants in the curare family if possible since allergic responses are relatively common.

▸ Use sedating drugs (e.g., benzodiazepines, antihistamines, and psychotropics) sparingly.

▸ Diprivan (propofol), Versed (midazolam), and Sublimase (fentanyl) are generally well tolerated.

▸ For local anesthesia, sparing use of lidocaine without epinephrine is recommended.

(Sources: Drs. Charles Lapp, Patrick Class, and Paul Cheney)

IMMUNIZATIONS

The use of immunizations such as flu vaccines remains controversial, with most practitioners favoring flu shots for CFS/FMS patients unless they have been poorly tolerated in the past. For those who choose to have annual flu shots, NSAIDs ahead of time may reduce side effects. Some practitioners have recommended administration in divided doses, but this practice may not confer immunity.

MEDICAL INSURANCE ISSUES

Medical insurance companies have largely taken over the practice of medicine, covering an increasingly restricted list of treatment interventions, and determining which treatments the patient can obtain. Patients must often fight for the "right" to obtain appropriate treatment. Many newer drugs that may be more effective (and more expensive) are unlikely to appear on insurance company formularies. Many beneficial treatments, including complementary medical practices, are noncovered services. Patients may be forced to use less effective interventions or pay out-of-pocket. When therapies not specifically mentioned as noncovered services in one's insurance contract are denied, patients must often serve as their own advocates in fighting for coverage for effective treatment.

Although a cure is not known and may never be discovered, treatment of CFS and FMS is available, and new medications are undergoing therapeutic trials. New drugs known as biological response modifiers offer exciting treatment possibilities. All of us are guinea pigs in the sense that every treatment we try is experimental. Future treatment efforts will be enhanced by our growing understanding of the neuroimmune network and by uncovering ways to influence immune and neurological functioning.

15

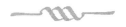

Coping with Chronic Illness

Being sick is hard work!

— *Susan Milstrey Wells, author of* A Delicate Balance:
Living Successfully with Chronic Illness

Our perceptions and coping techniques help define our experience of chronic illness. We learn the difference between hope and expectation in our futile search for the magic bullet. We wish for discovery of a cause and cure but learn to settle for anything that helps us to feel better and function more normally. We have no choice about being ill but have many options as to how to handle symptoms, losses, and limitations.

Self-care is an active rather than passive process, coming from "in here" rather than "out there." It requires giving up the attempt to control that which we cannot, focusing instead on the areas in which we do have choices. Opportunities to choose lie primarily in the realm of lifestyle modification: balancing activity and rest, examining our thought processes and self-messages, and learning to adapt to difficult circumstances. Coping means giving up the fairy-tale notion that life is fair or simple, as we reluctantly accept its difficulties and complexities. We develop realistic strategies for dealing with rotten circumstances. As researchers continue to seek effective treatments and (dare we hope?) a cure, we cannot afford to wait passively to be rescued. Despite feelings of helplessness and defeat at times, we remain our own best sources of effective coping strategies.

In patient surveys regarding all therapies, results have been mixed, yielding no consistently helpful treatment except self-care and lifestyle modification. Those who cope best with chronic illness identify what has helped: acceptance of the illness, altered lifestyle, cooperative relationships with treating professionals, a sense of meaning and purpose in life, self-nurturing, development of a realistically positive belief system, spirituality, support systems, and enhanced communication skills. Personal growth is one of the few benefits of being ill. Skilled coping allows us to remain as self-reliant as possible, maintaining a sense of adequacy and self-esteem. We do not need to embrace illness or passively resign ourselves to illness, but instead to learn from it while striving toward improved health and self-integration.

ACTIVITY-LEVEL MODIFICATIONS

Illness often tears one's lifestyle to shreds. We ricochet from one extreme to the other: from mad dashes to brutal crashes. When we begin to feel better, we overdo again, with the same results, ultimately learning that this cycle will continue until we accept moderation. Giving up the notion of doing it all—quickly and perfectly— allows us to balance priorities and slow down. I have hated this process, just as I dislike many things that are good for me. I may never come to like moderation, but this lesson in adaptation serves me well. I've decided not to stop living but to start living smarter and more flexibly.

Many of us are accustomed to being "on call" at all times: available to meet others' needs, to take care of things, to excel, to be busy. We've built our identities around taking care of others and we pride ourselves on constantly achieving, constantly giving. We don't recognize the inherent imbalance until we get sick, ultimately realizing that we've encouraged others to depend upon us as we indulged in the belief that we could work miracles. High expectations, self-pressure to do more and do it better, to push, to conquer and overcome obstacles, to work hard, never to disappoint, never to say "no"—this was normal! Anything less was unacceptable.

The opposite extreme, complete inactivity, is also harmful. Having nothing to do and no reason to wake up in the morning is to live a life devoid of meaning with little sense of purpose, value, or self-esteem. A sense of purpose and validity may be achieved through employment or meaningful activity.

Flexibility allows us to continue to function in accordance with constantly changing energy levels and abilities, whereas a fixed schedule may impose difficulties. "Lifestyle adjustment [means] getting hold of the rheostat of your life and winding it down to 60% from what it was set at before, which was sometimes at 120%," said Paul Cheney, M.D. (1987). "As you wind it down to 60%, your functional capacity goes way up."

"I've learned to stop instead of pushing," says Paula. "I've learned to back off. So the dishes and vacuuming don't get done. So what? I used to be a perfectionist; I had to be the best mother, the best teacher, the best wife, the best whatever. I had superwoman syndrome." By moderating, she regained some of what she had lost. Working part-time as a substitute teacher, Paula says, "I don't have to make an inspirational effort; I have no preplanning, and my days are short. While I'm working I usually feel better; I'm up; I'm doing something I enjoy doing. I make sure I take care of myself by resting and eating properly. When I stop, it's real easy to get depressed."

"I have a basketful of energy," she says. "That's all the energy I have in the world. If I waste my energy on anger, then I don't have the energy to do something else." Learning moderation, Paula moved from extremes toward a more comfortable center, stating, "It probably makes me an easier person to live with."

"My personal style won't change. I can't go from Type A to being totally mellow," says Bill. "I've had a lot of trouble with relaxation. Now I work when I'm able to and kick back more often." Not everyone has this degree of flexibility, but home-based work allows many freedoms.

Betty described learning to rest: "I make sure to rest—I mean bed rest. I had to learn how. My boss wants me back, but I need to give myself time. I won't push myself."

We need to regard energy as a checking account, one with an unknown and fluctuating balance. Writing too many checks without making significant deposits pushes us into credit reserve as we crash. Yet balancing work and rest is difficult because our physical and emotional status keeps changing. Some days we can do a few things; other days, nothing at all. Frequent rest periods between activities may rejuvenate us, but sometimes a full week of rest doesn't help. Pushing harder (overspending) makes matters worse. Adaptation to uncertainty doesn't mean giving in or being a wimp but developing a sensible approach to determining priorities: what to give up, what to continue, and what to deem optional. Chronic illness comes with warnings: Adjust your life, or it will overcome you. Push, and the illness will push back harder.

I once carried a full patient load as a psychologist, taught college classes, and lectured at seminars and workshops, while regretting that I didn't have time to do more. Once I became ill, I continued my busy schedule for as long as I could, becoming increasingly sicker. Tenacious and stubborn, I didn't want to give up anything. However, pushing proved futile. Confronted with a difficult choice between continuing until I crashed completely or modifying my activity level, I chose to cut back. By giving up part of what I loved to do, I mitigated the risk of losing it all. Monitoring and adjusting on a continuing basis, I am learning when to give up without giving in.

LIFESTYLE MODIFICATION

Here are a few adjustments that may make your illness easier to cope with:

> Practice moderation and self-pacing. Modify your activity level substantially, and choose activities wisely.

> Listen to your body, pay attention to its signals, and don't overdo unless you are prepared to pay the price.

> Do what you must do and let the rest go. Most "urgent" matters are less important than they seem at the moment, and most things can wait.

> Establish realistic priorities and goals in accordance with what is right for you rather than what you think you should do, or what you think others expect you to do.

> Do not set a deadline or time limit unless absolutely necessary, since time pressure is highly stressful. Don't berate yourself if progress is slow. Time doesn't count.

> Break down goals into small, short-term goals (e.g., tidying one drawer vs. organizing the kitchen). A seemingly overwhelming task can be accomplished in increments. Tackle each project in a series of specific small steps, for example, making one phone call or writing out one holiday card. If you tend to become absorbed, lose track of time, and overdo, use a timer

to limit how long you spend at a task. A two-hour task can often be accomplished more comfortably and productively in six twenty-minute chunks. Intersperse chores with rest periods. Measure progress by what you have done, not by what remains undone.

▶ Let go of excessive needs to accomplish and control. "If I can't do it, screw it!"

▶ Try to eliminate self-defeating behaviors such as trying to control what you cannot.

▶ Dump the "shoulds." No one is keeping score, and martyrs don't get medals. Allow the way you feel to determine how much you can do. Know your limits and the cost of exceeding them. "I've really worked on the shoulds and am learning not to let them rule my life," says Paula. "Realizing how many of my self-expectations and messages stem from external demands and manipulation helps me to talk less judgmentally to myself and to set realistic limits. When my mother says, 'If you were a good daughter, you would...,' I say, 'Then I'm not a good daughter,' which brings her up short. Then she'll realize what she's done. It took me a long time to learn to do it."

▶ Separate what you can control from what you cannot. Decide on a case-by-case basis whether to take an active or passive approach to a situation, determining what to fight and what to accept. Although we cannot change most events, we do choose our responses to them.

▶ Manage time effectively. Develop a sense of when you function best, and build your schedule accordingly. Plan extra time if things take longer than they used to. It's easier to add to a minimal schedule than to subtract from a hectic one.

▶ Get organized. Time invested in setting up systematic files and methods for accomplishing tasks will pay off later by making life easier.

▶ Pace yourself by interspersing tasks with rest periods.

▶ Use gadgets and shortcuts that make life easier: large-handled kitchen implements, cushions for support, pens and pads next to each telephone, catalog and Internet shopping, supermarkets and pharmacies that deliver.

> Be flexible to accommodate the unpredictable nature of your illness.

SELF-CARE

Make self-care your number one priority. Attend to basic needs: rest, nutrition, and appropriate activity. Without proper self-care, you are unable to do for others.

> Sleep and rest: There is no formula for determining the optimum rest/activity ratio because it varies unpredictably over time. Insufficient rest increases symptom severity and may prolong the course of the illness. Too little activity causes deconditioning, but most patients err on the side of overdoing rather than doing too little. Interspersing activity with frequent rest periods generally works best.

> Exercise if you are able. Start slowly and gently, increasing gradually. You are the best judge of how much you can tolerate without inviting a crash.

> Decrease stress in every way possible, particularly by reducing time pressure.

> Become well educated about your illness. Educate others about your illness if they are receptive.

> Continue to explore treatment options with realistic hopes for improvement.

> Attend to proper diet and nutrition.

> Stay in touch with the external world. Go outside when you can, even just in your backyard. Use assistive devices, such as a cane for support or balance, a wheelchair, or a motorized cart.

> Stay in touch with your internal world by keeping a journal. Identify personal strengths, and resolve old problems such as perfectionism, overly strong control needs, troublesome behavior patterns and relationship patterns of the past, unrealistic self-expectations, and irrational thought patterns. Learn what is enough and what is good enough.

> Avoid what is bad for you. Try to steer away from physically and emotionally stressful situations. Discover your exacerbation "triggers," and learn to stop and take care of yourself.

- Keep a calendar of symptoms, activities, life changes, and medications to see whether you can identify correlations or patterns.

- Treat yourself with care and respect. Self-criticism is hurtful and self-defeating, fostering fear and self-deprecation. Self-care is thus far the most potent tool in the medicine cabinet. We can and will endure this illness and deserve praise for coping as well as we have.

- Pamper yourself. Do things that make you feel good. Don't deny yourself pleasure because you're ill. It is not your fault, and you certainly don't deserve to be punished. Take a bubble bath or cuddle with your pet. Watch television. Read a good book if your brain is working—or a trashy one if it isn't. A former ice skater watches videotapes of skaters to keep in touch with her favorite activity. A woman who enjoys cooking spends most of the day in bed, getting up in time to cook dinner for her family. A "retired" bike rider had to give up strenuous activity but discovered her long-neglected guitar in the garage and began to play again. Identify what is soothing, perhaps a warm drink, pillows, flowers, and conversation.

- If you habitually attempt to rescue or control others, recognize the futility of pouring energy into "fixing" others. The only person whose behavior you can effectively change is your own. Continue to care *about* others, but stop trying to take care *of* them by doing for them what they should and need to do for themselves. You may feel initially as if you are abandoning them, but over time their capabilities will become apparent.

- Identify personal problems and seek solutions. If you are unable to determine the importance of issues, turning minor events into catastrophes, seek feedback and reassurance. Read self-help books, keep a journal, and consider psychotherapy with a CFS/FMS-knowledgeable psychologist or counselor.

- Work toward peace of mind rather than unattainable perfect wellness. Hope and positive beliefs will not fix us but can help us along the healing path.

- Learn to be gentle and kind to yourself: How would you treat a friend who was sick?

▶ Do something pleasant or fun each day. Consider hobbies, volunteer work, being in nature, self-pampering, meditation, exploration, music, playing a game, lighting candles, doodling, gardening, being with friends, and laughing. Try new things; discover new skills and pleasures. Life with chronic illness can be boring. If nothing makes you feel good, an assessment for depression is in order.

▶ Learn what to avoid, such as pushing yourself beyond reasonable limits; emotional, cognitive, or physical stressors; certain environments, foods, and chemicals; fad treatments that may be harmful; people who don't understand your illness or who are unduly critical of you; irrational thinking; people with overwhelming emotional needs or excessive negativity; and making unrealistic commitments.

RELATIONSHIPS AND COMMUNICATION

Here are some tips for communicating with the other people in your life:

▶ Don't apologize for your illness or limitations. They're not your fault.

▶ Ask others for positive input and encouragement.

▶ Do something for another person, even something small like sending a letter or card.

▶ Reestablish ties with friends. If you are not able to visit, call or e-mail to catch up on news.

▶ Seek out the people you enjoy. Spend time with people who are funny and uplifting. Avoid the "downers" and the "needies"—especially at times when you are down and needy.

▶ Learn to say no. Refusing a request is not the same as rejecting a person. You can be a good person without being a people pleaser. Set limits and do for others only what you are reasonably able to do.

▶ Make specific requests and delegate tasks that you cannot or should not perform. Others, too, have the right to say no and are responsible for their responses to your requests. You know the good feeling of helping others; grant others the opportunity to help you. Ask directly; don't hint, complain, or manipulate. "I'd appreciate your picking the kids up this afternoon" is more effective than "I'm so tired; how will I ever manage to pick up the kids?"

▸ Find support. Those who are ill speak your language, relate to your situation, and provide valuable understanding and support. Those who are well cannot fully understand but do add an outside perspective and keep you from getting totally caught up in the illness.

▸ Reach out to others: talk, hug, touch, love.

PLAY

Play is an important part of a well-balanced life. Here are a few ideas for increasing your sense of playfulness:

▸ Balance work and play. Being sick doesn't mean you have to be miserable all the time.

▸ Don't turn everything into a job; play and have fun, too.

▸ Find an activity that restores your sense of meaning even if you can do it only intermittently.

▸ Use your imagination to develop pastimes and projects that you can do despite your limitations.

▸ Explore new types of play: crafts, writing, drawing, collage, doodling, puzzles, computer or Internet games. Playing games may help cognition (keeping neural pathways active); choose those that fit your present cognitive abilities or stretch them a bit. Trying games that involve more sensory input or challenge than you can handle defeat the purpose, which is enjoyment of the process.

▸ Plan something to look forward to, a pleasant activity that is not likely to be jeopardized by a downward health swing.

▸ Laugh! Humor is a universal restorative and healing force with beneficial physiological effects including enhanced immunity, pain reduction, and decreased stress levels. Norman Cousins used humor as a coping and therapeutic tool during a serious illness, extolling the benefits of laughter in his books *Anatomy of an Illness* and *Head First*. "Illness is not a laughing matter," he wrote. "Maybe it ought to be."

COGNITIVE COPING

These techniques may help you cope with the cognitive aspects of your illness:

- Do one thing at a time. Multitasking is a thing of the past.
- Read small amounts at a sitting. Take time away, return to the task, and start by scanning what you have already read. New information is lost rapidly, typically within twenty minutes. Reinforce what you have learned, using as many senses and techniques as possible.
- If concentration or comprehension is difficult, take a break and try again later.
- Several brief study sessions are more effective than one long one.
- Take frequent breaks during cognitive tasks.
- Eliminate distractions and minimize sensory stimuli.
- When learning new material, try these tips:
  - Make things to be remembered stand out by highlighting them or writing in different colors.
  - Read a paragraph, pause, and state its main point out loud.
  - Use many senses: Read and repeat material aloud. Record what you say, and play it back.
  - Review frequently.
  - Create visual images of things you want to remember.
  - Memorizing new material may be easier when set to music, using a familiar tune.
  - If you become frustrated and unable to make sense of a task, leave it alone and return to it when you are rested. Trying to force a solution, like remembering a lost word, ensures that it will further elude you.
  - When reading, use an index card to jot down brief notes of relevant words or names, such as characters in a novel or plot basics. Use the card as a bookmark.
  - If you are unable to read books, read shorter, less complex matter, such as magazines or newspapers.
  - If you cannot read, listen to books on tape.

STRESS REDUCTION

Stress reduction techniques—including meditation, progressive muscle relaxation, self-hypnosis, healing imagery, breathing techniques, and affirmations or repetition of certain phrases—enhance well-being and coping capability while reducing stress and providing symptom relief. Benefits are felt both immediately and over time at the emotional, spiritual, and physiological levels.

Relaxation is a skill like any other that requires practice. Relaxation exercises are generally practiced once or twice a day for about twenty minutes. Find a distraction-free environment, turn off outside stimuli, lie down, get comfortable, close your eyes, and *be.* Experiment with techniques to determine what is most effective for you; you might use a prerecorded audiocassette or CD, or consult a stress management specialist or clinic.

Guided imagery is based on the theory that an individual's ability to imagine and feel a positive outcome can help to create it. It provides a time-out period to clear the mind and focus inward to develop insights, create peaceful feelings, and encourage self-healing, producing emotional and physiologic changes.

Biofeedback is a training process that takes place over a period of weeks or months. Monitoring such bodily functions as muscle tension and hand temperature indicates one's level of relaxation by offering feedback (e.g., noises or flashing lights) to signal progress toward the desired response as relaxation techniques are employed. The patient develops a sense of control over bodily functions that are usually beyond conscious control. Biofeedback is helpful for treating certain symptoms such as headache and body pain.

Meditation is the process of focusing one's attention on a bland stimulus in order to clear the mind and produce a sense of inner calm. Tuning out distractions and lowering body arousal brings a sense of stillness and peace, enhancing well-being and creating positive emotional and physiological changes. The type of meditation one practices is a matter of individual preference and effectiveness. Deep breathing, turning off the mind, and repeating phrases are some popular techniques. Benefits include relaxation, stress reduction, spiritual development, expansion of the mind, and heightened creativity.

Autogenic training, a form of relaxation that relies on passive concentration accompanied by repetition of certain phrases, helps to create bodily sensations, such as feelings of warmth and heaviness and slowed breathing. Mastering these highly structured exercises requires continual practice. The skills may be learned through individual or group instruction or materials used on one's own.

Hypnosis is achievement of an altered state of consciousness in which the unconscious mind plays a central role. Contrary to popular myth, the hypnotist has no special powers to convince the subject to perform silly or inappropriate acts. Tapping the neural links between mind and body, hypnosis is a wonderful tool for relaxation, pain reduction, stress management, and enhanced coping skills.

Massage increases relaxation, decreases pain, and improves circulation, among other positive physiological and emotional effects. Massage techniques are numerous; you must be comfortable with the type of massage and the massage therapist.

Exercise promotes cardiovascular fitness, strengthens muscles, combats depression, and increases flexibility, energy, and mental alertness by causing the production of energizing hormones called catecholamines. Exercise provides a time-out from daily problems, creates a greater sense of "normalcy," and may enhance immune functioning. However, exercise is not advisable for everyone, since individual tolerance varies significantly. Stretching exercises may be better tolerated. Medical advice, common sense, and a trial-and-error process will help you determine what is suitable. If you have not exercised in some time, start slowly, limiting your activity to a few minutes of stretching, yoga, tai chi, or water aerobics. Do not perform any exercises or stretches that cause pain or symptom exacerbation over the following twenty-four to forty-eight hours. Start slowly and gently; do not push.

NEW PERSPECTIVES

Don't let this illness make you look back. Look ahead with hope.
Look ahead to the great adventure of your new life, painful as it
may be, at times, and joyful at other times. See yourself as a
traveler whose journey has meaning beyond your understanding.

— Reg Moore

Live in the present. Illness presents limits and limitations for *right now*, not necessarily forever. You are not facing total, irrevocable deprivation. Life's only constant is its unpredictability, and most things are temporary. Your health may improve with self-care, treatment, and the passage of time. Examine and modify unrealistic notions to create a "new normal" based on how things are *now*. Slow down, live in the moment, and enjoy the ride when you can. Give yourself time just to be.

Stop making comparisons; quit comparing then with now. *Then* is irrelevant. Give up distorted memories of how perfect life once was, and live as well as you can. Do not compare yourself to others with the illness; when they are doing well, you wonder why you're not; when they're very ill, you worry about becoming that way yourself. Either way you lose—so don't play.

Reprogram your thinking. Feelings are based not on external events but on our interpretation of those events, that is, our self-messages. Recognize when you are unnecessarily harsh with yourself, allowing your internal critic to assign self-blame for all imperfections, imagined or real. Such statements as "I should accomplish more," "I shouldn't rely upon others," and "If I were fighting hard enough, I would be well by now" are harsh, irrational messages that cause self-esteem to plummet. Challenge and reformulate damaging messages. Many contain a grain of truth that has become distorted. "I'm just lazy" can become "I'm feeling fatigued." "I should accomplish more" can be replaced with "I wish I could do more, but that isn't realistic right now." "I can't handle anything" can become "It's difficult to cope when I'm feeling ill." Don't say anything to yourself that you wouldn't say to a close friend.

"Before, the house had to smell like Pine-Sol; everything had to be perfect," says Betty. When she discussed her "laziness" with her husband and her guilt about no longer maintaining a showcase home for her family, he said, "So what?" Her children didn't care either. Betty received her family's permission, and ultimately her own, to take better care of herself than of her house.

Dump blame—of yourself, someone else, or God. There is no sense to the prevalent notion that when something goes wrong, someone or something is to blame. Excrement happens, and it's not necessarily someone's fault.

Dump the notion that life is supposed to be fair. Where does this expectation originate—from movies, cartoons, fiction? Although we welcome a satisfying conclusion in which the good are rewarded and the bad are punished, such dynamics are not characteristic of real life. Bad things happen to good people; good things happen to bad people. Based on the notion of fairness, illness is viewed as a punishment for a wrongdoing, personal shortcoming, or bad thoughts. Fairness and illness have no connection.

Go easy during holidays. Strategize so the holidays can be enjoyable without inducing a postholiday crash. Trash unrealistic expectations (the Walton family syndrome); perfect families don't exist in real life. Don't knock yourself out. Tell others what you need, and ask them to pitch in. Use shortcuts, such as packaged or precooked meals. If others do not understand, don't allow their limitations to become your problems. Give up the martyr role and enjoy the holidays.

Count your blessings. Deprivations are obvious, but what are you grateful for? Is the glass half empty or half full? (George Carlin says the glass is too big.) Learn to appreciate the small stuff—the beauty of sunlight captured in a prism, a child's smile, a funny movie.

At times, we disregard the sensible stuff and say, "Screw it all. I give up. What's the point? Nothing is helping." These periodic tantrums are followed by a return to the reality that our decisions do affect well-being, both present and future, and we return to living sensibly, living within our limits. Periodic, minor rebellions are understandable and inevitable.

COPING WITH RELAPSES

Relapses may be caused by physical or emotional stress, trauma, overexertion, exposure to allergens or environmental chemicals, hormonal fluctuations, changes in weather and barometric pressure, or changes in medications—or in the absence of an identifiable trigger. The devastation is more pronounced when the relapse follows a period of improved health.

Identification and avoidance of relapse triggers can help prevent future relapses. During a relapse, further lifestyle modification is necessary. Self-care is especially important: additional resting and sleeping time, relaxation breaks, avoidance of stress, moderation of activities, use of heat and other therapies, and distracting activities. Replace such self-messages as, "I'll never feel better again" with rational statements such as, "This is a temporary setback and I can ride it out." A relapse is not forever, although it may feel like it. You've been there before and emerged; this cycle will repeat.

FEELINGS

Feelings defy logic; they cannot be seen and may be difficult to express, yet they're undeniably present. Our feelings vary unpredictably, interspersed with denial or numbness born of a need to push difficult emotions away. Many of us have been taught that hiding emotions, or better still, not having them in the first place, is a sign of maturity and strength. If we can't deny feelings, we attempt to rationalize them with elaborate explanations or apologies.

It is natural to have feelings and normal to express them. Rules to the contrary don't make sense. We have no choices about what feelings to have; as human beings, we experience all of them. Our rational minds will say, "No need to feel upset about *that*," while our emotions have other plans. We do have a choice, though, about how to deal with those emotions behaviorally—how we express them.

Emotions are not to be judged or justified. Sometimes we choose to conceal them, at least temporarily, but any strong feeling will ultimately need expression.

Fear regarding the illness and its unknowns is natural. Medical tests, treatments, strange symptoms, losses, and an unpredictable future are scary. Seek the two things that will help: information and reassurance. Talk with family, friends, and health care professionals about your fears.

Anger is considered the most unacceptable emotion. Most of us lack role models for the healthy expression of anger, a natural emotion that can be used constructively. We have seen anger turned into rage and used as a weapon. Angry feelings need not control us if we realize our options for dealing with them. Anger signals a problem that needs to be addressed and solved. When we are emotionally vulnerable, as we are during exacerbations, anger is close to the surface and can be easily triggered by minor events. Anger's intensity may be related to how sick you feel, not how big the problem is.

Why are we angry? We are angry that we're sick, deprived, in pain, unenergetic, and limited. We are angry that we are sick while other people are well and because we feel misunderstood by health care professionals, the media, and those close to us. We are angry because there is no cure and because we cannot will this illness to go away, no matter how good we are. We are angry because we've lost so much. We are angry when others don't really listen to us or hear us and because we often can't express ourselves as we would like to. We are angry because we are scared, lonely, and miserable. We are angry because we feel helpless to make ourselves well again. We are angry because our responsibilities and expectations for ourselves continue although our energy does not. We are often angry because we don't like ourselves or accept our situation very well.

We have good cause to be angry and need safe outlets for our anger; repressed anger may turn to bitter resentment or to depression. Because anger is a secondary response to a primary feeling (usually hurt or frustration), it is possible to identify its origin and express the feeling constructively rather than lashing out at a scapegoat.

Do something physical to "exorcise" the initial angry response, and then engage in rational problem solving. Take a time-out until the rage subsides—tear newspaper, throw darts or unbreakable objects, or yell out loud—alone. Once you have dumped the "hot" anger, try to identify the problems and feelings that may have triggered it. Allow your anger to help you identify problem issues and work through them. Express your anger in a way that isn't damaging to others.

Irritability, the overreaction to minor stimuli, is common in CFS and FMS, especially when we are on "overload." When this occurs, remove yourself from the situation, try to talk rationally to yourself about what's really going on, and apologize for inappropriate outbursts. Certain antidepressants help to diminish irritability.

Depression usually waxes and wanes, although it remains constant for some. Depression is a result of being ill, of suffering limitations and losses, and of distorted thinking that results in irrational self-messages. Feeling hopeless, helpless, and desperate, we may not be able to imagine ever feeling better again. We may feel unmotivated, resigned, and out of options. Sometimes, the depression occurs in

reaction to an event; at other times, it seems to swoop in unexpect-
edly, more difficult to accept because it's impossible to understand.
Abnormalities in neurotransmitter and cytokine levels can cause or
contribute to depression. Treatment with antidepressants can correct this biochemical problem, and talking with a friend or therapist
can bring relief.

Allow yourself to experience and feel the depression as it runs
its course. Denial and faking can prolong the depression. Cry and
feel sorry for yourself for a while. Tears are cathartic. You will
emerge from depression once you have gone through it. As difficult
as it is to believe during a depressive episode, depression is not forever. You really will feel okay again. If you become stuck, medications and psychotherapy can help.

Here are a few more suggestions for copies with depression:

▶ Identify other issues (problems, repressed emotions) that have
triggered the depression, and deal with them when you are
able.

▶ Enlist the support of others, or if you need to be alone, let others know that you need some time. (When you withdraw without explanation, people often assume you are angry at them.)

▶ Learn what you can from the depression; for some reason, the
most meaningful learning experiences are painful.

▶ Physical touch may help, as can some type of meaningful
activity if you are up to it.

▶ Talk or write about your feelings, even those that have been
discussed before. Talk to yourself, or talk with others. Let them
know that your intent is to express feelings and sort them out;
that you are not expecting to be rescued or fixed. Tell them
whether or not you want feedback; their responses may help
you to develop new perspectives, but unsolicited advice or
attempts at "fixing" frustrate both parties.

▶ Suicidal thoughts may result from chemical changes and from
how we view our circumstances. Sometimes it seems the only
way out of the pain. We may feel pushed in that direction by
those who trivialize or dismiss our illness, who do not or cannot understand. If you feel suicidal, talk with someone. Call a
suicide hotline if friends or family are unavailable.

HANDLING LOSS

No matter how fragile the human body, the human spirit can
take just about anything.

— *Cheri Register*, Living with Chronic Illness

The grieving process is difficult and painful but a necessary reaction to any significant loss. Healing cannot take place until the loss is mourned. Illness-related losses include energy, vitality, enthusiasm, good health, ability to perform responsibilities and activities, certain roles, pleasure, motivation, independence, predictability and control, financial security, self-esteem, relationships, others' former perceptions of us, jobs and careers, educational or training plans, leisure and social activities, plans, and dreams. We have lost vital parts of our lives and of ourselves.

There are several stages in the grieving process: denial, bargaining, anger, sadness/depression, and acceptance/adaptation. We may experience the stages in order, skip around, omit certain stages entirely, or return to one stage repeatedly. There is no right way to grieve, nor an easy one.

"This can't be happening to me. This illness can't be real." The **denial** stage is often experienced as general numbness, reflecting our inability to absorb and deal with painful experiences and enormous losses all at once. "Numbing out" allows us to absorb the impact of an overwhelming situation gradually. During this stage, we tend to overdo and then crash, often repeatedly, as we alternately deny and are reminded of our illness.

During the **bargaining** phase, we try to make deals with ourselves, our doctors, or God. We promise to "be good" in exchange for restoration of what we have lost. "If I eat vegetables, deny myself junk food, and follow my doctor's advice, maybe I'll get back my good health in return." This stage is generally brief; some do not experience it at all.

Anger! Faced with a situation that is unfair and beyond our control, with no known cause or responsible party, we don't understand how or why our lives have become devastatingly disrupted. There is no identified target at which to direct our anger. We feel misunderstood, maligned, and mistreated. Anger is natural and justified, but we have difficulty figuring out how to handle it and often lack role models for the nondestructive expression of anger. Anger may breed guilt; not only are we more dependent on others, but sometimes we are not even *nice* to them. Getting through the anger stage is a significant step toward emotional recovery.

Depression hits as we acknowledge the reality of our illness and its devastating effects. We experience feelings of hopelessness, helplessness, disappointment, isolation, and self-pity. During this stage, we may feel that our lives are over, we will never feel good again, we are totally useless, everything has been taken away, no one understands, and there is nothing left to live for.

Acceptance and adaptation. "Ultimately chronic [illness] becomes a background fact of life, not a foreground obsession," writes Karyn Feiden. Our losses become integrated into our lives. We give up trying to manipulate reality and accept the situation. We make peace instead of war. We adapt to a difficult situation and focus on what we can do, while remaining painfully aware of what we cannot do. New strengths emerge. We stop living in the "if onlys," with what should be, and learn to live with what is. As we realize that our illness does not define us, we begin to restructure our lives. We learn to live with limitations, with unpredictable and difficult symptoms, and we move forward. We become less afraid and better able to accept difficulties. We learn to be flexible, for our very survival depends upon our ability to bend and flow. No longer passive and stuck, we move forward, taking responsibility for the management of our lives. But our fears and doubts continue; acceptance remains a matter of degree.

Accepting CFS/FMS as a part of our lives doesn't mean we want or deserve it, but there it is. We may have to live with it indefinitely, but we can still live.

Acceptance means riding out the cycles—the ups and downs, the unfamiliar, the new and unwelcome, and the periods of respite.

Adaptation means learning to live with changed circumstances; it does *not* mean admitting defeat. We give up the miraculous hope that it will simply be gone some morning soon. We realize that we will have to coexist with a host of symptoms that limit our fun, relationships, and productivity. We then find a way to move on anyway, to continue our lives in a different mode. Rather than defining our "true" selves as our pre-illness selves, we acknowledge that things are different now and paint a different picture of ourselves and our lives.

The grieving process is lengthy and bumpy; there are no short-cuts. We bounce back and forth among stages, sometimes feeling we have finally adapted, only to find ourselves thrown back into anger, denial, or depression. Knowing that we have survived these stages before tempers the process, making us less overwhelmed the second, third, or fourth time around.

COUNSELING

It is not a sign of failure to seek a therapist but a willingness to grow.

— Stephanie Simonton

Despite the facts that biological and emotional illness are not separate entities and that people who need help are not necessarily insane, society continues to stigmatize emotional disorders. Those who are depressed or confused are often told to pull themselves together or to tough it out. It's still okay to have a hairdresser style your hair or a mechanic fix your car, but different rules apply to seeking help for emotional matters. Even those who are supportive of people with chronic illnesses may have difficulty understanding the need or desire for psychological or psychiatric help. (However, when illness is deemed "all in your head," you are *expected* to seek such care.)

Seeking help to cope with the emotional fallout of chronic illness is a sign of strength rather than weakness, implying a willingness to learn to cope more productively with illness-related issues: grieving, problem solving, adjustment issues, depression, anxiety, and the need to understand and balance one's life in new ways. The therapeutic setting provides a safe place to express feelings, focus on personal needs and growth, and ease the emotional pain of illness without feeling judged.

Seek out a psychiatrist, psychologist, or counselor who has been recommended by health care professionals, support groups, or other patients. See someone who is CFS/FMS-familiar so you are not placed in the defensive position of proving you are ill or educating the professional.

A good fit between therapist and client is essential. You should feel that your concerns are heard and taken seriously. If you are uncomfortable with a professional, attempt to work out the problems with the individual or seek help elsewhere. However, make sure your expectations are realistic. Providers take differing approaches to treatment, and therapy may be supportive, psychodynamic, cognitive behavioral, systems oriented, or more commonly eclectic, employing various approaches based upon patient needs. Although it is beyond the scope of this book to explain the various types of practice in depth, it is essential that you be comfortable with the type of therapy provided.

SUPPORT GROUPS

A profound sense of relief comes from meeting others who "speak the same language," says Susan Milstrey Wells. Large, information-oriented groups or smaller, emotional support groups serve different needs. Larger organizations often operate hotlines or help lines, have professional speakers at meetings, and publish newsletters. Smaller groups, typically more informal, are oriented toward interaction and emotional support. Shared feelings, coping suggestions, exchange of information, and the knowledge that others experience similar difficulties can be invaluable. Some groups address specific topics at each meeting, such as changes in identity and self-esteem, coping with losses and limitations, practical skills, lifestyle modification, dealing with significant others and people in the workplace, and obtaining quality health care.

Each support group has its own personality, and unfortunately some become bound in negativity. Participants may be bitter, using meetings as an opportunity to vent negative emotions and dwell on misfortune. Although this process may be cathartic at times, continued negativity tends to alienate those who seek positive support and help with problem solving. Such groups are best avoided since they are counterproductive and often depressing.

Although education about one's illness is important, we may become uncomfortably preoccupied or overwhelmed with illness-related information, needing to distance ourselves from materials and meetings. Each of us must find a comfortable balance between living in the illness and being a part of the world outside it.

TOWARD A NEW LIFE PHILOSOPHY

Illness offers us new opportunities whether we want them or not, forcing us to examine issues that would otherwise remain unexplored. No longer able to view the world in accustomed ways, we question the meaning of life—specifically, our own lives.

Our value systems change; we may become less materialistic and more oriented toward health, spirituality, and relationships with family and friends. We may become more loving, more aware of people and things around us, and fully alive—ironically at a time when we feel half dead.

Spirituality is an individual matter, whether in the sense of organized religion or development of one's own belief system through reading, talking with others, and meditating. Some find that religious/spiritual beliefs help them to endure the illness ordeal. Both traditional and nontraditional belief systems may offer great comfort.

We learn to rely less on the opinions and beliefs of others and more fully on our own convictions and the resources that have enabled us to cope, learn, and survive. We learn that self-approval holds great value.

No longer able to rely on former goals and life expectations, we learn to live in the moment. It is too late for yesterday, although we remain nostalgic for the way things used to be, and too soon for tomorrow—made especially unpredictable by radical fluctuations in health. Today is all we can work with.

Illness offers an opportunity to develop a new sense of purpose. A retired college professor who had always wanted to learn charcoal drawing now enjoys his newfound talent. Energies may be directed toward a cause: writing newsletter articles, facilitating or helping at support group meetings, or becoming politically involved.

As ability to function vacillates, our lives seem to gain and lose meaning. Everything is up for grabs; life becomes chaotic. Transformative insights and understandings often emerge from the chaos. In facing the challenge of leading meaningful lives despite severe limitations, our perceptions are permanently altered. We learn to identify and rid ourselves of extraneous baggage and focus on that which is most important. The process of learning to live and love more fully is necessary to our individual and collective survival.

Below, people with CFS and FMS share their new learning:

> I have new appreciation for things I overlooked in the past: a tree, a flower, a day of improved health.

I hate this illness, but I no longer hate myself for having it.

I am more compassionate to the suffering of others and to my own suffering.

I have learned the importance of self-care. I used to go until I dropped, and now I know it's a mistake.

The people who really care about me accept me as I am.

I realize the importance of solitude, quiet time, and meditation in many forms.

I keep things open-ended and try to be flexible.

I don't have to do what I did in the past to prove I am a good person.

My life was out of balance before I got sick, and I didn't even know it. I am looking for a new sense of balance.

I have met many wonderful people who have the same disorder, people I wouldn't have met otherwise.

I am learning how to prioritize—to deal with the important stuff and let the trivial stuff go.

Life is unpredictable, but I am more adaptable than I knew.

Illness is not my whole life, just one aspect of it.

My goals are to simplify, to meet my basic needs, and to be comfortable in my environment.

I created a "healing place" where I meditate.

I keep trying to remember that my self-worth is about who I am, not what I do.

I am better off without those who use me, who only value me for what I can do for them rather than who I am inside.

I may be a sick person, but I am still a person with value and self-worth.

I am learning to focus on taking care of myself rather than trying to fix everyone else.

I've quit telling myself how to feel.

I'm learning what really matters in life.

I can still live my life if I give up insisting that it be restored to just the way it was before I got sick. That's old stuff; it's gone.

Some people refuse to understand. I'm tired of wasting my time trying to convince them.

It's okay to need help—and to ask for it.

I have become a more spiritual person.

I hope they find a cure but I've learned not to expect a miracle.

I try to focus on what I can still do, rather than on my limitations.

I am learning to talk kindly to myself. I wouldn't take crap from anyone else, and I shouldn't tolerate it from myself, either.

I am coping pretty well with a lot of unwelcome situations.

I am learning patience and flexibility and am more resilient that I ever thought I could be.

HOPE

Unrealistic hope, and wishes turned into expectations, create disappointment and decrease our chances of developing realistic hope—the belief that we can endure and improve and that the way we feel in our most desperate moments will not persist forever. When hopeful, we believe that things can and will be better, albeit temporarily. We congratulate ourselves for making it this far, sometimes for getting out of bed at all, for being able to smile even fleetingly, for tolerating daily unpredictability and ambiguity. Hope and hopelessness, like day and night, are cyclical.

"Mentally, I think I can affect my health by working at it, thinking more positive things, using positive visualization. Who knows how it works, but I think we can," says Paula. "People with the will to live can overcome things that other people just give up on. The rest of us just lead lives of quiet desperation."

Hope and despair battle like archenemies in the face of chronic illness. Hope reigns briefly, later replaced by the periodic desperation that accompanies exacerbations. Hope flees in the face of isolation, depression, anxiety, and an inability to feel "normal." Loss of control and our inability to trust our body to respond predictably or productively cause doubt—in ourselves, in others, and in the notion that things can ever again be made right. How can we dare to be hopeful when everything seems to be going wrong? How can we maintain faith that all will be well when symptoms rage and emotions run wild?

We hear that "things could be worse"—true, but not particularly helpful. It's difficult to be Pollyanna-joyous about not having leprosy or cancer; we resent what we *do* have. Is it a crime to feel sorry for oneself? We speak of "pity parties," heaping guilt on top of self-pity on top of pain. From my journal:

> *I feel sorry for others who are ill; why shouldn't I feel sorry for myself sometimes? This is a terrible illness. Why shouldn't I complain? It's a cheap hobby. People say, "Keep your chin up." I can't always do that. I enjoy optimism, but when I'm sickest, hope disappears along with everything else that feels good. But I know I will feel better again, that the world will appear different...and I look forward to that time, knowing hope and measured optimism will return.*

So how do we "get" hope? By exploring and trying anything that might work: spiritual and philosophical beliefs; our way of regarding life, the world, our purpose; recreation; and our ability to find peace and happiness. We examine beliefs about life through reading, discussion, meditation, and self-exploration. We may not find ultimate conclusions or discover any earth-shattering cosmic truths, but we can discover inner sources of positive belief.

Exploration reveals new facets of our experiences and perceptions. The black-and-white "all good or all bad" approach blocks the open, creative perceptions of which we are all capable. Realistic optimism is the most sensible approach.

Oscar Wilde said, "We are all in the gutter, but some of us are looking at the stars."

Sometimes I am looking into the gutter; it's all I can see. At other times I raise my head in awe of the universe. My attitude fluctuates so often I could give myself whiplash. But I try to remember that even when I cannot see them, the stars are there. Sometimes clouds or urban lights get in the way—and sometimes the air is crystal clear and the heavens magical.

---∿∿---

16

Relationships:
The Balancing Act

When chronic illness disrupts our lives, it affects those with whom we are close as well. Lacking guidelines for such situations, we wonder how to help others understand—and whether it's even possible for them to have a true sense of what we experience. We don't know how much to disclose or when. We fear the consequences of being honest—of complaining too much or becoming too needy. We wonder how much they can tolerate before they explode or desert us. We fear that caring will crumble in the face of adversity.

Although we try to share our experience with others, we realize that the illness is ours alone. Others may be victims of the domino effect, but we bear the direct brunt. Illness inevitably changes us and others' perceptions of us. We need to know that they believe we are seriously ill, understand as best they can, and are willing to offer support and help.

Important people in our lives need to be educated regarding the illness and its effects through medical literature, magazine articles, support group publications, books, discussions, or support group meetings. Some will read extensively, while others are satisfied with a few articles presenting information accurately and concisely.

Communication about the illness and the resulting relationship changes is the key to coping productively as friends or significant others.

SUGGESTIONS FOR FAMILIES

Chronic illness disrupts a family's usual patterns and dynamics. All families develop ways of coping with stress, but a chronic illness presents the unique, lingering stressor of continuing disruption. Families that are cohesive, flexible, resourceful, and adaptable cope most successfully.

Talk about what's happening, even though you'd rather deny it. Discuss the shared problems of illness and its effects on the family as a whole and on individual family members without assigning blame. All family members need to develop an understanding of the illness, even young children.

Family members must be allowed to speak for themselves, rather than for one another, and all feelings must be accepted as valid. Trying to talk someone out of how she is feeling ("It isn't really that bad") invalidates feelings and shuts down productive communication. Empathize with others' feelings, even when you wish they didn't feel that way. When the ill family member says "I'm scared that I'll never recover," avoid knee-jerk responses like, "That's ridiculous—of course you will!" A more empathetic statement is more effective; for example, "It's natural to be frightened. Not knowing is very difficult." No one wants to be told how to feel.

Develop flexibility in the way the family functions. Brainstorm to seek solutions to new problems. When responsibilities are reassigned, each family member should be clear about what is expected.

In many families, one person is unofficially regarded as the caretaker, often the person who is now ill. As each family member assumes some caretaking responsibilities, the burden is divided and all learn valuable skills.

The patient should openly discuss limitations and problems rather than covering them up in an attempt to shield the family from difficulty and pain. However, the patient should avoid becoming overly dependent on other family members, especially young children. Primary support of a parent is an inappropriate burden for a child.

The family should avoid overprotecting and making assumptions about what the patient can do or would like to do. All should be involved in making family plans, with the understanding that the ill family member may not be able to participate.

Extended family members, neighbors, and others in the community can provide additional support and perhaps help with the added illness-imposed responsibilities.

The needs of all family members must be understood and respected. In addition to showing caring for the ill family member, each must consider personal well-being a priority.

Children often resent the limitations imposed on their lives by a parent's illness. They may react by becoming demanding or depressed, blaming themselves for the illness or family problems, or exhibiting behavior problems at home or school. They may be unaware of the connection between their behavior and the disruption of stability in their lives. Children need love and limits—both reassurance and acknowledgment of their difficulties and appropriate expectations and standards, with consequences for misbehavior. A parent's guilt or sadness about being ill should not serve as an excuse for condoning a child's misbehavior. Individual or family therapy helps when problems increase or do not resolve over time.

Express caring for one another openly through words and gestures. Touch, hug, and be sensitive to one another's needs. Acknowledge feelings. Express hope. Let all family members know that they are valuable and helpful to the family. The challenge of illness can create new strength, growth, and closeness.

◆◆ Grief and Mourning ◆◆

Couples and families, as well as people with CFS or FMS, experience numerous losses: changes in family roles, activities, finances, familiar patterns, and division of responsibilities. Some families grieve together, others go through the process individually, and some remain in denial, unable to accept unwanted changes and feelings.

Grieving and rebuilding allow new strengths and interests to emerge. Seeing the humor in a situation relieves tension and provides a break from the pain. Laughter and tears express the comedies and tragedies of life, allowing a release of feelings.

SUGGESTIONS FOR CAREGIVERS AND SIGNIFICANT OTHERS

Be a helper rather than a rescuer. A rescuer tries to "make it all okay," an exercise in futility rather than heroism. A helper's task is to provide assistance as needed. Unsolicited advice is often perceived as insensitive intrusion. You can be most helpful by making observations and offering assistance without pressure.

Productive communication about effects of the illness tears down barriers. Assertive communication requires appropriate and direct expression of ideas, feelings, and needs: making and refusing requests, voicing concerns, and making direct statements rather than hinting. Open communication allows honest exchanges that enhance self-esteem and closeness.

BEING SINGLE WITH CFS OR FMS

Enduring illness as a single person is a mixed bag. "If I don't do it, it doesn't get done," says Dana. "I wish I had the comfort and support of a partner." Those who face illness without partner or family involvement lack help with chores and responsibilities. Shouldering the financial burden alone is difficult and frightening. Some are forced to live with grown children or with parents. On the other hand, singles living alone do not have to take others' expectations or needs into account when making decisions or keeping odd hours.

Those who are dating or seeking a permanent relationship must deal with uncertainty, fear of rejection, and decisions about what and when to disclose. The illness should not be kept a secret, but disclosing detailed information too soon can scare some people away. In a middle ground between that extreme and hiding is a more comfortable level of disclosure that will work best. New relationships are always risky, and most do not last, even without chronic illness. If the new person in your life is unable or unwilling to deal with your illness, you would probably rather know sooner than later.

If a primary relationship is not feasible for you right now, don't isolate yourself. Remain in contact with the outside world as much as possible by attending meetings, going to the library, taking a class, seeing a movie, and staying in touch with friends and family. Vary your friendships among the healthy and the ill.

In "Living Alone with CFIDS," Tamara Lewis wrote:

> *Shockingly, the world has shrunk down to the size of my apartment. And my body is no longer the vehicle with which I move through life. Rather, it is my life. . . . I am no longer expected anywhere by two o'clock or even by Tuesday. And I live alone, so no one's coming home for dinner—and I don't bump into anyone on the way to the bath-room. So, I can go days without seeing anyone. And I begin to feel*

unreal. . . . No one sees me staring lifelessly at the walls. No one sees me toss through another sleepless night. No one sees me lying on the floor crying. My illness and I are like an unsolved crime—no eyewitnesses.

When the relentlessness of the illness has finally gotten to me, I am without good judgment. I can't tell what's wrong and I can't tell what I need. It is at those moments that I most need someone to walk into the room and state the obvious: "Turn on the lights. Eat something. Call your doctor." It is those moments when living alone is most painful.

When we do reach out, we don't always know what we seek or how to verbalize our needs. Singles lack a sounding board, a contact to help them live vicariously in the outside world, and a reality-check source—but ultimately we all face the illness alone, with or without a partner.

WHEN A CHILD IS ILL

Children need to understand their illnesses and be assured it is not their fault. They need age-appropriate information and opportunities to talk about their experiences and questions. Offer reassurance, but don't withhold the truth. Ask them about their feelings: Do they feel left out of important activities? Ignored by their peers? Burdensome to the family? Different, not okay? Unable to do "normal" things? Are there ways for other family members to help?

Adjust your expectations of the child in accordance with a realistic, objective assessment of strengths and impairments in cognitive and physical functioning. Unrealistically high expectations will make the child feel like a constant failure. Unrealistically low expectations allow the child to dodge appropriate responsibilities and standards of acceptable behavior. Flexibility allows expectations to fluctuate with the illness.

If school attendance is a problem, consider part- or full-time home instruction. Educate the child's teacher, principal, guidance counselor, and nurse about CFS/FMS, particularly its cognitive effects, and work cooperatively to develop a flexible and appropriate learning plan. If you encounter resistance from the school administration, pursue the matter assertively with the help of health care providers and support or advocacy groups.

Illness may prolong a child's dependence on the family; this is especially problematic in adolescence. Discuss this problem openly. Allow the child maximum but reasonable autonomy in making decisions.

Make coping suggestions to your child. Some respond well to guided imagery and art therapy for self-expression and healing. Because children have not yet acquired adult constraints, they are often more responsive to imagery than adults.

Be attentive to other children in the family. If they are resentful about the "privileged" status of the ill child (fewer responsibilities, more attention), allow them to express their feelings appropriately, in a manner that is not destructive, demeaning, or blaming.

Treat the ill child as normally as possible. Try not to make too many special exceptions. Genuine illness can be used manipulatively. Be aware of any tendency to "baby" or rescue the child, to "make up" for the illness with inappropriate favors or privileges. You can ease, but not compensate for, the child's losses and burdens.

Children, especially teenagers, may attempt to deny health problems. They need to know that denial won't help, that facing illness is painful but that they are strong enough to do so and will have the family's support. Allow them to express their feelings, including those that don't make sense, and to grieve. Allow them to experience and accept illness in their own way.

Try to plan enjoyable activities and allow the child to interact with friends as much as possible. Peer relationships are extremely important to kids; don't be insulted when peer contact takes precedence over family activities.

Children are very adaptable and often handle hardships amazingly well. Like all of us, they need frequent signs of support and encouragement.

RELATIONSHIPS IN THE WORKPLACE

If you are able to continue working, there have probably been changes in your attendance record, work hours, procedures, and relationships with employer and coworkers. It is not wise to hide or lie about your illness. In the long run, a cover-up is difficult to sustain, and greater problems may ensue if your health status is discovered later on. If illness does not interfere with your ability to work, however, there may be no reason to volunteer health information.

There are no official guidelines for handling this situation; it is a matter of individual preferences and judgment.

Many employers are quite understanding of illness-related special needs; some even request information about the illness. Others are less tolerant. The work setting and your responsibilities might not offer the flexibility you need right now. If you are unable to meet the requirements of your present job, consider alternatives: switch to a less demanding job, cut back on work hours, telecommute, take a leave of absence, or explore disability benefits if necessary. If you are able to perform the basic duties of your job but need assistance due to special needs, the Americans with Disabilities Act (ADA) requires that your employer make reasonable accommodations so that you may continue working. If difficulties arise, consult an attorney who specializes in labor law.

Some of your symptoms will become apparent to coworkers; again, you must decide what and when to disclose. You may want to give them general information about your illness, explaining its effects on you, including impairments and fluctuations in health status, mood, and functioning. Encourage them to ask questions. Expect that some coworkers will be understanding and supportive, and some will not.

RELATIONSHIPS WITH FRIENDS

Friendships vary in tolerance of illness-related issues. Some continue relatively unchanged, some become closer, and some dissolve. A balance of ill and healthy friends offers both the support only others with your illness can provide as well as contact with the outside world. Characteristics of friendships vary, with some revolving around shared interests or activities and others based on common traits or professions. Some are just for fun—humor, movies, leisure activities. Deeper relationships involve more intimate sharing. Having a variety of friends reduces boredom and loneliness.

Relationships vary in tolerance and flexibility, tolerance for change, and the ability to survive the increased ongoing needs of an individual with chronic illness. In close friendships, it is essential to discuss the impact of your present needs on the relationship. In more distant relationships, such in-depth discussions may strain relationship boundaries. Even though illness is a major factor in your life, you will need to make decisions about how much discussion of the illness is appropriate in each of your relationships.

Friends will not always know how to respond to your statements about your illness. They may think you are exaggerating and respond with disbelief. If their reactions are consistently disappointing, you may need to confront them or even sever the relationship.

The pain, energy crunch, and isolative tendencies that often accompany CFS/FMS make friendships difficult. Not everyone can understand or tolerate alternating needs for distance and closeness. If you are fortunate, most of your friendships will last, but not all relationships can survive the toll of chronic illness.

WHEN THEY DON'T UNDERSTAND

Never try to teach a pig to sing. It's a waste of your time and
it annoys the pig.

— Unknown

Not everyone will be receptive or supportive. It's not just difficult for healthy individuals to understand what we are going through; it's impossible. They may try to understand, or think they understand, but they cannot fully understand. Their misperceptions may be unintentionally hurtful.

Healthy individuals do experience similar symptoms, although less frequently and severely. Such statements as "I get tired, too" and "You're not the only one who's forgetful" cause us to feel discounted. Trying to convince skeptics usually proves futile.

ABOUT SUICIDE: SUGGESTIONS FOR FRIENDS AND FAMILY

During times of desperation, many with chronic illness have considered suicide a possible route for escaping their great physical and emotional pain. Although relatively few follow through with their plans, the incidence of suicide is significantly higher among the chronically ill than the general population. Suicidal talk or behavior should always be taken seriously.

Discouraging relapses may lead to the irrational thinking (which seems quite real and logical at the time) that improvement can never take place, life is too painful to endure, no one cares, and no hope exists. Trying to talk a suicidal person out of being pessimistic is usually ineffective, but you can help by listening. Keep communication going. Allow the person to do most of the talking as you pay careful attention. To avoid the risk of alienation, be supportive but not unrealistically optimistic. Ask what you can do to help. Stay with the person until you feel certain that the danger has passed. If you need to leave for a period of time, it is often wise to find someone to be with the patient. Suggest resources such as counseling, group therapy, or contact with others who are ill. Once the initial feelings are expressed and you feel the timing is right, help the person identify reasons to live, to hope. If depression is severe and does not lift, hospitalization may be appropriate.

AN OPEN LETTER FROM A PATIENT
TO A FRIEND

Dear friend,

I know my illness puts pressure on both of us and strains our relationship. Don't give up on me! Please try to be patient. I have unpredictable mood swings; please don't take them personally. Sometimes I'm so depressed I want the whole world to go away and I don't want to talk to anyone. I just need to pull back until I am ready to interact productively again.

Let's talk together about the changes in me and the changes in our relationship. I know you've noticed them. Please tell me about your life, too, even if I forget to ask. Illness is a very self-absorbed state, but I still care about you. If I forget to show my caring, please let me know, gently. Your needs matter to me a lot, but sometimes mine get in the way.

I need lots of attention right now, lots of caring. I don't want to overwhelm you with my needs but sometimes they overwhelm me. I don't expect you to rescue me and make it all better, but I hope you're willing to listen while I express thoughts, emotions, and needs. Sometimes I'll need your feedback. As I attempt to express my needs, tell me if I'm not being clear or if I'm expecting too much.

There are times I think I can't get through this. Please remind me that I'm strong and that I've gotten through so far. Tell me you believe in me.

Our relationship is uneven and unbalanced. I don't feel good about being the one with greater needs. I don't expect to be babied or coddled, but I often need a lot of attention and caring. I sometimes feel like a burden and wonder if you just tolerate me to be nice. I know better; this is my insecurity talking. I wish I could repay you somehow, even though you probably don't expect it.

Please continue to stay in touch and invite me to do things with the understanding that I wish I could join you but may have to respond with "maybe" or "no." Try to realize that what seems to you like minor exertion is a major effort for me. When I'm not doing well, such an effort can deplete my energy resources and may further jeopardize my health. I miss doing things with you but need to be very careful about my activity level.

I both love and hate it when you tell me I'm looking good. Please don't assume that means I'm feeling good. And when you ask how I am, I'll answer honestly but will try to be concise.

I know you can't always be available for me, and I'll try to understand when you have conflicting needs of your own. Illness has helped me to realize the importance of feeling cared about. Thank you for being my friend.

AN OPEN LETTER FROM A PATIENT TO A SPOUSE/PARTNER

Dear significant other,

Please understand that I am going through a horrible ordeal. I feel terrible about inflicting my illness on you. I know that you're affected by my changes, and I wish it were otherwise. I don't want to be ill.

I feel guilty about my inability to shoulder former responsibilities at work and at home, dumping more on you. I wish I could do more or know in advance what I will be capable of each day. I worry that you think I'm lazy or trying to dodge responsibilities I dislike, but that's not it. Sometimes I just can't, and other times I know it would be a mistake to use up all my energy on a minor thing and then have to give up something more important.

I want to know that I can trust you and that you will be available to listen and try to understand. And I'll try to understand that you can't always be available.

At times my feelings are irrational. My moods are erratic, and I get angry for no apparent reason, or way out of proportion to the trigger. This is part of my illness, and I'll try to keep it under control. I don't mean to direct the anger and frustration at you, but I will sometimes fail. If my mood swings become too hard to take and you feel ready to explode, please tell me so, gently. Maybe one of us can leave the scene, and we can talk about it later when we're both calmer.

Sometimes I need to talk about these irrational feelings. Just listen, okay? Please don't tell me how to feel or how not to feel. You can't "fix" my feelings. Please don't judge them; just accept and acknowledge them. When you say such things as, "Your illness must be terribly frustrating for you," I feel understood and comforted. But don't tell me you know how I feel. You don't and you can't; no one can know exactly what this is like for me. And when I cry, don't try to make me stop. Please let me cry—I'll feel better later.

I know I complain a lot. It helps to relieve tension. If my complaining strains your tolerance, please tell me so. I won't like hearing it and may not handle it well, but I really do understand that you need to distance yourself from my complaints.

I need to work at making clear requests so that you'll know what I need. It's not your job to mind read—it's my responsibility to ask for what I want. This is difficult for me; it's easier for me to meet others' needs than to admit my own and ask that they be met.

Don't try to talk me out of my symptoms or remind me that they're not as bad as they could be or not as bad as they were. I know I need to stay hopeful, but if you take an optimistic role when I feel pessimistic, I feel as if you don't understand me and won't validate my feelings.

I know you don't understand why I'm sick. Neither do I. Let's stay away from blame and acknowledge our feelings of helplessness.

Don't give up your whole life for me. Please continue to do the things that are important to you. I won't always be able to do them with you, so do them alone or with a friend. Sometimes I resent my limitations and your freedom, but I'll try to keep a healthy perspective. If you put your life on hold because of my illness, I'll feel guilty and your resentment will build. I appreciate your invitations to do things as a reminder that you still value my company. Please don't assume what I can or can't do; ask, and I'll answer you honestly. I hope you will understand that when I say "no," it's not because I don't want to but because I can't or shouldn't.

I know I'm not the way I used to be. I'm trying to learn from my illness, from these changes, and you can help. We can't pretend that things are the way they were or that they'll ever be the same again. But as we change and grow, I want us to grow together rather than apart. Let's keep the lines of communication open. When I need to withdraw, I'll try to let you know so you won't take it personally. Please do the same for me. Don't just pull away; explain to me that you need distance temporarily so I'm less inclined to feel abandoned.

Because we're both experiencing losses, we need to grieve. Some of our grieving will be solitary and some of it shared. Let's acknowledge what we've lost by mourning together.

Please don't try to make my decisions for me. If you see me wearing down and think I should rest, I value your observations and suggestions, but dislike being told what I should do. I need to take care of myself and you can help, but don't try to take over. Your encouragement helps me to do a better job of taking care of myself.

When you acknowledge my difficulties and my strengths, I might have trouble believing what you say, but I need to hear it. Tell me you think I'm brave, that I'm fighting hard, that I'm weathering this calamity well. Tell me you still love and value me, and why. Small tokens help—a flower, a phone call, a card.

Sometimes I may be unable to hear you or I may even push you away when I'm hurting, especially at times when I can't love myself. I'll try not to hurt you, but if I do, please understand that I don't mean to reject you.

I know our sexual relationship has changed and that we both miss the way it was. My lack of energy and sexual interest is a result of my illness and not a rejection of you. I need to remain close with you in every possible way. Hugs and cuddling are comforting and reassuring to me.

These are rough times for us. I appreciate the efforts you've made to help me to cope and to be comfortable. I know I've been difficult to live with. At times you have been too. If we can get through these times together, our relationship will become stronger—something I want very much.

AN OPEN LETTER FROM A HEALTHY
SPOUSE/PARTNER TO A PATIENT

Dear _____,

I know your illness-related needs can be overwhelming and that you have difficulty coping. Please try to see that I'm going through a hard time, too. I almost feel as if I shouldn't have needs, but your illness affects me as well, very deeply. I care about you, and when you hurt and I can't fix it, then I hurt too.

I wish I knew how to make you better, and I feel helpless because I cannot. Sometimes I give you unwanted advice. My intention is to be helpful, and I don't know what else to give or do. I'll try not to take over your care or tell you what's best for you. I don't want you to be dependent on me any more than you have to be.

Please tell me what you need. When you hold back, I become frustrated because I can't figure out your needs. If you ask for something specific, I have the option of saying "yes" or "no." But you have to ask.

I take what you say seriously, even though some of it doesn't make sense to me. Please take what I say seriously as well, even when I don't make sense to you.

There are times when I just don't understand. You seem crazy, or lazy, or as if you no longer care about *my* needs. I know it isn't true, but I can't help my feelings. I guess sometimes you need to feel sorry for yourself. I feel sorry for myself, too.

Sometimes you dump on me when you're especially tired or grouchy. I understand this in my head, but it still hurts. I feel as if you're blaming me for your illness and expecting me to fix it. I'd do anything I can to help you, but I can't make it go away. Please try not to lash out. If something is really bothering you, let's talk about it at a good time.

When I do something that's helpful, let me know. I need feedback and acknowledgment from you. I'm doing an awful lot right now. I need to know that you notice and appreciate what I do.

I love you. I need other friends and family in my life as well. I hope that my time with them won't cause you to feel left out when you're not well enough to participate. I may become overly involved in work and other activities because of my need for a time-out. I'm trying to balance our needs, and just as you need to take care of yourself, I need to take care of myself. I still need to see friends, exercise, play, and deal with job stresses, family needs, and my own health concerns.

I agree that we should continue to make decisions together, even though I may have to carry them out alone. I'll try not to be a martyr or a dictator. If I'm making too many decisions without your input and you feel left out, please tell me.

Sometimes I think you should do things differently in order to get better. When I ask you to try some special treatment, diet, or positive thinking, it's because I'm trying to help. Sometimes I even get mad at your doctor, thinking that with adequate care you'd get better.

Although I try not to burden you with the way I feel, I don't want to pretend I have no bad feelings about this. I feel afraid, hurt, vulnerable, angry, and sad. Sometimes I become angry with you for being sick, although rationally I know it's not your fault.

When you are depressed or lie in bed staring into space, I feel abandoned. Sometimes I think this illness has taken over your life, and I'm not very important anymore. I need to know that I'm still important to you.

Let's do some fun things together. I know your energy is limited, but we need some time off from the gloom. Let's figure out what we can do to enjoy each other. Save some of your precious energy for *us*, even if it's just to watch a movie together and share some popcorn.

We can get through this together. Despite the pain and the struggles, let's not forget how much we mean to each other.

17

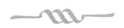

Conclusion

The important thing is not to stop questioning.

— *Albert Einstein*

Chronic illnesses, and those who have them, remain unpopular. Despite high-tech medical gains and breakthroughs in other areas, we lack a basic understanding of the pathophysiology of chronic illnesses that afflict millions of people. Studies to date have been numerous but often limited, flawed, and contradictory, since many illness definitions, study procedures, and outcome measures are not standardized. While we continue to wait for answers—causes, markers, and effective therapies, if not a cure—studies and informal trials yield tentative conclusions that remain matters of scientific debate. We grope in darkness for pieces of a complex puzzle.

Given the magnitude of the problem, relatively little has been done to solve it. Penny-wise and pound-foolish, we repeat the HIV/AIDS phenomenon, ignoring serious and prevalent chronic illnesses and refusing to take action until the problems have grown to epidemic proportions. Meanwhile, illnesses such as CFS and FMS exact a huge toll in disability benefits, medical expenses, and loss of productivity and wages, often during patients' prime work years. Those who are disabled are unable to contribute to the national economy, drawing from it instead.

As a nation, we are fickle and inconsistent with our spending. American taxpayers will spend an estimated 1.3 billion dollars for the 2002 Winter Olympics, 4 billion dollars for an International Fertilizer Development Center, 5 million dollars for an insect rearing facility in Mississippi, and 3.5 billion dollars to refurbish the Vulcan Monument in Alabama, according to Senator John McCain. Yet, of the fifty-two National Institutes of Health Research Initia-

tives/Programs of Interest for the fiscal years 1998, 1999, and pro-
jections for 2000, CFS and FMS are numbers fifty-one and fifty-two
in allocated funding: last on the list. The CDC has misspent a large
portion of the funds allocated by congress for CFS research, but the
populace is apparently unaware and unconcerned.

As the nation looks the other way, our numbers and needs are
swelling. CFS and FMS will be taken seriously once quantifiable
markers and causes have been identified, a near-impossible task
without adequate research funding. Not to make such illnesses as
CFS and FMS strong national priorities is both inhumane and
financially foolish. We boast a huge federal budget, national research
institutes, state-of-the-art health-care resources, outstanding media
involvement and coverage of health issues, and a humanitarian philosophy, while hypocritically turning a deaf ear to the cries of those
afflicted with chronic illnesses. Pet projects are clearly a higher priority than the alleviation of human suffering.

CFS and FMS need to be taken seriously and granted the same
legitimacy as other illnesses in the public eye and in medical circles.
We need to take the politics out of medicine. We need well-
designed multidisciplinary studies that focus on cause(s), markers,
treatments, and sick children and adolescents, rather than repetitive studies proving that our illnesses are "real." We need new case
definitions and accurate, credible names that reflect the debilitation associated with FMS and CFS. We need to study the overlaps
and links among chronic illnesses. We need to educate physicians
about CFS and FMS and how to be open-minded about what they
do not yet understand. We need to hold insurance companies
accountable, insisting that they deliver what they sell. Above all,
we need reasons to hope.

We have been patient long enough. History teaches us that
minority groups are not granted their rights until they have made
noise or become destructive. In order to be granted their rights,
blacks burned ghettos, feminists burned bras, and ACT UP made
noise about HIV/AIDS. National and local support groups have
been reasonable and effective advocates, but their voices have
largely been ignored. We need an aggressive campaign to accomplish our goals, a vocal, insistent equivalent of ACT UP. We need
dramatic action to draw attention to the severity of CFS and FMS,
the numbers of people who are ill, and the tremendous individual

and societal toll. The squeaky wheel gets the grease. Silently out-raged for years, we've been too passive and too ill to squeak. Although physically debilitated and financially compromised, we need to make noise. We need to write letters to those in a position to help, including government representatives and agencies as well as the private sector. We must educate others by prodding the media, continuing to develop and implement educational pro-grams, increasing fund-raising efforts, and encouraging our signifi-cant others to become more involved.

The cause(s) of FMS and CFS will ultimately be found, as will a cure or at least helpful therapies. In the meantime, we must net-work with others, stay informed and united, and continue to seek the support of the media, the medical community, our elected rep-resentatives, and the public.

We do have valuable allies: knowledgeable and compassionate health practitioners, researchers, spokespersons, and organizations that have done an admirable job of standing up for us when we are too ill to stand on our own. At the risk of professional ostracism, dedicated health professionals have diagnosed and treated us, defending us against those who do not take our debilitation and dis-abilities seriously. Significant others have made countless contribu-tions to the quality of our lives.

In ways we previously could not have imagined, FMS and CFS affect every aspect of our lives, including relationships; careers; activities; self-image; and the ability to think, reason, and learn. The ongoing challenge of learning to accept and live with chronic illness is our primary responsibility.

Our lives are filled with contradictions: We are fragile yet resilient; we crumble and rebuild, fight and retreat. We make progress; we lose ground. We feel better; we crash. We endure a journey like no other; our tenacity expresses the triumph of the human spirit over adversity.

Illness is not a detour but a journey along a bumpy road. It's not time out from real life; it IS real life. Our lives are not the way they once were, but they are the lives we have now. We must dump the "before and after" comparisons, work with what we've got, and con-tinue to live our lives, albeit in a modified fashion.

I have grown during the time I have been ill, and I have learned lessons that come from grappling with painful challenges. Of course,

I would prefer to be well and make do with less personal growth—but since I don't have that choice, I've decided to make the best of it in my own way, continuing to enjoy life when I can and to endure it when I must. I hope you will do the same.

Illness has spurred me to examine the meaning of life in general, and of my life in particular. Susan Levine, M.D., described CFS as "a silent illness" that "robs people of their day-to-day sanity." Altering everything from relationships to my ability to think coherently, illness can *borrow* my sanity, but it can't *have* it. Tomorrow I may think differently, but my wish is to have many more hopeful and productive days like today. I can live with that.

Chronic Fatigue Syndrome/ Fibromyalgia Syndrome Symptom Checklist

Indicate **on a scale of 1 to 10** the severity of each symptom, with 10 being the most severe and frequent. Use the past sixty days as a general guide. If you do not have the symptom, leave the space blank.

____ Fatigue, made worse by physical exertion or stress
____ Activity level decreased to less than 50 percent of preillness activity level
____ Recurrent flulike illness
____ Sore throat
____ Hoarseness
____ Tender or swollen lymph nodes (glands), especially in neck and underarms
____ Shortness of breath with little or no exertion
____ Frequent sighing
____ Tremor or trembling
____ Severe nasal allergies (new or worsened)
____ Cough
____ Night sweats
____ Low-grade fevers
____ Feeling cold often
____ Feeling hot often
____ Cold extremities (hands and feet)
____ Low body temperature (below 97.6°)
____ Low blood pressure (below 110/70)
____ Heart palpitations
____ Dryness of eyes and/or mouth
____ Increased thirst
____ Symptoms worsened by temperature changes
____ Symptoms worsened by air travel
____ Symptoms worsened by stress

Pain

_____ Headache
_____ Tender points or trigger points
_____ Muscle pain
_____ Muscle twitching
_____ Muscle weakness
_____ Paralysis or severe weakness of an arm or leg
_____ Joint pain
_____ Temporomandibular Joint (TMJ) syndrome
_____ Chest pain

Eyes and Vision

_____ Eye pain
_____ Changes in visual acuity (frequent changes in ability to see well)
_____ Difficulty with accommodation (switching focus from one thing to another)
_____ Blind spots in vision

Sensitivities

_____ Sensitivities to medications (unable to tolerate a "normal" dosage)
_____ Sensitivities to odors (e.g., cleaning products, exhaust fumes, colognes, hair sprays)
_____ Sensitivities to foods
_____ Alcohol intolerance
_____ Alteration of taste, smell, and/or hearing

Urogenital

_____ Frequent urination
_____ Painful urination or bladder pain
_____ Prostate pain
_____ Impotence
_____ Endometriosis
_____ Worsening of premenstrual syndrome (PMS)
_____ Decreased libido (sex drive)

Gastrointestinal

_____ Stomach ache; abdominal cramps
_____ Nausea
_____ Vomiting
_____ Esophageal reflux (heartburn)
_____ Frequent diarrhea
_____ Frequent constipation
_____ Bloating; intestinal gas
_____ Decreased appetite

_____ Increased appetite
_____ Food cravings
_____ Weight gain (_____ lbs)
_____ Weight loss (_____ lbs)

Other

_____ Rashes or sores
_____ Eczema or psoriasis
_____ Aphthous ulcers (canker sores)
_____ Hair loss
_____ Mitral valve prolapse
_____ Cancer
_____ Dental problems
_____ Periodontal (gum) disease

General Neurological

_____ Light-headedness; feeling "spaced out"
_____ Inability to think clearly ("brain fog")
_____ Seizures
_____ Seizure-like episodes
_____ Syncope (fainting) or blackouts
_____ Sensation that you might faint
_____ Vertigo or dizziness
_____ Numbness or tingling sensations
_____ Tinnitus (ringing in one or both ears)
_____ Photophobia (sensitivity to light)
_____ Noise intolerance

Equilibrium/Perception

_____ Feeling spatially disoriented
_____ Dysequilibrium (balance difficulty)
_____ Staggering gait (clumsy walking; bumping into things)
_____ Dropping things frequently
_____ Difficulty judging distances (e.g., when driving; placing objects on surfaces)
_____ "Not quite seeing" what you are looking at

Sleep

_____ Hypersomnia (excessive sleeping)
_____ Sleep disturbance: unrefreshing or nonrestorative sleep
_____ Sleep disturbance: difficulty falling asleep
_____ Sleep disturbance: difficulty staying asleep (frequent awakenings)
_____ Sleep disturbance: vivid or disturbing dreams or nightmares
_____ Altered sleep/wake schedule (alertness/energy best late at night)

Cognitive

_____ Difficulty with simple calculations (e.g., balancing checkbook)
_____ Word-finding difficulty
_____ Saying the wrong word
_____ Difficulty expressing ideas in words
_____ Difficulty moving your mouth to speak
_____ Slowed speech
_____ Stuttering; stammering
_____ Impaired ability to concentrate
_____ Easily distracted during a task
_____ Difficulty paying attention
_____ Difficulty following a conversation when background noise is present
_____ Losing your train of thought in the middle of a sentence
_____ Difficulty putting tasks or things into proper sequence
_____ Losing track in the middle of a task (remembering what to do next)
_____ Difficulty with short-term memory
_____ Difficulty with long-term memory
_____ Forgetting how to do routine things
_____ Difficulty understanding what you read
_____ Switching left and right
_____ Transposition (reversal) of numbers, words and/or letters when you <u>speak</u>
_____ Transposition (reversal) of numbers, words and/or letters when you <u>write</u>
_____ Difficulty remembering names of objects
_____ Difficulty remembering names of people
_____ Difficulty recognizing faces
_____ Poor judgment
_____ Difficulty making decisions
_____ Difficulty following _simple written_ instructions
_____ Difficulty following _complicated written_ instructions
_____ Difficulty following _simple oral_ (spoken) instructions
_____ Difficulty following _complicated oral_ (spoken) instructions
_____ Difficulty integrating information (putting ideas together to form a complete picture or concept)
_____ Difficulty following directions while driving
_____ Becoming lost in familiar locations when driving
_____ Feeling too disoriented to drive

Mood/Emotions

_____ Depressed mood
_____ Suicidal thoughts
_____ Suicide attempts
_____ Feeling worthless
_____ Frequent crying

_____ Feeling helpless and/or hopeless
_____ Inability to enjoy previously enjoyed activities
_____ Increased appetite
_____ Decreased appetite
_____ Anxiety or fear with no obvious cause
_____ Panic attacks
_____ Irritability; overreaction
_____ Rage attacks: anger outbursts with little or no cause
_____ Abrupt, unpredictable mood swings
_____ Phobias (irrational fears)
_____ Personality changes

© copyright 2001 by Katrina H. Berne, Ph.D.
Permission to copy for personal use is granted, with the provision that
attribution to copyright holder appears.

Resources

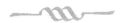

CAUTIONS ABOUT USING THE INTERNET

Authors and Organizations

Know the source of the information. Is the author a researcher, physician, organization, patient, or health writer? Is the author credentialed or otherwise qualified to provide accurate information?

Are references or documentation (e.g., a bibliography) provided?

Is the article intended as fact or opinion?

How current is the information?

What is the reputation of the organization? Does it have an advisory board, and if so, who serves on it? How is the organization funded?

Are products promoted? Are sales tactics reasonable or pushy and somewhat suspect?

Research Articles

Who conducted the study? Was it published in a peer-reviewed journal? Has the study been sponsored by a group that might influence its results?

How many patients were studied? What criteria were used to select the participants? Was a control group (nonpatients) used for comparison? How similar was the control group to the patient group in terms of age, gender, race, etc.?

Is the study randomized, double-blind, placebo-controlled?

What outcome measures were used? (How did the researchers determine criteria for improvement?)

Are the results statistically significant?

Could other factors (variables) have influenced the outcome?

If a treatment study, were long-term results included? Were side effects of the treatment discussed? Were the benefits of treatment sufficient to offset side effects and costs?

If a study of causation, are assumptions being made? Is correlation assumed to imply causation?

Was follow-up done on the patients to see if the results lasted over time? Does the study seem reasonable, objective, and unbiased?

At present, websites offering medical information are not regulated for accuracy, proper disclosures, or ethical practices, including privacy, accountability, identification of sources of information, links to other sites, and methods of contacting the parent organization and registering consumer complaints.

With these caveats, the following resources are offered as a sampling of tools for individual exploration but not as an endorsement of their contents. Please consult with experienced, credentialed professionals in making decisions regarding treatment and other important issues.

INFORMATIONAL RESOURCES

Chronic Fatigue Syndrome

American Association for Chronic Fatigue Syndrome (AACFS)
c/o Harborview Medical Center
PO Box 359780
Seattle WA 98104   (206) 521-1932   Website: www.aacfs.org

The CFIDS Association of America, Inc.
PO Box 220398
Charlotte NC 28222-0398   (800) 442-3437
Resource line: (704) 365-2343   Website: www.cfids.org

The CFIDS Support Network of America (CSN)
(*See* "The CFIDS Association of America")

CFS Information International   Website: www.cfs.inform.dk/

CFS News (Co-Cure)   Website: www.cfs-news.org/

Massachusetts CFIDS Association (CFS & FM)
PO Box 690305
Quincy MA 02269-0305   (617) 471-5559
Website: www.masscfids.org

National CFIDS Foundation
103 Aletha Rd.
Needham MA 02492   (781) 449-3535
Website: www.NCF-NET.org

Fibromyalgia

American College of Rheumatology (ACR)
1800 Century Pl., Ste. 250
Atlanta GA 30345   (404) 633-3777
Website: www.rheumatology.org

The American Fibromyalgia Syndrome Assoc., Inc. (AFSA)
6380 Tanque Verde Rd., Ste. D
Tucson AZ 85715   (520) 733-1570   Website: www.afsafund.org

Arthritis Foundation National Office
PO Box 7669
Atlanta GA 30326   (404) 872-7100   Website: www.arthritis.org

Fibromyalgia Management Association (FMA)
PO Box 8119
Minneapolis MN 55408-0119   (800) 328-9493
E-mail: info@cuddleewe.com   (763) 424-1104

Fibromyalgia Network
P.O. Box 31750
Tucson AZ 85751   (800) 853-2929   (520) 290-5508
Website: www.fmnetnews.com

National Fibromyalgia Awareness Campaign (NFAC)
2415 N. River Trail Rd, Ste. 200
Orange CA 92865   (714) 921-0150
Website: www.fmaware.com

National Fibromyalgia Partnership (NFP)
140 Zinn Way
Linden VA 22642-5609   (866) 725-4404
Website: www.fmpartnership.org

National Fibromyalgia Research Association
PO Box 500
Salem OR 97308   Website: www.teleport.com/~nfra

Oregon Fibromyalgia Foundation (OFF)   Website: www.myalgia.com

CFS/FMS

About.com: Chronic Fatigue Syndrome/Fibromyalgia
Website: http://chronicfatigue.about.com/mbody.htm

CEFCA Support Group (CFIDS, FM, related illnesses)
PO Box 341533
Los Angeles CA 90034
Website: www2.interaccess.com/montage/cefca/

CFIDS and Fibromyalgia Health Resource
2040 Alameda Padre Serra, Ste. 101
Santa Barbara CA 93103   (800) 366-6056
Website: www.immunesupport.com

Chronic Fatigue Syndrome & Fibromaylgia Exchange (Co-Cure)
Website: www.co-cure.org

Colorado HealthNet Fibromyalgia and Chronic Fatigue Syndrome Center
Website: www.coloradohealthnet.org/site/idx_fibro.html

National Chronic Fatigue Syndrome and Fibromyalgia Association
(NCFSFA)
PO Box 18426
Kansas City MO 64133   (816) 313-2000

Canada

The ME Association of Canada
246 Queen St., Ste. 400
Ottawa Ontario K1P 5E4   (613) 563-1565   Website: www.mecan.ca

The Nightingale Research Foundation
121 Iona St.
Ottawa Ontario K1Y 3M1   (613) 728-9643

National ME/FM Action Network (ME, FM, GWS & MCS)
3836 Carling Ave., Hwy 17B
Nepean Ontario K2H 7V2   (613) 829-6667
Website: www3.sympatico.ca/me-fm.action/

ORGANIZATIONS FOR PROFESSIONALS

The American Association for Chronic Fatigue Syndrome (AACFS)
PO Box 895
Olney MD 20830   (206) 521-1932   Website: aacfs.org

Association of Rheumatology Health Professionals (ARHP)
c/o Lori Clovis
1800 Century Pl., Ste. 250
Atlanta GA 30345   (404) 633-3777
Website: www.rheumatology.org/arhp/index.html

Medical Professionals With CFIDS
c/o Gail Dahlen, R.N.
50 Cecil Ave.
Indianapolis IN 46219

Medical Professionals/Persons With CFIDS (MPWC)
PO Box 144
Hinsdale NY 14743

Professionals with CFS/ME: M/PWC-ME, Inc.
PO Box 8
Fairmont MN 56031

RELATED DISORDERS

Allergy

American Academy of Asthma, Allergy, and Immunology
611 East Wells St.
Milwaukee WI 53202   (800) 822-2762   (414) 272-6071
Website: www.aaaai.org

Asthma and Allergy Foundation of America (AAFA)
1233 20th St., NW, Ste. 402
Washington DC 20036   (800) 727-8462   Website: www.aafa.org

Food Allergy and Anaphylaxis Network
10400 Eaton Pl., Ste. 107
Fairfax VA 22030   (800) 929-4040
Website: www.foodallergy.org

Anxiety and Panic Disorders

Anxiety Disorders Association of America
11900 Parklawn Dr., Ste. 100
Rockville MD 20852   (301) 231-9350   Website: www.adaa.org

Anxiety Disorders Education Program   (800) 64-PANIC (647-2622)

National Institute of Mental Health (NIMH)   (301) 443-4513
(See listing under "Government Health Agencies.")

Arthritis

Arthritis Foundation (See listing under "Fibromyalgia.")

Arthritis National Research Foundation
200 Oceangate, Ste. 400
Long Beach CA 90802   (800) 588-2873
Website: www.curearthritis.com

Johns Hopkins: Arthritis News
Website: www.hopkins-arthritis.com

Balance Disorders

Dizziness and Balance Disorders Association of America
1015 NW 22nd Ave.
Portland OR 97210   (800) 227-5726   (503) 229-7348

Vestibular Disorders Association (VEDA)
PO Box 4467
Portland OR 97208   (800) 837-8428   (503) 229-7705
Website: www.vestibular.org

Candidiasis

About.com: Candida/Yeast Sensitivity
Website: http://allergies.about.com/cs/yeastsensitivity/

Candidiasis: MedLine Plus Health Information, NIH
Website: www.nlm.nih.gov/medlineplus/candidiasis.html

Depression

National Depressive and Manic-Depressive Association
730 N. Franklin St., Ste. 501
Chicago IL 60610   (800) 826-3632   (312) 642-0049
Website: www.ndmda.org

National Foundation for Depressive Illness, Inc.
PO Box 2257
New York NY 10116   (800) 239-1265
Website: www.depression.org

National Institute of Mental Health: Depression
Website: www.mentalhealth.com/fr20.htm

National Suicide Hotline   (800) SUICIDE (784-2433)

SAVE—Suicide Awareness Voices of Education
Minneapolis MN 55424   (952) 946-7998   Website: www.save.org

Dysautonomia

National Dysautonomia Research Foundation
421 W. Fourth St., Ste. 9
Red Wing MN 55066   (651) 267-0525   Website: www.ndrf.org

Endometriosis

The Endometriosis Association
8585 N. 76th Pl.
Milwaukee WI 53223   (414) 355-2200
Website: www.endometriosisassn.org

The Endo/CFIDS Data Project
PO Box 501
Hillsborough NC 27278

Gulf War Syndrome

Gulf War Illness Site, Department of Defense
5113 Leesburg Pike, Ste. 901
Falls Church VA 22041   (800) 497-6261
Website: www.gulflink.osd.mil

Gulf War Veterans Resource Pages   Website: www.gulfweb.org

Gulf War Vets   (800) 749-8387
Website: www.va.gov/health/environ/persgulf.htm

National Gulf War Resource Center
1224 M St., NW
Washington DC 20005   (202) 628-2700, ext. 162
Website: www.gulfwar.org/Resource_Center

Headache

About.com: Headaches/Migraine
Website: http://headaches.about.com

American Academy of Neurology
1080 Montreal Ave.
St. Paul MN 55116   (651) 695-1940   Website: www.aan.com

American Council for Headache Education (ACHE)
19 Mantua Rd.
Mt. Royal NJ 08061   (856) 423-0258
Website: www.achenet.org

National Headache Foundation   (888) NHF-5552 (643-5552)
Website: www.headaches.org

World Headache Alliance
208 Lexington Rd.
Oakville Ontario L6H 6L6, Canada   (905) 257-6229
Website: www.w-h-a.org

Interstitial Cystitis

Interstitial Cystitis Association (ICA)
51 Monroe St., Ste. 1402
Rockville MD 20850   (301) 610-5300   Website: www.ichelp.org

Irritable Bowel Disorders

The Crohn's and Colitis Foundation of America
386 Park Ave. S., 17th Fl.
New York NY 10016-8804   (800) 932-2423   (212) 685-3440
Website: www.ccfa.org

International Foundation for Functional Gastrointestinal Disorders
(IFFGD)
PO Box 170864
Milwaukee WI 53217   (888) 964-2001   (414) 964-1799
Website: www.iffgd.org

Lupus (Systemic Lupus Erythematosus, or SLE)

American Lupus Society
260 Maple Ct., Ste. 123
Ventura CA 93003-3512   (800) 331-1802   (805) 339-0443
Website: www.healthy.net/pan/cso/cioi/TALS.HTM

The Lupus Foundation of America, Inc. (LFA)
1330 Piccard Dr., Ste. 200
Rockville MD 20850-4303   (800) 558-0121   (301) 670-9292
Website: www.lupus.org

Lyme Disease

Lyme Disease Foundation
One Financial Plaza,18th Fl.
Hartford CT 06103   800-886-LYME   (860) 525-2000
Website: www.lyme.org

Lyme Disease Resource Center (LDRC)
PO Box 707
Weaverville CA 96093   Website: www.lymedisease.org

Mitral Valve Prolapse

The Mitral Valve Prolapse Center
880 Montclair Rd., Ste. 370
Birmingham AL 35213   (800) 541-8602   (205) 592-5765
Website: www.mvprolapse.com/center.htm

Advocate Health Care: Mitral Valve Prolapse Syndrome
Website: www.advocatehealth.com/healthinfo/articles/heartcare/common/mvpsynd.html

Multiple Chemical Sensitivities

American Academy of Environmental Medicine
7701 East Kellogg, Ste. 625
Wichita KS 67207   (316) 684-5500   Website: www.aaem.com

Chemical Injury Information Network
PO Box 301
White Sulphur Springs MT 59645   (406) 547-2255
Website: www.ciin.org

National Environmental Health Association (NEHA)
720 S. Colorado Blvd., Ste. 970-S
Denver CO 80245   (303) 756-9090   Website: www.neha.org

MCS Referral & Resources
508 Westgate Rd.
Baltimore MD 21229   (410) 362-6400   Website: www.mcsrr.org

Multiple Sclerosis

Multiple Sclerosis Foundation, Inc.
6350 North Andrews Ave.
Fort Lauderdale FL 33309   (888) MSFOCUS (673-6287)
Website: www.msfacts.org   (954) 776-6805

National M.S. Society
733 Third Ave.
New York NY 10017   (800) 344-4867   (212) 986-3240
Website: www.nmss.org

Pain

American Academy of Pain Management
4700 W. Lake
Glenview IL 60025   (847) 375-4731   Website: www.painmed.org

American Chronic Pain Association
PO Box 850
Rocklin CA 95677   (916) 632-0922
Website: www.members.tripod.com/~Widdy/ACPA.html#who

American Pain Society
4700 W. Lake Ave.
Glenview IL 60025   (847) 375-4715
Website: www.ampainsoc.org

HealthCentral.com: Pain
Website: www.healthcentral.com/Centers/OneCenter.cfm?Center=Pain-
    Management

The National Foundation for the Treatment of Pain
1330 Skyline Dr., #21
Monterey CA 93940   (831) 655-8812   Website: www.paincare.org

Partners Against Pain
Website: www.partnersagainstpain.com

Restless Legs Syndrome

RLS Foundation, Inc.
PO Box 7050
Rochester MN 55902   Website: www.rls.org

Post-Polio Syndrome

Harvest Center Post-Polio Library
Website: http://members.aol.com/harvestctr/Library

Polio Connection of America
PO Box 182
Howard Beach NY 11414   (718) 835-5536
Website: http://idt.net/~1066

Polio Network (IPN)
4207 Lindell Blvd, #110
St. Louis MO 63108   (314) 534-0475
Website: www.post-polio.org

Prostatitis

American Prostate Society
7188 Ridge Rd.
Hanover MD 21076   (410) 859-3735   Website: www.ameripros.org

Prostatitis Foundation   (888) 891-4200
Website: www.prostatitis.org

Psychological/Psychiatric Disorders

American Psychiatric Association
1400 K St., N.W.
Washington DC 20005   (202) 682-6000   Website: www.psych.org

American Psychological Association
750 1st St., N.E.
Washington DC 20002   (202) 336-5500   Website: www.apa.org

Sjögren's Syndrome

National Sjögren's Syndrome Association
366 North Broadway, Ste. PH-W2
Jericho NY 11753   (800) 475-6473   (516) 933-6365
Website: www.sjogrens.org

Sleep

American Academy of Sleep Medicine
6301 Bandel Rd. NW, Ste. 101
Rochester MN 55901   (507) 287-6006   Website: www.asda.org

National Sleep Foundation
1367 Connecticut Ave., N.W., Ste. 200, Dept. V-1
Washington DC 20036   Website: www.sleepfoundation.org

Syringomyelia/Chiari Syndrome

American Syringomyelia Alliance Project (ASAP)
PO Box 1586
Longview TX 75606-1586   (800) ASAP-282 (272-7282)
Website: www.asap4sm.com (903) 236-7079

World ACM Association
31 Newtown Woods Rd.
Newtown Square PA 19073 (610) 353-4737
Website: www.pressenter.com/~wacma/

Temporomandibular Joint Dysfunction

Jaw Joints and Allied Musculoskeletal Disorders Foundation, Inc. (JJAMD)
The Forsyth Institute
140 Fenway
Boston MA 02115   (617) 267-9020   Website: www.tmjoints.org

The TMJ Association, Ltd.
PO Box 26770
Milwaukee WI 53226   Fax: (414) 259-3223
Website: www.tmj.org

Tinnitus

American Tinnitus Association
PO Box 5
Portland OR 97207   (800) 634-8978   (503) 248-9985
Website: www.ata.org

Thyroid Disorders

American Thyroid Association, Inc.
PO Box 1836
Falls Church VA 22041   (800) 542-6687   Website: www.thyroid.org

Thyroid Foundation of America, Inc.
350 Ruth Sleeper Hall – RSL 350
Parkman St.
Boston MA 02114   (800) 832-8321   (617) 726-8500
Website: http://myweb.clark.net/pub/tfa/

Vulvodynia

National Vulvodynia Association (NVA)
PO Box 4491
Silver Spring MD 20914   (301) 299-0775   Website: www.nva.org

The Vulvar Pain Foundation
PO Drawer 177
Graham NC 27253   (910) 226-0704 (Tues/Thurs)
Website: www.vulvarpainfoundation.org

Other Disorders

American Autoimmune-Related Diseases Association, Inc. (AARDA)
22100 Gratiot Ave.
E. Detroit MI 48021   (810) 776-3900
or 750 17th St., N.W.
Washington DC 20006   (202) 466-8511   Website: www.aarda.org

Center for Complex Infectious Diseases
3328 Stevens Ave.
Rosemead CA 91770   (626) 572-7288   Website: www.ccid.org/

Galaxy Directories to disorders
Website: www.galaxy.com/cgi-bin/dirlist?node=53510

HealthAtoZ   Website: www.healthatoz.com/

Healthweb   Website: http://healthwwweb.org

Medical Information Network (InfoMIN)
Website: www2.rpa.net/~lrandall/

Medical Information site links (Emory University)
Minann, Inc.
PO Box 582
Glenview IL 60025   Website: www.gen.emory.edu/

National Organization for Rare Disorders, Inc. (NORD)
PO Box 8923
New Fairfield CT 06812   (800) 999-6673   203-746-6518
Website: www.rarediseases.org

US Dept Health & Human Services: Healthfinder
Website: healthfinder.gov

WebMD   Website: www.webmd.com

TREATMENT

Pharmaceuticals

RxList—The Internet Drug Index (Health Central)
Website: www.rxlist.com

MedicineNet   Website: www.medicinenet.com

U.S. Pharmacopoea
12601 Twinbrook Pkwy.
Rockville MD 20852   (800) 822-8772   (301) 881-0666
Website: www.usp.org

Pharmaceuticals: Assistance Programs

Each drug company has its own eligibility requirements for assistance, often including ineligibility for Medicaid, lack of private insurance covering outpatient medicine, and financial need.

* Most require that a physician make initial contact.

Academy for Health Services Research and Health Policy
1801 K St., N.W.
Washington DC   (202) 292-6700
Website: www.statecoverage.net

FamiliesUSA: The Voice for Healthcare Consumers
Website: www.FamiliesUSA.org

Medicare Savings Programs for low-income seniors
(800) MEDICARE (633-4227)
or call your local Medicare office

*The Medicine Program
PO Box 515
Doniphan MO 63935   (573) 996-7300
Website: www.themedicineprogram.com

*NeedyMeds
c/o Libby Overly
PO Box 2372
Washington DC 20013   Website: www.needymeds.com

*Pharmaceutical Manufacturer's Association (PMA)
(800) PMA-INFO (762-4636)
for a PMA Directory of Prescription Drug Programs call: (573) 778-1118

*Pharmaceutical Research and Manufacturers of America
1100 Fifteenth St., N.W.
Washington DC   (202) 835-3400
Website: www.phrma.org/searchcures/dpdpap/

*Rx Assist   (877) 844-8442   Website: www.rxassist.org

Online Pharmacies

When ordering medications online, look for companies certified as Verified Internet Pharmacy Practice Sites, or VIPPS, by the National Association of Boards of Pharmacy.

Destination Rx: Online pharmacies: web price comparison
3530 Wilshire Blvd., Ste. 10
Los Angeles CA 90010   (213) 365-5721
Website: www.DestinationRx.com

Drug Trials

CenterWatch (industry- and government-sponsored drug trials)
Website: www.centerwatch.com

NIH drug trials   Website: nih.gov/health/trials/index.htm

COMPLEMENTARY/ALTERNATIVE MEDICINE

Acupuncture

National Certification Commission for Acupuncture and Oriental Medicine
11 Canal Center Plaza, Ste. 300
Alexandria VA 22314   (703) 548-9004   Website: www.nccaom.org

Traditional Chinese Therapies: Acupuncture Resources
Website: www.medicalacupuncture.org

Biofeedback

Association for Applied Psychophysiology and Biofeedback
  and Biofeedback Certification Institute of America
10200 W. 44th Ave., Ste. 304
Wheat Ridge CO 80033   (303) 422-8436
Website: www.aapb.org   Website: www.bcia.org

Herbal Medicine

American Botanical Council
PO Box 201660
Austin TX 78720   (512) 926-4900
Website: www.herbalgram.org

Herb Research Foundation
1007 Pearl St., Ste. 200
Boulder CO 80302   (303) 449-2265   Website: www.herbs.org

Herbweb (The CRC Ethnobotany Desk Reference of selected herbs)
Website: www.herbweb.com

Homeopathy

National Center for Homeopathy
801 North Fairfax, Ste. 306
Alexandria VA 22314   (877) 624-0613   (703) 548-7790
Website: www.homeopathic.org

North American Society of Homeopaths
1122 East Pike St., #1122
Seattle WA 98122   (206) 720-7000
Website: www.homeopathy.org

Naturopathy

American Association of Naturopathic Physicians
8201 Greensboro Dr., Ste. 300
McLean VA 22102   (703) 610-9037
Website: www.naturopathic.org

Nutrition

American Dietetic Association
216 W. Jackson Blvd.
Chicago IL 60606-1600   312-899-0040 Website: www.eatright.org

CONSUMER RESOURCES

Protection and Advocacy, Inc., a federal agency that provides services for the disabled, including children: Consult business white pages or see Department of Health and Human Services in the Federal Government section of your telephone book.

Your State Department of Education

Advocacy

C-ACT (CFIDS Activation Network) (*See* "Chronic Fatigue Syndrome: The CFIDS Association of America.")

CFIDS Activation Network (CAN)
PO Box 345
Larchmont NY 10538   (212) 627-5631
or
720 Balboa St.
San Francisco CA 94118

Minann, Inc.
(See listing under "Chronic Illnesses and Other Disorders.")

National Fibromyalgia Awareness Campaign (NFAC)
(See listing under "Fibromyalgia.")

RESCIND
9812 Falls Rd., Ste. 114-270
Potomac MD 20854   Fax: (after 6 P.M. ET) (301) 983-5644
E-mail: MAY12@American.edu

San Francisco CFIDS Task Force
3543 18th St., #20
San Francisco CA 94110   (415) 525-6415

CHILDREN AND ADOLESCENTS

National Information Center for Children and Youth with Disabilities
(NICHCY)
PO Box 1492
Washington DC 20013   (800) 999-5599

CFIDS Youth Alliance (See listing under "Chronic fatigue syndrome:
CFIDS Association of America.")

Support Givers

Family Caregiver Alliance
690 Market St., Ste. 600
San Francisco CA 94104   415-434-3388   Website: www.caregiver.org

National Family Caregivers Association
10400 Connecticut Ave., #500
Kensington MD 20895   (800) 896-3650
Website: www.nfcacares.org

National Parent to Parent Support and Information System
PO Box 907
Blue Ridge GA 30513   (800) 651-1151   (706) 632-8822

Well Spouse Foundation
30 E. 40th St.
New York NY 10016   (800) 838-0879   (212) 685-8815
Website: www.wellspouse.org

GOVERNMENT HEALTH AGENCIES

American Federation for Medical Research (AFMR)
227 Massachusetts Ave., NE, Ste. 302
Washington DC 20002   (202) 543-7032   Website: www.afmr.org

Centers for Disease Control and Prevention (CDC)
1600 Clifton Rd.
Atlanta GA 30333   (800) 311-3435   (404) 639-3534
Website: www.cdc.gov

National Center for Complementary & Alternative Medicine (NCCAM) of
the NIH
OCAM Clearinghouse
PO Box 8218

Silver Spring MD 20907-8218   (888) 644-6226
Website: http://nccam.nih.gov

National Institute of Allergy and Infectious Diseases (NIAID)
Office of Communications
Bldg. 31, Rm. 7A-50
31 Center Dr. MSC 2520
Bethesda MD 20892   (301) 496-5717   Website: www.niaid.nih.gov

National Institute of Arthritis and Musculoskeletal and Skin Diseases
(NIAMS)
National Institutes of Health
NIAMS Clearinghouse
1 AMS Circle   (301) 495-4484
Bethesda MD 20892-3675   (877) 22-NIAMS (226-4267)
Website: www.nih.gov/niams/healthinfo/fibrofs.htm

National Institutes of Health (NIH)
Clinical Center Communications
9000 Rockville Pike
Bldg. 10, Rm. 1C255
Bethesda MD 20892   (301) 496-5717   Website: www.nih.gov

National Institute of Mental Health (NIMH)
6001 Executive Blvd., Rm. 8184, MSC 9663
Bethesda MD 20892   (301) 443-4513   Website: www.nimh.nih.gov

National Library of Medicine of the National Institutes of Health
Website: www.nlm.nih.gov

Web Medline Searches

Occupational Safety and Health Administration (OSHA)
(202) 219-8148

U.S. Department of Labor
200 Constitution Ave., N.W.
Washington DC 20210   Website: www.osha.gov

Office of Disease Prevention and Health Promotion   (800) 336-4797

National Health Information Center
PO Box 1133
Washington DC 20013   Website: http://odphp.osophs.dhhs.gov/

CONSUMER AGENCIES

Federal Consumer Information Center
PO Box 100
Pueblo CO 81002   (800) 688-9889
Website: www.pueblo.gsa.gov

Federal Trade Commission
CRC-240
Washington DC 20580   (877) 382-4357   Website: www.ftc.gov

The Food and Drug Administration (FDA)
Consumer Affairs and Information
5600 Fishers Ln., HFC-110
Rockville MD 20857   (301) 443-3170   Website: www.fda.gov

MEDWATCH (FDA)   (800) 332-1088
Website: www.fda.gov/medwatch.
Report adverse reactions to untested substances, such as herbal remedies
and vitamins:

National Council Against Health Fraud (private, non-profit)
PO Box 141
Fort Lee NJ 07024   (201) 723-2955   Website: www.ncahf.org

The U.S. Postal Service
Chief Postal Inspector
475 L'Enfant Plaza
Washington DC 20260   Website: www.usps.com
to report mail fraud: Website: www.usps.com/postalinspectors/fraud/

DISABILITY AND ASSISTANCE

Americans with Disability Act: ADA Home Page
U.S. Department of Justice
PO Box 66118
Washington DC 20035-6118   (800) 514-0301
Website: www.usdoj.gov/crt/ada/adahom1.htm

CFS/FMS/ME WebRing: Disability
Website: www.cfids-me.org/disinissues/

Clearinghouse on Disability Information   (202) 334-8241

U.S. Department of Education
Switzer Bldg., Rm. 3132
Washington DC 20202-2524
Website: www.arcat.com/index.cfm

Disability, Social Security, and Financial Aid
Government Entitlement Services
22144 W. Nine Mile
Southfield MI 48034   (800) 628-2887
or 23930 Michigan Ave.
Dearborn MI 48124

Independent Living Centers (704) 375-3977
Website: www.jik.com/ilcs.html
300 centers located in all 50 states (listings by state)

Job Accommodation Network (JAN)
West Virginia University
PO Box 6080
Morgantown WV 26506-6080   (800) 526-7234

Medicare   (800) 633-4227   Website: www.medicare.gov

Medicare Rights Center
1460 Broadway, 11th Fl.
New York NY 10036   Website: www.medicarerights.org

National Council on Independent Living
1916 Wilson Blvd.
Arlington VA 22201   (703) 525-3406   Website: www.ncil.org

National Health Law Program
2639 S. La Cienega Blvd.
Los Angeles CA 90034   (310) 204-6010   Website: www.healthlaw.org

National Library Service for the Blind and Physically Handicapped
Library of Congress
1291 Taylor St., NW
Washington DC 20011   (202) 707-5100   Website: www.loc.gov/nls

National Organization of Social Security Claimants Representatives
(NOSSCR)
6 Prospect St.
Midland Park NJ 07432-1691   (800) 431-2804
Website: www.nosscr.org

New Freedom Initiative   Website: www.disability.gov

Social Security Administration (SSA)
Office of Public Inquiries
6401 Security Blvd., Room 4-C-5 Annex
Baltimore MD 21235-6401   (800) 772-1213   Website: www.ssa.gov

U.S. Equal Employment Opportunity Commission (EEOC)
1801 L St., N.W.
Washington DC 20507   (800) 669-4000   (202) 663-4900
Website: www.eeoc.gov

COMPUTER NETWORKING

CFS/ME Computer Networking Project
PO Box 11347
Washington DC 20008-0567
E-mail: cfsme@sjuvm.stjohns.edu

CFS/ME Computer Networking Project: Resources on CFS
Website: www.ncf.carleton.ca/ip/social.services/cfseir/CFSEIR.HP.html

Institute for Health Care Research & Policy, Georgetown University
listings by state: Website: www.georgetown.edu/research/ihcrp/hipaa

INFORMATION ABOUT PHYSICIANS

American Board of Medical Specialties
1007 Church St., Ste. 404   (847) 491-9091
Evanston IL 60201-5913   (866) ASK-ABMS (275-2267)
to check board certification:
    health care entities   Website: www.certifacts.org
    consumers   Website: www.abms.org

American Medical Association (AMA)
Department of Physician Data Services
515 N. State St.
Chicago IL 60610   (800) AMA-3211 (members only)
Website: www.ama-assn.org

CFS & FM Good Doctor List (Co-Cure)
Website: www.co-cure.org/good-doc.htm
listed by state and by country

CFS & FMS resources (AOL Server listing of electronic resources)
Website: http://members.aol.com/cfslists/

Federation of State Medical Boards
Federation Pl.
400 Fuller Wiser Rd., Ste. 300
Euless TX 76039-3855   (817) 868-4400   Website: www.fsmb.org

Pain & Policy Studies Group
University of Wisconsin
406 Science Dr., Ste. 202
Madison WI 53711-1068   (608) 263-7662
Website: www.medsch.wisc.edu/painpolicy

Glossary

ABBREVIATIONS OF TERMS

ACTH	adrenocorticotropin hormone
AED	anti-epileptic drug
ALS	amyotrophic lateral sclerosis
ANA	antinuclear antibodies
ANS	autonomic nervous system
CBT	cognitive behavioral therapy
CFIDS	chronic fatigue and immune dysfunction disorder
CFS	chronic fatigue syndrome
CMV	cytomegalovirus
CNS	central nervous system
CRH	corticotropin releasing hormone
CS	cervical stenosis
CSF	cerebrospinal fluid
CT	computerized tomography
DHEA	dehydroepiandrosterone
EBV	Epstein-Barr virus
ECG	electrocardiogram
EEG	electroencephalogram
EFA	essential fatty acid
EI	environmental illness
EMG	electromyography
FM/FMS	fibromyalgia/ fibromyalgia syndrome
FSS	functional somatic syndromes
GAD	generalized anxiety disorder
GI	gastrointestinal
GH	growth hormone
GWS, GWI	Gulf War Syndrome or Gulf War illness; aka Persian Gulf syndrome or illness

HHV-6, -7	human herpes virus 6 (or 7), particular strains of herpes-viruses
HIV/AIDS	human immunodeficiency virus/acquired immunodeficiency disorder
HPA	hypothalamic-pituitary-adrenal axis
IBD	inflammatory bowel disease
IBS	irritable bowel syndrome
IC	interstitial cystitis
IGF-I	insulin-like growth factor I
IM	intramuscular (injection)
ITT	insulin tolerance test
IV	intravenous
MAO-I	monoamine oxidase inhibitor
MCS	multiple chemical sensitivities
MDD	major depressive disorder
ME	myalgic encephalomyelitis
MRI	magnetic resonance imaging (brain scan)
MS	multiple sclerosis
NK	natural killer cells
NMH	neurally mediated hypotension
NSAID	nonsteroidal anti-inflammatory drug
OA	osteoarthritis
OI	orthostatic intolerance
OTC	over-the-counter (medications, etc.)
PCR	polymerase chain reaction for detection of viruses and bacteria
PET	positron emission tomography
PLMS	periodic limb movements during sleep
POTS	positional (or postural) orthostatic tachycardia
PPS	postpolio syndrome
PRN	as needed
PVFS	postviral fatigue syndrome
PWC	Person with CFS/CFIDS/ME/FMS
PWF	Person with fibromyalgia syndrome
Q-EEG	quantitative electroencephalogram
RA	rheumatoid arthritis

RLS	restless legs syndrome
Rx	by prescription
SLE	systemic lupus erythematosus (lupus)
SPECT	single photon emission computed tomography
SS	Sjögren's syndrome
SSDI	Social Security Disability Income
SSI	Supplementary Security Income
SSRI	selective serotonin reuptake inhibitor
TCA	tricyclic antidepressant
TF	transfer factor
TMD	temporomandibular joint dysfunction/disorder
TPI	trigger point injection
TRH	thyrotropin releasing hormone
TSH	thyroid stimulating hormone
YPWC	Young Person with CFS/CFIDS/ME/FMS

GOVERNMENT AGENCIES

CDC	Centers for Disease Control and Prevention
NIAID	National Institutes of Allergies and Infectious Disease
NIH	National Institutes of Health
NIAMS	National Institute of Arthritis and Musculoskeletal and Skin Diseases
SSA	Social Security Administration

Bibliography and Recommended Reading

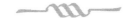

Chronic Fatigue Syndrome

Ali, M. *The Canary and Chronic Fatigue*. Life Span Press, 1994.

Bell, DS. *Faces of CFS: Case Histories of Chronic Fatigue Syndrome*. MZR Publishing, 2000.

Bell, D. *The Doctor's Guide to Chronic Fatigue Syndrome: Understanding, Treating, and Living with CFIDS*. Addison Wesley Longman, 1994.

Bell, DS, Robinson T, Robinson MZ. *A Parents' Guide to CFIDS: How to Be an Advocate for Your Child with Chronic Fatigue Immune Dysfunction Syndrome*. Haworth, 1999.

Berne, KH. *CFIDS Lite: Chronic Fatigue Immune Dysfunction Syndrome with $1/3$ the Seriousness*, 1990. Orders: BHB Communications, 2207 East Ivy, Mesa, AZ 85213, ($10.00, including s/h)

Brotherston, NE. *Adolescence and Myalgic Encephalomyelitis/Chronic Fatigue Syndrome: Journeys with the Dragon*. Haworth, 2000.

Conley, EJ. *America Exhausted: Breakthrough Treatments of Fatigue and Chronic Fatigue Syndrome* (revised edition). Vitality Press, 1998.

Courmel, K, Goldstein J. *A Companion Volume to Dr. Jay A. Goldstein's Betrayal by the Brain: A Guide for Patients and their Physicians*. Haworth, 1997.

Demitrack, MA, Abbey SE (eds.). *Chronic Fatigue Syndrome: An Integrative Approach to Evaluation and Treatment*. Guilford, 1996.

Friedberg, F. *Coping with Chronic Fatigue Syndrome: Nine Things You Can Do*. New Harbinger, 1995.

Friedberg, F, Jason LA. *Understanding Chronic Fatigue Syndrome: An Empirical Guide to Assessment and Treatment*. American Psychological Association, 1998.

Goldstein, JA. *Chronic Fatigue Syndromes: The Limbic Hypothesis*. Haworth, 1993.

Goldstein, JA. *Betrayal by the Brain: The Neurologic Basis of Chronic Fatigue Syndrome, Fibromyalgia Syndrome, and Related Neural Network Disorders.* Haworth, 1996.

Hyde, B (ed.). *The Clinical and Scientific Basis of Myalgic Encephalomyelitis/Chronic Fatigue Syndrome.* The Nightingale Research Foundation, 1992.

Jenkins, R, Mowbray JF (eds.). *Post-Viral Fatigue Syndrome.* Wiley, 1991.

Johnson, H. *Osler's Web: Inside the Labyrinth of the Chronic Fatigue Syndrome Epidemic.* Crown, 1996.

Klimas, NG, Patarca R (eds.). *Clinical Management of Chronic Fatigue Syndrome: Clinical Conference, American Association of Chronic Fatigue Syndrome.* Haworth, 1996. (Published simultaneously as the *Journal of Chronic Fatigue Syndrome*, v. 1, no. 3–4)

Munson, P. *Voices from the Hidden Epidemic of Chronic Fatigue Syndrome.* Haworth, 2000.

Natelson, B. *Facing and Fighting Fatigue: A Practical Approach.* Yale University Press, 1998.

Patarca-Montero, R. *Concise Encyclopedia of Chronic Fatigue Syndrome.* Haworth, 2000.

Rosenbaum, ME, Susser M. *Solving the Puzzle of Chronic Fatigue Syndrome.* Life Science Press, 1992.

Teitelbaum, J. *From Fatigued to Fantastic!* Avery, 1996.

Verillo, EF, Gellman LM. *Chronic Fatigue Syndrome: A Treatment Guide.* Quality Medical Publishing, 1998.

Fibromyalgia and Chronic Pain

Arnold, C. *Pain: What Is It? How Do We Deal with It?* Morrow, 1986.

Backstrom, G, Rubin BR. *When Muscle Pain Won't Go Away* (revised edition). Taylor, 1998.

Bigelow, SL. *Fibromyalgia: Simple Relief Through Movement.* Wiley, 2000.

Catalano, EM. *The Chronic Pain Control Workbook.* New Harbinger, 1987.

Cunningham, C. *The Fibromyalgia Relief Handbook.* United Research, 2000.

Davies, C. *The Trigger Point Therapy Workbook: Your Self-treatment Guide for Pain Relief.* New Harbinger, 2001.

Hammerly, M. *Fibromyalgia: The New Ingetrative Approach: How to Combine the Best of Traditional and Alternative Therapies.* Adams Media Corp., 2000.

Hulme, JA. *Fibromyalgia: A Handbook for Self Care & Treatment.* Phoenix Publishing, 1995.

Marcus, NJ. *Freedom from Chronic Pain.* Simon & Schuster, 1994.

Pellegrino, MJ. *The Fibromyalgia Survivor.* Anadem, 1995.

Pellegrino, MJ. *Fibromyalgia: Managing the Pain.* Anadem, 1997.

Pellegrino, MJ. *Understanding Post-Traumatic Fibromyalgia: A Medical Perspective.* Anadem, 1999.

Pellegrino, MJ. *Inside Fibromyalgia with Mark J. Pellegrino, MD.* Anadem, 2001.

Prudden, B. *Pain Erasure, the Bonnie Prudden Way.* Random House, 1982.

Russell, IJ (ed.). *Clinical Overview and Pathogenesis of the Fibromyalgia Syndrome, Myofascial Pain Syndrome, and Other Pain Syndromes.* Haworth, 1997. (Published simultaneously as the *Journal of Musculoskeletal Pain* 1996, v. 4, no. 1–2)

Wallace, DJ, Wallace JB. *Making Sense of Fibromyalgia: A Guide for Patients and Their Families.* Oxford University Press, 1999.

Williamson, ME, Nye DA. *Fibromyalgia: A Comprehensive Approach: What You Can Do about Chronic Pain and Fatigue.* Walker, 1996.

CFS & FMS

Chalmers, A, Littlejohn GO, Salit IE, Wolfe F (eds.). *Fibromyalgia, Chronic Fatigue Syndrome, and Repetitive Strain Injury: Current Concepts in Diagnosis, Management, Disability, and Health Economics.* Haworth, 1995. (Published simultaneously as the *J. of Musculoskeletal Pain* v. 3, no. 2)

Skelly, M, Helm A. *Alternative Treatments for Fibromyalgia and Chronic Fatigue Syndrome: Insights from Practitioners and Patients.* Hunter House, 1999.

Coping with Chronic Illness

Collinge, W. *Recovering from Chronic Fatigue Syndrome: A Guide to Self-Empowerment.* Berkley, 1993.

Conant, S. *Living with Chronic Fatigue: New Strategies for Coping With and Conquering CFS.* Taylor, 1990.

Dion, S. *Write Now: Maintaining a Creative Spirit While Homebound and Ill.* Puffin Foundation, 1993. Orders: S. Dion, 432 Ives Ave., Carneys Point, NJ 08069.

Donoghue, PJ, Siegel ME. *Sick and Tired of Feeling Sick and Tired: Living with Invisible Chronic Illness.* Norton, 2000.

Dorian, JS. *Above and Beyond: 365 Meditations for Transcending Chronic Pain and Illness.* Penguin, 1996.

Ediger, B. *Coping with Fibromyalgia.* LHR Publications, 1991.

Epstein, DM. *The 12 Stages of Healing: A Network Approach to Wholeness.* Amber-Allen, 1994.

Feiden, K. *Hope and Help for Chronic Fatigue Syndrome.* Fireside, 1992.

Fransen, RN, Russell IJ. *The Fibromyalgia Help Book: A Practical Guide to Living Better with Fibromyalgia.* Smith House, 1997.

Gardiser, K, Kerry K (eds.). *We Laughed We Cried: Life with Fibromyalgia.* KMK Associates, 1995.

Jacobs, PD. *500 Tips for Coping with Chronic Illness.* Reed, 1995.

Jeffreys, T. *The Mile-High Staircase.* Auckland: Hodder and Stoughton, 1982. Orders: Waiake Wordsmiths, PO Box 35-0429, Browns Bay, Auckland 10, New Zealand.

Kabat-Zinn, J. *Full Catastrophe Living: Using the Wisdom of Your Body and Mind to Face Stress, Pain and Illness.* Dell, 1990.

Kelly, J, Devonshire R, Romano T. *Taking Charge of Fibromyalgia.* Fibromyalgia Educational Systems, 1998.

Kenny, T. *Living with Chronic Fatigue Syndrome: A Personal Story of the Struggle for Recovery.* Thunder's Mouth Press, 1994.

Lewis, KS. *Successful Living with Chronic Illness.* Avery, 1985.

Pitzele, SK. *We Are Not Alone: Learning to Live with Chronic Illness.* Workman, 1985.

Register, C. *Living with Chronic Illness: Days of Patience and Passion.* Bantam, 1987.

Shepherd, C. *Living with ME: The Chronic/Post-Viral Fatigue Syndrome.* Vermilion, 1998.

Skloot, F. *The Night-Side: CFS and the Illness Experience.* Line Press, 1996.

Starlanyl, DJ. *The Fibromyalgia Advocate: Getting the Support You Need to Cope.* New Harbinger, 1998.

Starlanyl, DJ, Copeland MA. *Fibromyalgia and Chronic Myofascial Pain Syndrome: A Survival Manual* (2nd edition). New Harbinger, 2001.

Stearns, AK. *Living Through Personal Crisis.* Thomas More Press, 1984.

Sternbach, RA. *Mastering Pain: A Twelve-Step Program for Coping with Chronic Pain.* Ballantine, 1987.

Strubbe-Wittenberg, J. *The Rebellious Body: Reclaim Your Life from Environmental Illness or Chronic Fatigue Syndrome.* Plenum Insight Books, 1996.

Taylor, S, Epstein R. *Living Well with a Hidden Disability: Transcending Doubt and Shame and Reclaiming Your Life.* New Harbinger, 1999.

Wells, SM. *A Delicate Balance: Living Successfully with Chronic Illness.* Plenum, 1998.

Williamson, ME. *The Fibromyalgia Relief Book: 213 Ideas for Improving Your Quality of Life.* Walker, 1998.

Caregivers and Families

Kay, P, Williams B. *The Caregiver's Manual.* Citadel Press, 1995.

Kievman, B. *For Better or for Worse: A Couple's Guide to Dealing with Chronic Illness.* Contemporary Books, 1989.

National Family Caregivers Association. *The Resourceful Caregiver.* Mosby Press, 1996.

Pellegrino, M. *The Fibromyalgia Supporter,* Anadem, 1997.

Pitzele, SK. *Kind Words for Caring People: Daily Affirmations for Caregivers.* Health Communications, 1993.

Samples, P. *Daily Comforts for Caregivers.* Fairview Press, 1999.

Simonton, S. *The Healing Family: The Simonton Approach for Families Facing Illness.* Bantam, 1985.

Strong, M. *Mainstay: For the Well Spouse of the Chronically Ill.* Little, Brown & Co, 1988.

Vanderzalm, L. *Finding Strength in Weakness: Help and Hope for Families Battling Chronic Fatigue Syndrome.* Zondervan, 1995.

Disability

Chalmers, et al. "Prognostic indicators of disability after a work-related musculoskeletal injury," and "Disability—A medical-legal concept—The physician's role," in *Fibromyalgia, Chronic Fatiuge Syndrome, and Repetitive Strain Injury* (see under "Fibromyalgia," above).

Klimas, NG, Patarca R (eds.). *Disability and Chronic Fatigue Syndrome: Clinical, Legal and Patient Perspectives.* Haworth Press, 1997. (Published simultaneously as *J. of Chronic Fatigue Syndrome,* v. 3, no. 4)

Morton, DA, Sherman S (eds.). *Nolo's Guide to Social Security Disability: Getting and Keeping Your Benefits.* Nolo, 2001.

National Organization of Social Security Claimants Representatives (NOSSCR). *Social Security Disability and SSI Claims: Your Need for Representation* and *Preparing for your Social Security Disability or SSI Hearing* (pamphlets). NOSSCR, 6 Prospect St., Midland Park NJ 07432-1691; (800) 431-2804; www.nosscr.org.

Ross, JW. *Social Security Disability Benefits: How to Get Them! How to Keep Them!* Ross, 1984.

Smith, DM. *Disability Evaluation in a Nutshell, a Three-Minute Guide to Effective Medical Reports.* Physicians' Disability Services, 2000.

Smith, DM. *Disability Workbook for Social Security Applicants: Managing Your Application for Social Security Disability Insurance Benefits* (5th ed). Physicians' Disability Services, 2000.

Social Security Administration. Pamphlets about Social Security Disability and Supplementary Security Income benefits. Obtain at local SS offices; (800)772-1213; or www.ssa.gov/pubs/englist.html.

Healing, Wellness, and Medical Care

Balch, JF, Balch PA. *Prescription for Nutritional Healing* (2nd ed). Avery, 1997.

Borysenko, J. *Minding the Body, Mending the Mind.* Addison-Wesley, 1987.

Borysenko, J. *Guilt Is the Teacher, Love Is the Lesson.* Warner, 1990.

Chopra, D. *Quantum Healing.* Bantam, 1990.

Chopra, D. *The Path to Love: Spiritual Strategies for Healing,* Three Rivers Press, 1998.

Cousins, N. *Anatomy of an Illness as Perceived by the Patient.* Norton, 1979.

Kastner, M. *Alternative Healing.* Halcyon Publishers, 1993.

Levinson, HL. *Phobia Free.* Evans, 1986.

Locke S, Colligan D. *The Healer Within: The New Medicine of Mind and Body.* New American Library, 1986.

MacFarlane, EB, Burstein P. *Legwork: An Inspiring Journey through a Chronic Illness* [multiple sclerosis]. Scribner, 1994.

Matthews-Simonton, S, Simonton OC, Creighton JL. *Getting Well Again.* Bantam, 1980.

Mizel, SB, Jaret P. *The Human Immune System: The New Frontier in Medicine.* Simon and Schuster, 1986.

Siegel, BS. *Love, Medicine and Miracles.* Harper and Row, 1986.

Siegel, BS. *Peace, Love and Healing.* Harper and Row, 1989.

Tyler, VE. *The Honest Herbal: A Sensible Guide to the Use of Herbs and Related Remedies (3rd ed.).* Pharmaceutical Products Press, 1993.

Weil, A. *Health and Healing* (revised edition). Houghton Mifflin, 1988.

Weil, A. *Natural Health, Natural Medicine.* Houghton Mifflin, 1990.

Other

American Psychiatric Association. *Diagnostic and Statistical Manual of Mental Disorders (DSM-IV).* 1994.

Duff, K. *The Alchemy of Illness.* Bell Tower, 1994.

Goldenberg, DL. *Chronic Illness and Uncertainty: A Personal and Professional Guide to Poorly Understood Syndromes.* Dorset, 1996.

Kilburn, KH. *Chemical Brain Injury.* Van Nostrand Reinhold/John Wiley, 1997.

Roessler, R., Decker N. *Emotional Disorders in Physically Ill Patients.* Kluwer Academic Publishers, 1986.

Rooney, AA.. *Mr. Rooney Goes to Work* (orig. broadcast 5 July 1977). In *A Few Minutes with Andy Rooney.* Warner, 1981.

Rooney, AA.. *Pieces of My Mind.* Avon, 1982.

Sampson, R, Hughes P. *Breaking Out of Environmental Illness: Essential Reading for People with Chronic Fatigue Syndrome, Allergies, or Chemical Sensitivities.* Bear, 1997.

Selye, H. *Stress Without Distress.* New York: Signet, 1974.

Sontag, S. *Illness as Metaphor.* Farrar, Straus and Giroux, 1977.

BIBLIOGRAPHY: PERIODICALS

Aaron LA, Buchwald D. Review of the evidence for overlap among unexplained clinical conditions [abstract]. *Ann Intern Med* 1 May 2001; 134(9):868–81.

Ablashi DV, Berneman Z., et al. Kutapressin inhibits in vitro infection of human herpesvirus type 6. *Clin Infect Dis* 1994:18,S113.

Ablashi DV, Eastman HB, et al. Frequent HHV-6 reactivation in multiple sclerosis (MS) and chronic fatigue syndrome (CFS) patients. *J Clinical Virology* 1 May 2000;16(3):179–191.

Abraham GE, Flechas JD. Management of fibromyalgia: Rationale for the use of magnesium and malic acid. *J Nutritional Medicine* 1992;3:49–59.

Amir M, Kaplan Z, et al. Posttraumatic stress disorder, tenderness and fibromyalgia. *J Psychosom Res* 1997 Jun; 42(6):607–13.

Ammen J, Acupuncture: Targeting chronic pain. Online chat: www.Lahey.org, 18 May 2000.

Arthritis Foundation. *Bulletin on the rheumatic diseases.*

Bagge E, Bengtsson BA, et al. Low growth hormone secretion in patients with fibromyalgia—a preliminary report on 10 patients and 10 controls. *J Rheumatol* 1998 Jan;25(1):145–8.

Bakshi R. Highlights from the Fifth Annual Meeting of the Americas Committee for Treatment and Research in Multiple Sclerosis (ACTRIMS), 2000 October 15. Medscape Neurology: <www.medscape.com/Medscape/Neurology/journal/2000/v02.n06/mn1205.baks/mn1205.baks.html>; accessed 1 December 2000.

Baldwin CM, Bell IR, O'Rourke MK. Odor sensitivity and respiratory complaint profiles in a community-based sample with asthma, hay fever, and chemical odor intolerance. *Toxicol Ind Health* 1999 Apr–Jun;15(3–4):403–9.

Barker E, Fujimura, SF, et al. Immunologic abnormalities associated with chronic fatigue syndrome. *Clin Inf Diseases* 1994;18:S136–141.

Barsky AJ, Borus JF. Functional somatic syndromes. *Annals of Internal Medicine*. 1 June 1999;130:910–921.

Bastien S. Neuropsychological deficits in chronic fatigue syndrome [lecture]. Bel Air, CA: Chronic Fatigue Syndrome: Current Theory and Treatment, 19 May 1991.

Bates DW, Buchwald D, et al. Clinical laboratory test findings in patients with chronic fatigue syndrome. *Arch Intern Med* 9 Jan 1995; 155(1):97–103.

Bazelmans E, Bleijenberg G, et al. Levels of activity and fatigue after extreme exercise in chronic fatigue syndrome (CFS). Cambridge, MA, Research Conf AACFS, 10–11 Oct 1998.

Behan PO, Chaudhuri A, et al. The symptoms of chronic fatigue syndrome are related to abnormal ion channel function. Cambridge, MA, Research Conf AACFS, 10–11 Oct 1998.

Bell DS. Chronic fatigue syndrome in children. *J CFS* 1995;1(1):9–33.

Bell DS. Chronic fatigue syndrome in children and adolescents: A review. *Focus & Opinion: Peds* 1995;1:412–420.

Bell DS. Diagnosis of chronic fatigue syndrome in children and adolescents: Special considerations. *J CFS* 1995;1(3/4):29–36.

Bell DS. Illness onset characteristics in children with Chronic Fatigue Syndrome and Idiopathic Chronic Fatigue. *J CFS* 1997;3(2):43–51.

Bell DS, Bell KM, Cheney PR. Primary juvenile fibromyalgia syndrome and chronic fatigue syndrome in adolescents. *Clin Infect Dis* 1994 Jan;18:S21–S23.

Bell IR, Baldwin CM, Schwartz, GE. Illness from low levels of environmental chemicals: Relevance to chronic fatigue syndrome and fibromyalgia. *Am J Med*. 1998; 105(3A):74S–82S.

Bell IR, Schwartz GE, et al. Individual differences in neural sensitization and the role of context in illness from low-level environmental chemical exposures. *Environ Health Perspect* 1997 Mar;105:457–466

Bennett RM. The fibromyalgia syndrome: Myofascial pain and the chronic fatigue syndrome, in *Textbook of Rheumatology* (4th ed.), edited by Kelley WN, Harris ED, Ruddy S, Sledge CB. 1993:471–483.

Bennett RM. Fibromyalgia: The commenest cause of widespread pain. *Compr Ther* 1995;21:6, 269–275.

Bennett RM. Fibromyalgia, chronic fatigue syndrome, and myofascial pain. *Curr Opin Rheumatol* 1998 10:95–103

Bennett RM. Emerging concepts in the neurobiology of chronic pain: Evidence of abnormal sensory processing in fibromyalgia. *Mayo Clin Prac* 1999;74:385–398.

Bennett RM. The scientific basis for understanding pain in fibromyalgia. <http://www.myalgia.com/Scientific%20basis.htm>, accessed 30 Apr 2001.

Bennett RM, Clark SC, Walczyk J. A randomized, double-blind, placebo-controlled study of growth hormone in the treatment of fibromyalgia. *AJM* 1998;104:227–231.

Bennett RM, Cook DM, et al. Hypothalamic-pituitary-insulin-like growth factor-1 axis dysfunction in patients with fibromyalgia. *J Rheum* 1997;24(7):1384–89.

Berg D, Berg LH, Couvaras J. Is CFS/FM due to an undefined hypercoagulable state brought on by immune activation of coagulation? Does adding anticoagulant therapy improve CFS/FM patient symptoms? [Lecture abstract]. M.E./CFS Scientific Conference, Sydney, Australia, 24–26 February 1999.

Blomkvist V, Evengård B, et al. On symptoms and life events surrounding the onset of chronic fatigue syndrome. [Lecture abstract] Cambridge, MA, AACFS Research Conf 10 Oct 1998.

Borenstein D. Sjögren syndrome: Epidemiology, diagnostics, and management. American College of Rheumatology 1999 Annual Scientific Meeting, November 13–17.

Bottero P. Rickettsia and chlamydia in patient psychopathology: A diagnostic and a therapeutic report. [lecture abstract] Sydney, Australia, M.E./CFS Scientific Conference 24–26 February 1999.

Bou-Holaigah I, Rowe PC, et al. The relationship between neurally mediated hypotension and the chronic fatigue syndrome. *JAMA* 1995 Sep;247:961–967.

Braden GL. Phoenix, AZ. Update on inflammatory bowel disease. 64th American College of Gastroenterology Annual Scientific Meeting [online: Medscape.com] 17 October 1999.

Bradley LA, et al. Pain complaints in patients with fibromyalgia vs. chronic fatigue syndrome. *Current Rev Pain* 2000;4:148-57, published in *CFIDS Chronicle* 2001 Winter;2(1):11.

Branco JC, Tavares V, et al. HLA studies in fibromyalgia. *J Musculoskeletal Pain* 1996;4(3),21–27.

Brehio R, Sievering C. The search for a test, part one. *CFIDS Chronicle* 2000 Winter;13(1):5–7

Brown DB, Managing sleep disorders. *Clinician Reviews* 1999;9(10):51–54, 57–58, 60, 63–64, 69.

Bruno RL. Paralytic versus "non-paralytic" polio: A distinction without a difference? *American Journal of Physical Medicine and Rehabilitation* 2000;79:1–9.

Bruno RL, Creange S, et al. Elevated plasma prolactin and EEG slow wave power in post-polio fatigue: Implications for a dopamine deficiency underlying post-viral fatigue syndromes. *J CFS* 1998;4:61–76.

Bruno RL, Creange SJ, Frick NM. Parallels between post-polio fatigue and chronic fatigue syndrome: A common pathophysiology? *Am J Med* 1998;105(3A):66S–73S.

Bruno RL, Creange S, et al. Polioencephalitis and the brain fatigue generator model of post-viral fatigue syndromes. *J CFS* 1998;4:61–76.

Buchwald D. FM and CFS: similarities & differences. *Rheum Dis Clin North Am* 1996 May;22(2):219–43.

Buchwald D, Garrity D. Comparison of patients with chronic fatigue syndrome, fibromyalgia, and multiple chemical sensitivities. *Arch Internal Med* 1994 September;154:2049–2053.

Buchwald D, Komaroff AL. Review of laboratory findings for patients with chronic fatigue syndrome. *Rev Infect Dis* 1991 Jan–Feb;13:S12–S28.

Buchwald, D, Pascualy, et al. Sleep disorders in patients with chronic fatigue. *Clin Infect Dis* 1994; 18:S68–72.

Buchwald D, Pearlman T, et al. Functional status in patients with chronic fatigue syndrome, other fatiguing illnesses, and healthy individuals. *Am J Med* 1996 Oct;171:364–370.

Burnet R, Scroop G, et al. Serum potassium and hormone responses to exercises in Chronic Fatigue Syndrome. [Lecture abstract] Sydney, M.E./CFS Scientific Conference, 24–26 February 1999.

Burrascano JJ. *The New Lyme Disease: Diagnostic hints and treatment guidelines for tick-borne illnesses* (12th ed.)1998, published on LymeNet with permission from the author.

Buskila D. Fibromyalgia, chronic fatigue syndrome, and myofascial pain syndrome. *Curr Opin Rheumatol* 1999 Mar;11(2):119–126.

Buskila D, Neumann L, et al. Familial aggregation in the fibromyalgia syndrome. *Semin Arthritis Rheum* 1996 Dec;26(3):605–11.

Buskila D, Neumann L, et al. Increased rates of fibromyalgia following cervical spine injury. A controlled study of 161 cases of traumatic injury. *Arthritis Rheum* 1997 Mar;40(3):446–452.

Buskila D, Neumann L. Fibromyalgia syndrome (FM) and nonarticular tenderness in relatives of patients with FM. *J Rheumatol* 1997 May;24(5):941–944.

Buskila D, Odes LR, et al. Fibromyalgia in inflammatory bowel disease. *J Rheumatol* 1999 May;26(5):1167–71.

Caffery BE, Josephson JE, and Samek MJ. The ocular signs and symptoms of chronic fatigue syndrome. J Am Optometry Assoc 1994; 65(3),187–191.

Calabrese LH, Davis ME, Wilke WS. Chronic fatigue syndrome and a disorder resembling Sjögren's syndrome: Preliminary report. Clin Infect Dis 1994;18:S28–31.

Caro X. Is there an immunologic component to the fibrositis syndrome? [lecture]. Los Angeles: CFS and FM: Pathogenesis and Treatment 1990 Feb.

Carpman V. Chemical warfare: CFIDS, multiple chemical sensitivity and silicone implant disorder. CFIDS Chronicle 1993 Fall:33–41.

Carpman V. CFIDS treatment: The Cheney Clinic's strategic approach. CFIDS Chronicle 1995 Spr:38–45.

Carter BD, Edwards JF, et al. Screening instruments for psychiatric morbidity in CFS. R Soc Med 1998 Jul;91(7):365–8.

Chaudhuri A, Behan PO. Neurological dysfunction in chronic fatigue syndrome, J CFS, 2000;6:3/4:51–68.

Cheney PR. CFS: A current perspective [lecture]. Bel Air, CA: CFS: Current theory and treatment, 18 May 1991.

Cheney PR, Lapp CW. The diagnosis of chronic fatigue syndrome. CFS DysPatch 1993 Mar/Apr;3(2),1–8.

Chester AC, Levine PH. Concurrent sick building syndrome and chronic fatigue syndrome: Epidemic neuromyasthenia revisited. Clin Infect Dis 1994;18:S43–8.

Chiari malformations and syringomyelia. <www2.mc.duke.edu/depts/medicine/medgen/chiari.html>, accessed 1 July 1999.

Childs ND, Could infections be behind chronic Lyme disease? Medscape Skin & Allergy News 1999;30(8):13.

Clauw DJ. Fibromyalgia: More than just a musculoskeletal disease. Am Fam Physician 1 Sep 1995;52(3):843–851.

Clauw DJ. The pathogenesis of chronic pain and fatigue syndromes, with special reference to fibromyalgia. Med Hypotheses 1995;44:369–378.

Cleare AJ, Bearn J, et al. Contrasting neuroendocrine responses in depression and chronic fatigue syndrome. J Affect Disord 18 Aug 1995;34(4):283–928.

CNN & Time, with Jeff Greenfield & Bernard Shaw. Sick and tired, aired 24 October 1999, 9:00 P.M. ET.

Coyle C, Wernick R. Systemic lupus erythematosus: Recognizing the clinical signs. Hospital Medicine 1999;35(3):48–54.

Crean EA. CFIDS and anesthesia: What are the risks? CFIDS Chronicle. Winter 2000;13(1):11–13.

Crofford LJ. The hypothalamic-pituitary-adrenal stress axis in FM and CFS. *J Rheumatol* 1998, 57:S67–71.

Crofford LJ, Demitrack MA. Evidence that abnormalities of central neurohormonal systems are key to understanding FM & CFS. *Rheum Dis Clin North Am* 1996 May;22(2):267–284.

DeBecker P, Dendale P, et al. Autonomic testing in patients with chronic fatigue syndrome. *Am J Med* 1998;105(3A):22S–26S.

DeFreitas E, Hilliard B, et al. Retroviral sequences related to human T-lymphotropic virus type II in patients with chronic fatigue immune dysfunction syndrome. *Proceed Natl Acad Sci* 1991 Apr; 88:2922–2926.

DeLuca J, Johnson SK, et al. Cognitive functioning is impaired in patients with chronic fatigue syndrome devoid of psychiatric disease. *J Neurol Neurosurg Psychiatry* 1997 Feb;62(2):151–155.

De Meirleir K, Campine I, et al. RNase L dysfunction disorder (R.E.D.D.) in CFS [lecture summary]. Cambridge, MA, Research Conf AACFS, 10–11 Oct 1998.

Demitrack MA. Neuroendocrine aspects of chronic fatigue syndrome: A commentary. *Am J Med* 1998;105(3A):11S–14S.

Demitrack MA, Crofford LJ. Evidence for and pathophysiologic implications of hypothalamic-pituitary-adrenal axis dysregulation in FM & CFS. *Ann N Y Acad Sci* 1 May 1998;840:684–697.

Demitrack MA, Dale JK, et al. Evidence for impaired activation of the hypothalamic-pituitary-adrenal axis in patients with chronic fatigue syndrome. *J Clin Endocrinol Metab* 1991 Dec;73(6);1224–1234.

Dimitrov M, Grafman J. Neuropsychological assessment of chronic fatigue syndrome. *J CFS* 1997 3(4):31–42.

Dinan TG, Majeed T, et al. Blunted serotonin-mediated activation of the hypothalamic-pituitary-adrenal axis in CFS. *Psychoneuroendocrinology* 1997 May;22(4):261–267.

DiPino RK, Kane RL. Neurocognitive functioning in CFS [Review]. *Neuropsychol Rev* 1996 Mar;6(1):47–60.

Doebbeling BN, Clarke WR, et al. Is there a Persian Gulf War syndrome? Evidence from a large population-based survey of veterans and nondeployed controls. *AJM* 15 Jun 2000;108(9):695–704.

Ellenbogen RG, Armonda RA, et al. Toward a rational treatment of Chiari I malformation and syringomyelia. *Neurosurg Focus* 2000;8(3).

English TL. Skeptical of skeptics. *JAMA* 21 Feb 1991;265(8):964.

Fennell PA. The four progressive stages of the CFS experience: a coping tool for patients. *J CFS* 1995; 1(3/4): 69–79.

Fischler B, D'Haenen H, et al. Comparison of $^{99}Tc^m$-HMPAO SPECT scan between CFS, major depression NS healthy controls: An exploratory study of clinical correlates of regional cerebral blood flow. *Neuropsychobiology* 1996;34(4):175–83.

Friedberg F, Jason LA. Chronic fatigue syndrome and fibromyalgia: Clinical assessment and treatment. *J Clin Psychol*, 2001, 57(4);433–55.

Friedberg F, Krupp LB. A comparison of cognitive behavioral treatment for chronic fatigue syndrome and primary depression. *Clin Infec Dis* 18, 1994, S105–110.

Fudenberg HH. Immunotherapy of chronic fatigability immune dysregulation syndrome [lecture]. Los Angeles: CFS and FM: Pathogenesis and Treatment, 1990 Feb.

Fukuda K, Nisenbaum R, et al. Chronic multisymptom illness affecting Air Force veterans of the Gulf War. *JAMA* 16 Sep 1998;280(11):981–988.

Fukuda K, Straus SE, et al. The chronic fatigue syndrome: a comprehensive approach to its definition and study. International Chronic Fatigue Syndrome Study Group. *Ann Intern Med* 15 Dec 1994;121(12):953–959.

Geddes BJ, Summerlee AJS. The emerging concept of relaxin as a centrally acting peptide hormone with hemodynamic actions. *J Neuroendocrinology*, 1995;7:411–417.

Giovengo SL, Russell IJ, Larson AA. Increased concentrations of nerve growth factor in cerebrospinal fluid of patients with fibromyalgia. *J Rheumatol* 1999 Jul;26(7):1564–1569.

Glacy SD. Myofascial pain: One of the most common causes of pain. *Pain Management Newsletter* 1997 Fall.

Glaser R, Kiecolt-Glaser JK. Stress-associated immune modulation: relevance to viral infections and CFS. *AJM* 28 Sep 1998;105(3A):35S–42S.

Glass RT. The human/animal interaction of chronic fatigue and immune dysfunction syndrome: A look at 127 patients and their 463 animals. *Medical Professionals With CFIDS News* 1998 Spring:3(2).

Goldberg MJ. Chronic fatigue syndrome in children and adults and its connection to ADHD. For Parents of Sick & Worn-Out Kids at <http://home.bluecrab.org/~health/sickids.html>, accessed 25 Oct 2001.

Goldenberg DL. Psychiatric and psychologic aspects of fibromyalgia syndrome. *Rheum Dis Clinics of N Amer* 1989 Feb;15:1:105–114.

Goldenberg DL. Psychological symptoms and psychiatric diagnosis in patients with fibromyalgia. *J of Rheumatology* 1989;16(supp 19):127.

Goldenberg DL. A controlled study of tender points in patients with chronic fatigue syndrome [lecture]. Los Angeles: CFS and FM: Pathogenesis and Treatment, 1990 Feb.

Goldenberg DL. Fibromyalgia and chronic fatigue syndrome: Are they the same? *J Musculoskeletal Med* 1990;7:19.

Goldenberg DL. Fibromyalgia, chronic fatigue, and myofascial pain syndromes. *Current Opinion Rheum* 1992;4:247–257.

Goldenberg DL, Simms RW, et al. High frequency of fibromyalgia in patients with chronic fatigue seen in a primary care practice. *Arthritis Rheum* 1990;*33*(3):381–387.

Goldstein JA. Presumed pathogenesis and treatment of the chronic fatigue syndrome/fibromyalgia complex [lecture]. Los Angeles: CFS and FM: Pathogenesis and Treatment 1990 Feb.

Goldstein JA. Chronic fatigue syndrome. *Female Patient* 1991 Jan;16(1):39–50.

Goldstein JA, Mena, I, et al. The assessment of vascular abnormalities in late life chronic fatigue syndrome by brain SPECT: Comparison with late life major depressive disorder. *J CFS* 1995;1(1):55–79.

Hill NF, Tiersky LA, et al. The fluctuation and outcome of CFS over time [lecture summary]. Cambridge, MA, AACFS Research Conf AACFS 10–11 Oct 1998.

Horvath SB, Peterson DL, Suhadolnik RJ. Characterization of Rnase L dysfunction in peripheral blood mononuclear cell extracts from patients with Chronic Fatigue Syndrome. [lecture abstract] Cambridge, MA, AACFS Research Conf 10–11 Oct 1998.

Gonzalez MB, Cousins JC, Doraiswamy PM. Neurobiology of CFS. *Prog Neuropsychopharmacol Biol Psych* 1996 Jul;20(5):749–59.

Grinspoon L (ed.). Sleep Disorders—Parts I and II. *Harv Ment Health Lett*, 1994 Aug and Sept;*11*(2):1–4; (3):1–5.

Haley RW, Kurt TL, Hom J. Is there a Gulf War syndrome? Searching for syndromes by factor analysis. *JAMA* 1997;277(3):215–222.

Hansen HC. Treatment of chronic pain with antiepileptic drugs: A new era. *South Med J* 1999; 92(7):642–649.

Harvard Health Letter. Fibromyalgia syndrome: Feeling more pain. 1999 Oct:4–5.

Hickie IB, Lloyd A, et al. The psychiatric status of patients with the Chronic Fatigue Syndrome. *Brit J Psychiatry* 1990;156:534–540.

Hickie IB, Scott EM, et al. Somatic distress: developing more integrated concepts. *Curr Opin Psychiatry* 1998 Mar;11(2):153–158.

Holmes GP, Kaplan JE, et al. Chronic Fatigue Syndrome: a working case definition. *Ann Intern Med* 1988 Mar;108(3):387–389.

Hooper, J. A new germ theory. *Atlantic Monthly* 1999 Feb.

Hotopf M, David A, et al. Role of vaccinations as risk factors for ill health in veterans of the Gulf War: A cross sectional study. *BMJ* 20 May 2000;320:1363–1367.

Ichise M, Salit IE, et al. Assessment of regional cerebral perfusion by ^{99}Tc^m-HMPAO in chronic fatigue syndrome. *Nucl Med Comm* 1992 Oct;13(10):767–772.

Iger LM. The MMPI as an aid in confirming a chronic fatigue syndrome diagnosis [lecture]. Los Angeles, CFS and FM: Pathogenesis and Treatment 1990 Feb.

Iger L. The MMPI as an aid to CFS diagnosis. *CFIDS Chronicle*, 1990 Spring/Summer:35–38.

Iger LM. Cognitive restructuring with the CFS patient [lecture]. Bel Air, CFS: Current Theory and Treatment 19 May 1991.

Iger LM. Changes on the chronic fatigue syndrome profile with the MMPI-2 [lecture]. Bel Air, CA, Chronic Fatigue Syndrome and the Brain Symposium, 26 Apr 1992.

Jaret P. Our immune system: The wars within. *Natl Geogr* 1986; 169:702–735.

Jason LA, Richman JA, et al. Politics, science, and the emergence of new disease: The case of Chronic Fatigue Syndrome. *Am Psychol* 1997 Sept;52(9):973–983.

Jason LA, Richman JA, et al. A community-based study of chronic fatigue syndrome. *Arch Intern Med* 11 Oct 1999;159(18):2129–2137.

Jason LA, Wagner L, et al. Estimating the prevalence of Chronic Fatigue Syndrome among nurses. *Am J Med* 1998;105(3A):91S–93S.

Jeschonneck M, Grohmann G, Sprott H. Abnormal microcirculation and temperature in skin above tender points in patients with fibromyalgia. *Rheumatology* 2000 Aug;39 (8):917–21.

Johnson H. Journey into fear: The growing nightmare of Epstein-Barr virus [Parts 1 & 2]. *Rolling Stone* 1987 Jul 16:56–63,139–141 and Aug 13:42–46,55–57.

Jordan KM, Ayers PM, et al., Prevalence of fatigue and chronic fatigue syndrome-like illness in children and adolescents. *J CFS*;6(1):3–21.

Jorge CM, Goodnick PJ. Chronic fatigue syndrome and depression: Biological differentiation and treatment. *Psychiatric Annals* 1997 May;27(5):365–371.

Kaplan RF, Jones-Woodward L, et al. Neuropsychological deficits in Lyme disease patients with and without other evidence of central nervous system pathology. *Appl Neuropsych* 1999;6(1):3–11.

Klekamp J, Batzdorf U, et al. The surgical treatment of Chiari I malformation, *Acta Neurochir* 1996.

Klimas NG, Fletcher MA, et al. A Phase I trial of autologous ex vivo expanded lymph node derived cells as immunomodulatory therapy in CFS [summary]. Cambridge, MA, Research Conf AACFS 1998 Oct.

Klimas NG, Patarca R (eds.). Disability and chronic fatigue syndrome: Clinical, legal and patient perspectives. *J CFS* 1997;3(4):1–109.

Klimas NG, Salvato FR, et al. Immunologic abnormalities in chronic fatigue syndrome. *J Clin Microbiol* 1990 Jun;28(6):1403–1410.

Komaroff AL. Clinical crossorads: A 56-year-old woman with chronic fatigue syndrome. *JAMA* 1997;278(14):1179–1185.

Komaroff AL, Buchwald DS. Chronic fatigue syndrome: an update, *Annu Rev Med* 1998;49:1–13.

Komaroff AL, Fagioli LR, et al. Health status in patients with chronic fatigue syndrome and in general population and disease comparison groups. *AJM* 1996 Jan;101:281–290.

Komaroff AL, Fagioli L, et al. An examination of the working case definition of chronic fatigue syndrome. *AJM* 1996 Jan;100(1):56–64.

Krilov LR, Fisher M, et al. Course and outcome of chronic fatigue in children and adolescents. *Pediatrics* 1998 Aug; 102(2 Pt 1):360–6.

LaManca JJ, Sisto SA, et al. Influence of exhaustive treadmill exercise on cognitive functioning in CFS. *AJM* 28 Sep 1998;105(3A):59S–65S.

Lange G, Wang S, et al. Neuroimaging in chronic fatigue syndrome. *AJM* 1998;105(3A):50S–53S.

Lapp CW. Chronic Fatigue Syndrome is a real disease. *North Carolina Family Physician* 1992;43(1):6–11.

Lapp CW. Management of Chronic Fatigue Syndrome in children: A practicing clinician's approach. *J CFS* 1997;3(2):59–76.

Larson A, Giovengo A, et al. Changes in the concentrations of amino acids in the cerebrospinal fluid that correlate with pain in patients with fibromyalgia: Implications for nitric oxide pathways. *Pain* 2000;87:201–211.

Leal-Cerro A, Povedano R, et al. The growth hormone (GH)-releasing hormone - GH - insulin-like growth factor-1 axis in patients with fibromyalgia syndrome. *Journal Clin Endo & Metab* 1999 Sept; 84(9):3378–3381.

Lerner AM, Zervos M, et al. Hypothesis: A unified theory of the cause of chronic fatigue syndrome. *Infectious Diseases in Clinical Practice* 1997;6:239–243.

Lentz MJ, Landis CA, et al. Effects of selective slow wave sleep disruption on musculoskeletal pain and fatigue in middle aged women. *J Rheumatol* 1999 Jul;26(7):1586–92.

Levin AS, Byers VS. Environmental illness: A disorder of immune regulation, in *State of the Art Reviews: Occup Med.* Philadelphia: Hanley and Belfus 1987;669–81.

Levine PH. Epidemiologic advances in CFS. *J Psychiatr Res* 1997 Jan–Feb; 31(1):7–18.

Levine PH. Chronic fatigue syndrome comes of age. *AJM* 1998 Sept;105 (3A):S1–S6.

Levine PH. What we know about chronic fatigue syndrome and its relevance to the practicing physician. *AJM*. 1998;105(3A):100S–103S.

Livingston JS. "No other illness like this one: Dr. Bell finds dramatic abnormalities in CFIDS," column, about.com, <http://chronicfatigue.about.com/health/chronicfatigue/library/weekly/aa0 72600b.htm>, 26 Jul 2000, accessed 20 Oct 2000.

Lloyd AR. Chronic fatigue and chronic fatigue syndrome: Shifting boundaries and attributions *AJM*, 1998 105(3A):7S–10S.

Lloyd A, Gandevia S, et al. Cytokine production and fatigue in patients with chronic fatigue syndrome and healthy control subjects in response to exercise. *Clin Infect Dis* 1994;18:S142–146.

Lloyd A, Hickie IB, et al. A double-blind, placebo-controlled trial of intravenous immunoglobin therapy in patients with chronic fatigue syndrome. *AJM* 1990;89:561–568.

Lloyd AR, Hickie IB, Loblay RH. Illness or disease? The case of chronic fatigue syndrome. *MJA* 2000; 172:471–472.

Loveless MO. Chronic immunologic activation and CFS [lecture]. Bel Air, CA: CFS: Current Theory and Treatment 18 May 1991.

Loveless MO, Lloyd A, Perpich R. Summary of public policy and Chronic Fatigue Syndrome: A perspective. *Clin Inf Dis* 1994;18:S163–65.

MacDonald JA. Arnold Chiari malformation. <www.uchc.edu>, updated 1998 Jan, accessed 1990 Jun.

Marchesani RB. Crimson crescents facilitate CFS diagnosis. *Inf Dis News* 1992 Nov;5(11):1,3.

Martin WJ. Detection of viral sequences using the polymerase chain reaction [lecture]. Los Angeles, CFS and FM: Pathogenesis and Treatment 1990 Feb.

Martin WJ. Stealth viruses: Nature's biological weapons program [lecture summary], Sydney, M.E./CFS Scientific Conference 1999 Feb 24–26.

Martin WJ. Bacteria related sequences in a simian cytomegalovirus-derived stealth virus culture. *Exp Mol Path* 1999;66:8–14.

Masterson M. The poison within (special series). *AZ Republic* 1989, Jan 29–Feb 3.

Matthews DA, Manu P, Lane TJ. Evaluation and management of patients with chronic fatigue syndrome. *Am J Med Sci* 1991;302(5):269–277.

McCain J. McCain condemns $356 million in 'pet projects.' <www.senate.gov/~mccain/legbran.htm>, 19 Sep 2000, accessed 12 Sep 2001.

McCain J. Foreign operations appropriations for fiscal year 2001, <www.senate.gov/~mccain/for01ap.htm>, 21 Jun 2000, accessed 12 Sep 2001.

McDermott JH, Motyka TM. Expert column: Assessing the quality of botanical preparations. Medscape Pharmacology, www.medscape.com, 2000.

McKenzie R, O'Fallon A, et al. Low-dose hydrocortisone for Rx of CFS: A randomized controlled trial. *JAMA* 23-30 Sep 1998;280(12):1061–1066.

Mena I. Study of cerebral perfusion by NeuroSPECT in Patients with CFS [lecture]. Bel Air, Chronic Fatigue Syndrome: Current Theory and Treatment 1991 May.

Mena I. Cerebral hypoperfusion in late life chronic fatigue syndrome and late life depression. *CFIDS Chronicle* 1993 Summer:53.

Moldofsky HD. Sleep, neuroimmune and neuroendocrine functions in fibromyalgia and chronic fatigue syndrome. *Advances in Neuroimm* 1995;5:39–56.

Moldofsky H, Lue FA, et al. Disordered circadian sleep-wake neuroendocrine and immune functions in chronic fatigue syndrome [lecture summary]. Cambridge, MA, AACFS Research Conf 1998 Oct.

Moore R, Finding new meaning in life through spiritual focus. *CFIDS Chronicle* 2000 Winter;13(1):28.

Moorkens G. Endocrine and metabolic aspects of the chronic fatigue syndrome [doctoral thesis]. Belgium, Antwerp University, 2000 March.

Moorkens G, Berwaerts J, et al. Characterization of pituitary function with emphasis on GH secretion in the chronic fatigue syndrome. *Clin Endocrinol (Oxf)* 2000 Jul;53(1):99–106.

Morelli J. Glucosamine/chondroitin products not measuring up: New research raises troubling quality control questions. *WebMD Medical News*, <http://my.webmd.com/content/article/1728.56163>, 2 April 2000.

Morriss R, Sharpe M, et al. Abnormalities of sleep in patients with the chronic fatigue syndrome. *BMJ* 1 May 1993;306(6886):1161–1164.

Natelson BH, LaManca JJ, et al. Immunologic parameters in chronic fatigue syndrome, major depression, and multiple sclerosis. *AJM* 1998;105(3A):43S–49S.

National Fibromyalgia Research Association. Fibromyalgia abstracts: Selected journal articles 1995.

National Institutes of Health, Research Initiatives/Programs of Interest, <http://www.best.com/~cfids/nihresearch.gif>, accessed 30 August 2001.

Neeck G, Riedel W. Thyroid function in patients with fibromyalgia syndrome. *J Rheumatol* 1992 Jul;19(7):1120–1122.

Nelson PK. Fingerprint "loss"—Is it a sign of CFIDS? *CFIDS Chronicle* 1994 Fall:49–50.

Nicolson GL, Nasralla M, et al. Mycoplasmal infections in chronic illnesses: Fibromyalgia and chronic fatigue syndromes, Gulf War illness, HIV-AIDS and rheumatoid arthritis. *Medical Sentinel* 1999;4:172–176.

Nye DA. A physician's guide to fibromyalgia syndrome. Missouri Arthritis Rehabilitation Research and Training Center, <www.hsc.missouri.edu/fibro/fm-md.html> 1997, accessed 25 Mar 1998.

Ohliger PC, Legal matters: New accreditation program for health websites, *Drug Benefit Trends* 2001,13(4):21–22, <www.medscape.com/SCP/DBT/2001/v13.n04/dbt1304.03/ohli/dbt1304.o hli01.html>, accessed 25 May 2001.

Oldendick R, Coker AL, et al. Population-based survey of complementary and alternative medicine usage, patient satisfaction, and physician involvement. *South Med J* 2000;93(4):375–381.

Older SA, Battafarano DF, et al. The effects of delta wave sleep interruption on pain thresholds and fibromyalgia-like symptoms in healthy subjects; correlations with insulin-like growth factor I. *J Rheumatol* 1998 Jun;25(6):1180–1186.

Pall ML. Elevated, sustained peroxynitrite levels as the cause of chronic fatigue syndrome. *Med Hypotheses* 2000;54:115–125.

Pall ML. New Theory on Explanations for Chronic Fatigue Syndrome, ImmuneSupport.com: <http://www.immunesupport.com/library/showarticle.cfm?ID=2976>, 13 Feb 2001, accessed 15 Feb 2001.

Patarca-Montero R, Klimas NG, Fletcher MA. Immunotherapy of chronic fatigue ayndrome: Therapeutic interventions aimed at modulating the Th1/Th2 cytokine expression balance. *J CFS* 2001;8(1):3–37.

Peckerman A, LaManca JJ, et al. CFS severity is related to reduced stroke volume and diminished blood pressure responses to mental stress [lecture summary]. Cambridge, AACFS Research Conf 1998 Oct.

Pepper CM, Doscher C, et al. Comparison of the psychiatric and psychological profiles of patients with chronic fatigue syndrome, multiple sclerosis, and major depression. *Clin Inf Dis* 1994;18:S86.

Pepping J. DHEA: Dehydroepiandrosterone. *Am J Health-Syst Pharm* 2000;57(22):2048–2056.

Peterson DL. Chronic fatigue syndrome and disability (editorial). *J CFS* 1997;3(4):5–7.

Peterson D. Phoenix, CFS Assoc of AZ [Lecture] 1991 May.

Peterson PK, Pheley A, et al. A preliminary placebo-controlled crossover trial of fludrocortisone for CFS. *Arch IM* 27 Apr 1998;158(8):908–14.

Pillemer SR (ed.), *The fibromyalgia syndrome: Current research and future directions in epidemiology, pathogenesis and treatment*, Haworth, published as *J Musculoskeletal Pain* 1994;2(3).

Potzanick W, Kozol N. Ocular manifestations of chronic fatigue and immune dysfunction syndrome. *Optom Vision Sci* 1992;69(10):811–814.

Reid S, Wessely S. Somatoform disorders. *Current Opinion in Psychiatry Datum* 1999;12(2):163–168.

Reilly PA, Littlejohn GO. Fibromyalgia and chronic fatigue syndrome. *Curr Op Rheum* 1990;2:282–290.

Rigden S. Entero-hepatic resuscitation program for CFIDS. *CFIDS Chronicle* 1995 Spring:46–49.

Rook GA, Zumla A, et al. Gulf War syndrome: Is it due to a systemic shift in cytokine balance towards a Th2 profile? *Lancet* 21 Jun 1997; 349(9068):1831–1833.

Rowe PC, Calkins H. Neurally mediated hypotension and Chronic Fatigue Syndrome. *AJM* 1998;105(3A):15S–21S.

Rowe P, Bou-Holaigah I, et al. Is neurally mediated hypotension an unrecognized cause of chronic fatigue? *Lancet* 1995;345:623–624.

Rubin P. Phoenix, CFS Association of Arizona [lecture] 6 Sep 1998.

Russell IJ. Biochemical abnormalities in fibromyalgia syndrome. *J Musculoskeletal Pain* 1995 May.

Russell IJ. Neurochemical pathogenesis of fibromyalgia. *J Rheumatol* 1998;57:63–66.

Russell IJ. Advances in fibromyalgia: possible role for central neurochemicals. *Am J Med Sci* 1998 Jun;315(6):377–84.

Russell IJ, Michalek JE, et al. Serum amino acids in fibrositis/fibromyalgia syndrome. *J Rheumatol* 19 Nov 1989:158–63.

Sandman C. Is There a CFS Dementia? [lecture transcript]. *CFIDS Chronicle* 1991 Spring:105–108.

Sandman C. It's all in your head: Well, indeed it is.... [lecture]. Bel Air, Chronic Fatigue Syndrome and the Brain Symposium 1992 May.

Sandman CA, Barron JL, et al. Memory deficits associated with chronic fatigue syndrome. *Biol Psychiatry*, 1993;33:618–623.

Schuster MM, Crowell MD, et al. Irritable bowel syndrome (IBS): Examining new findings and treatments. Medscape, <http://www.medscape.com/CMECircle/Gastroenterology/2000/CME01/pnt-CME01.html>, 26 Oct 2000, accessed 28 Oct 2000.

Schwartz RB, Garada BM, et al. Detection of intracranial abnormalities in patients with chronic fatigue syndrome: Comparison of MR imaging and SPECT. *Am J Roentgenol* 1994;162:935–941.

Schwartz RB, Komaroff AL, et al. SPECT imaging of the brain: Comparison of findings in patients with chronic fatigue syndrome, AIDS dementia complex, and major unipolar depression. *Am J Roentgenol* 1994;162:943–951.

Scott LV, Dinan TG. Urinary free cortisol excretion in CFS, major depression & in healthy volunteers. *J Affect Disord* 1998 Jan;47(1-3):49–54.

Servatius RJ, Tapp WN, et al. Impaired associative learning in CFS. *Neuroreport* 20 Apr 1998;9(6):1153–7.

Sharpe M. Cognitive behavior therapy for CFS: Efficacy and implications. *AJM* 1998;105(3A):104S–109S.

Sriram S, Mitchell W, Stratton C. Multiple sclerosis associated with *chlamydia pneumoniae* infection to the CNS. *Neurology* 1998 Feb;50:571–572.

Sisto SA, LaManca JJ, et al. Cardiovascular responses during a cognitive stressor before and after exercise in chronic fatigue syndrome vs. sedentary healthy subjects [lecture transcript]. Cambridge, AACFS Research Conf 1998 Oct.

Sperber AD, Carmel S, et al. The sense of coherence index and the irritable bowel syndrome. A cross-sectional comparison among irritable bowel syndrome patients with and without coexisting fibromyalgia, irritable bowel syndrome non-patients, and controls. *Scand J Gastroenterol* 1993 Mar;34(3):259–63.

Stewart J, Weldon A, et al. Neurally mediated hypotension and autonomic dysfunction measured by heart rate variability during head-up tilt testing in children with chronic fatigue syndrome. *Clin Auton Res* 1998 Aug; 8(4):221–30.

Straus SE, Dale JK, et al. Acyclovir treatment of the chronic fatigue syndrome: Lack of efficacy in a placebo-controlled trial. *N Engl J Med* 1998;319:1692–1697.

Strayer DR, Carter WA, et al. Long-term improvements in patients with chronic fatigue syndrome treated with Ampligen. *J CFS* 1995;1(1):35–53.

Strayer DR, Carter WA, et al. A controlled clinical trial with a specifically configured RNA drug, Poly(I)-Poly ($C_{12}U$), in chronic fatigue syndrome. *Clin Infect Dis* 1994;18:S88–95.

Strayer DR, Carter WA, et al. Durability of therapeutic beneift with Ampligen® treatment of chronic fatigue syndrome (CFS) as measured by the Karnofsky Performance Score (KPS) [lecture summary]. Cambridge, AACFS Research Conf 1998 Oct.

Streeten DH, Anderson GH Jr. The role of delayed orthostatic hypotension in the pathogenesis of chronic fatigue. *Clin Auton Res* 1998 Apr;8(2):119–24.

Streeten D, Bell D. Circulating blood volume in CFS. *J CFS* 1998;4(1):3–11.

Suhadolnik RJ. 2-5A Synthetase pathway. Testimony at congressional briefling on chronic fatigue and immune dysfunction syndrome, 16 May 1997.

Suhadolnik RJ, Peterson DL, et al. Biochemical evidence for a novel low molecular weight 2-5A-dependent RNase L in chronic fatigue syndrome. *J Interferon and Cytokine Res* 1997;17:377–385.

Thorson K. Coping with illness uncertainties. *Fibromyalgia Network* 1999 Oct;47:1–3.

Tirelli U, Chierichetti F, et al. Brain positron emission tomography (PET) in CFS: preliminary data. *AJM* 28 Sep 1998;105(3A):54S–58S.

Torpy DJ, Papanicolaou DA, et al. Responses of the sympathetic nervous system and the hypothalamic-pituitary-adrenal axis to interleukin-6: a pilot study in fibromyalgia. *Arthritis Rheum.* 2000 Apr;43(4):872–880.

Tougas G. The autonomic nervous system in functional bowel disorders. *Can J Gastroenterol* 1999 March;13:15A–17A.

Ulett GA, Han J, Han S. Traditional and evidence-based acupuncture: History, mechanisms, and present status. *South Med J* 1998;91(12):1115–1120.

Unwin C, Blatchley N, et al. Health of UK servicemen who served in Persian Gulf war. *Lancet* 16 Jan 1999;353(9148):169–178.

Vallings R. Report on the second world congress on chronic fatigue syndrome and related disorders: Towards effective diagnosis and treatment in the 21st century. *J CFS* 2000;6(3-4):3–21.

Vollmer-Conna U, Hickie IB, et al. Intravenous immunoglobulin is ineffective in the treatment of patients with CFS. *AJM* 1997 Jul;103(1):38–43.

Vollmer-Conna U, Wakefield D, et al. Cognitive deficits in patients suffering from CFS, acute infective illness or depression. *Br J Psychiatry* 1997 Oct;171:377–381.

Wallace DJ, Shapiro S, Panush RS. Update on fibromyalgia syndrome. *Bulletin on the Rheumatic Diseases* 1999;48(5):1–4.

Wearden A, Appleby L. Cognitive performance & complaints of cognitive impairment in CFS. *Psychol Med* 1997 Jan;27(1):81–90.

Weinstein SM, Laux LF, et al. Physicians' attitudes toward pain and the use of opioid analgesics: Results of a survey from the Texas Cancer Pain Initiative. *South Med J* 2000;93(5):479–487.

White KP, Speechley M, et al. Co-existence of chronic fatigue syndrome with fibromyalgia syndrome in the general population. A controlled study. *Scand J Rheumatol* 2000;29(1):44–51.

White KP, Speechley M, et al. The London fibromyalgia epidemiology study: comparing the demographic and clinical characteristics in 100 random community cases of fibromyalgia versus controls. *J Rheumatol* 1999 Jul;26(7):1577–1585.

Whiteside TL, Friberg D. Natural killer cells and natural killer cell activity in CFS. AJM 28 Sep 1998;105(3A):27S–34S.

Williamson M. Dysregulation spectrum syndrome: The tie that binds a host of illnesses. Fibromalgia Times, 1998 Summer.

Wilson RB, Gluck OS, et al. Antipolymer antibody reactivity in a subset of patients with fibromyalgia correlates with severity. J Rheumatol 1999 Feb;26(2):402–407.

Wise CM. Systemic lupus erythematosus: Clinical manifestations and diagnosis. Clin Rev Southern Association for Primary Care 1998 Summer:29–33.

Wolfe F, et al. The American College of Rheumatology 1990 criteria for the classification of fibromyalgia: Report of the multicenter criteria committee. Arthritis Rheum 1990;33:160.

Wolfe F, Anderson J, et al. Health status and disease severity in fibromyalgia: results of a six-center longitudinal study. Arthritis Rheum 1997 Sep;40(9):1571–1579.

Wolfe F, Anderson J, et al. Work and disability status of persons with fibromyalgia. J Rheumatol 1997 Jun;24(6):1171–1178.

Wolfe F, Russell IJ, et al. Serotonin levels, pain threshold, and fibromyalgia symptoms in the general population. J Rheumatol 1997 Mar;24(3):555–559.

Yazici Y, Gibofsky YA. A Diagnostic approach to musculoskeletal pain. Clin Cornerstone 1999;2(2):1–7.

Yirmiya R. Depression in medical illness: The role of the immune system. West J Med 2000;173(5):333–336.

Yirmiya R., et al. Cytokine secretion linked to emotional and cognitive disturbances. Arch Gen Psychiatry 2001;58:445–452.

Yue SK. Relaxin: Its role in the pathogenesis of fibromyalgia [lecture summary]. Tempe, AZ, 1997 Dec 5–6.

Yunus MD. Psychological aspects of fibromyalgia syndrome—a component of the dysfunctional spectrum. Bailleres Clinical Rheumatology 1998;8(811)–837.

Yunus M. Are fibromyalgia and other chronic conditions associated? ImmuneSupport.com, 8 June 2000: <http://www.immunesupport.com/Library/showarticle.cfm?ID=1406>, accessed 12 Dec 2000.

Zhang O, Natelson BH, et al. Altered immune status in Gulf veterans with chronic fatigue syndrome [lecture summary]. Cambridge, AACFS Research Conf 1998.

Index

TO ORDER OTHER BOOKS AND AUDIOTAPES BY KATRINA BERNE

CFIDS LITE: Chronic Fatigue (Immune Dysfunction) Syndrome with 1/3 the Seriousness. *(Paperback book ... illustrated ... 110 pages)* Chronic illness is no laughing matter, but humor can help us keep a healthy perspective on living with CFS and FMS. The jokes, riddles, limericks, and cartoons in *CFIDS Lite* help to combat pain, depression, and isolation. Perhaps laughter *is* the best medicine.

AUDIOTAPES (Narrated by the author)

UNDERSTANDING CHRONIC FATIGUE SYNDROME (90 minutes): For CFS patients and others. Information about symptoms, diagnosis, relapses and remissions, causal theories, treatment options, and resources.

UNDERSTANDING FIBROMYALGIA (90 minutes): For FMS patients and others. Information about symptoms, diagnosis, suspected causes, course of the illness, treatment options, and resources.

FOR THOSE WHO CARE (90 minutes): For spouses, partners, family members, friends, and co-workers. **Side 1:** Information about CFS/FMS and their impact on relationships. **Side 2:** Techniques for helping patients and enhancing relationships: communicating about the illness, giving and receiving emotional support, setting reasonable limits, coping with symptoms and limitations, handling guilt and disappointment, and affirming both partners.

CHRONIC ILLNESS AND SELF-ESTEEM (90 minutes): Addresses illness-related sources of low self-esteem: changed abilities, appearance, and productivity; altered self-image and self-expectations. Offers techniques for enhancing self-image and confidence, developing realistic, affirming self-talk, explaining limitations, and making necessary lifestyle changes without guilt.

NEUROCOGNITIVE ASPECTS OF CFS AND FMS (90 minutes): Addresses concerns about neurological and cognitive dysfunction such as short-term memory deficit; spatial disorientation; brain fog; difficulty using words and numbers; sensory overload; difficulty with concentration, comprehension, and sequencing. Includes strategies for improving cognition.

RELAXATION AND STRESS REDUCTION (60 minutes): Side 1: Daytime. Relaxation exercise for use as an adjunct to medical treatment to promote healing, reduce stress, create positive imagery, and help to mobilize the body's own healing and energy-producing potential. **Side 2: Evening.** Relaxation exercise designed to reduce anxiety, bring about a sense of peace and balance, and help to achieve sound sleep.

Ordering Information ** (see note below)

CFIDS Lite—special price—limited supply $8.00
Understanding Chronic Fatigue Syndrome $10.00
Understanding Fibromyalgia $10.00
For Those Who Care $10.00
Chronic Illness and Self Esteem $10.00
Neurocognitive Aspects of CFS and FMS $10.00
Relaxation and Stress Reduction $10.00

Shipping/handling: $2.50 for the first item; $1.00 for each additional item.
These materials may be ordered from:
BHB PUBLICATIONS, 2207 E. Ivy, Mesa, AZ 85213 or online at
www.LivingWithIllness.com.

** Please send all orders for items on this page and make checks payable to:
BHB Publications — not to Hunter House

Hunter House books on
CFS/FMS, SELF-CARE AND HERBAL CARE *pg. 1*

ALTERNATIVE TREATMENTS FOR FIBROMYALGIA AND CHRONIC FATIGUE SYNDROME: Insights from Practitioners and Patients *by* Mari Skelly

> Many people suffering from fibromyalgia and CFS are unable to find effective treatment and relief. This book combines interviews with practitioners of alternative therapies—including acupuncture, massage therapy, chiropractic, psychotherapy, and energetic healing—with personal stories from patients. These offer a firsthand look at symptoms, treatments, struggles and successes, lifestyle adaptations and medicine, diet, and activity regimens that might help others. There are also sections on obtaining health insurance and Social Security disability.

288 pages ... Paperback $15.95 ... Hardcover $25.95

THE ART OF GETTING WELL: A Five-Step Plan for Maximizing Health When You Have a Chronic Illness *by* David Spero, R.N., Foreword by Martin L. Rossman, M.D.

> Self-management programs have become a key way for people to deal with chronic illness. In this book, David Spero brings together the medical, psychological and spiritual aspects of getting well in a five-step approach: slow down and use your energy for the things and people that matter — make small, progressive changes that build self-confidence — get help and nourish the social ties that are crucial for well-being — value your body and treat it with affection and respect — take responsibility for getting the best care and health you can.

224 pages ... Paperback $15.95 ... Hardcover $25.95

CHINESE HERBAL MEDICINE MADE EASY: Natural and Effective Remedies for Common Illnesses *by* Thomas Richard Joiner

> Chinese herbal medicine is an ancient system for maintaining health and prolonging life. This book demystifies the subject, with clear explanations and easy-to-read alphabetical listings of more than 750 herbal remedies for over 250 common illnesses ranging from acid reflux and AIDS to breast cancer, pain management, sexual dysfunction, and weight loss. Whether you are a newcomer to herbology or a seasoned practitioner, you will find this book a valuable addition to your health library.

432 pages ... Paperback $24.95 ... Hardcover $34.95

All prices subject to change

WOMEN LIVING WITH MULTIPLE SCLEROSIS

by Judith Lynn Nichols and Her Online Group of MS Sisters

Judith Nichols was first diagnosed with MS in 1976 and cofounded an online support group of women who helped each other cope with the day-to-day challenges of MS. In this book, members of the group share intimate, emotional accounts of their experiences with MS. Some stories are painful, some are funny, often they are both. The range of deeply personal concerns includes family reactions to the diagnosis, workplace issues, sexuality and spirituality, depression and physical pain, loss of bladder and bowel control, and assistive devices and helpful tools. All topics are discussed freely and frankly, in the way closest friends do.

288 pages ... Paperback $13.95

LIVING BEYOND MULTIPLE SCLEROSIS: A Women's Guide

by Judith Lynn Nichols and Her Online Group of MS Sisters

This sequel to *Women Living with Multiple Sclerosis* focuses on transcending the effects of MS. This book shares the same engaging, conversational tone as the first book. In addition to providing more time, energy and sanity-saving techniques, this book talks about ways to live beyond the limitations MS imposes. Topics include the newest treatments for MS and how to maximize their benefits; household accessibility, safety, and remodeling; tips for choosing and using assistive devices; how to prepare applications for Social Security Disability and insurance benefits.

288 Pages ... Paperback $14.95

WHEN PARKINSON'S STRIKES EARLY: Voices, Choices, Resources and Treatment

by Barbara Blake-Krebs, M.A., & Linda Herman, M.L.S.

This book details the physical, emotional and social struggles faced by young people with Parkinson's and the roads to self-empowerment that can be found through the support and resources of the PD global community. Topics include the complex array of PD symptoms and the side effects of medications; the unique impact early onset PD has on individuals and society; and current surgery options as described by former patients. The book includes a listing of resources and grassroots advocacy ideas. *All royalties will be donated to PD research.*

288 pages ... Paperback $15.95 ... Hardcover $25.95

To order see last page or call (800) 266-5592

ORDER FORM

10% DISCOUNT on orders of $50 or more —
20% DISCOUNT on orders of $150 or more —
30% DISCOUNT on orders of $500 or more —
On cost of books for fully prepaid orders

NAME

ADDRESS

CITY/STATE   ZIP/POSTCODE

PHONE   COUNTRY (outside of U.S.)

TITLE	QTY	PRICE	TOTAL
Chronic Fatigue Syndrome... (paperback)		@ $15.95	

Prices subject to change without notice

Please list other titles below:

		@ $	
		@ $	
		@ $	
		@ $	
		@ $	
		@ $	
		@ $	
		@ $	

Check here to receive our book catalog ☐   free

Shipping Costs
By Priority Mail: first book $4.50, each additional book $1.00
By UPS and to Canada: first book $5.50, each additional book $1.50
For rush orders and other countries call us at (510) 865-5282

TOTAL _____
Less discount @____%   (_____)
TOTAL COST OF BOOKS _____
Calif. residents add sales tax _____
Shipping & handling _____
TOTAL ENCLOSED _____
Please pay in U.S. funds only

☐ Check ☐ Money Order ☐ Visa ☐ MasterCard ☐ Discover

Card #_____ Exp. date_____

Signature_____

Complete and mail to:
Hunter House Inc., Publishers
PO Box 2914, Alameda CA 94501-0914
Website: www.hunterhouse.com
Orders: (800) 266-5592 or email: ordering@hunterhouse.com
Phone (510) 865-5282 Fax (510) 865-4295

CFS-R2 9/2002